THE GANGLIOSIDOSES

THE
GANGLIOSIDOSES

Edited by
Bruno W. Volk and Larry Schneck
Kingsbrook Jewish Medical Center
and
State University of New York
Downstate Medical Center
Brooklyn, New York

PLENUM PRESS · NEW YORK AND LONDON

Library of Congress Cataloging in Publication Data
Main entry under title:

The Gangliosidoses.

Includes bibliographical references and index.
1. Gangliosidoses. I. Volk, Bruno W. II. Schneck, Larry. [DNLM: 1.
Gangliosides. 2. Lipid metabolism, Inborn errors. 3. Lipoidosis. WD205.G5 G197]
RC632.L5G36   616.3'99   75-11708
ISBN-13: 978-1-4615-8728-6   e-ISBN-13: 978-1-4615-8726-2
DOI: 10.1007/978-1-4615-8726-2

© 1975 Plenum Press, New York
Softcover reprint of the hardcover 1st edition 1975

A Division of Plenum Publishing Corporation
227 West 17th Street, New York, N.Y. 10011

United Kingdom edition published by Plenum Press, London
A Division of Plenum Publishing Company, Ltd.
Davis House (4th Floor), 8 Scrubs Lane, Harlesden, London, NW10 6SE, England

CONTRIBUTORS

Masazumi Adachi, M.D., Sc.D. • Chief of Neuropathology, Isaac Albert Research Institute of the Kingsbrook Jewish Medical Center and Clinical Professor of Pathology, State University of New York, Downstate Medical Center, Brooklyn, New York

Daniel Amsterdam, Ph.D. • Chief of Microbiology, and Head, Human Cell Biology Program, Birth Defects Center, Isaac Albert Research Institute of the Kingsbrook Jewish Medical Center, Brooklyn, New York

Stanley M. Aronson, M.D. • Dean of Medical Affairs, Brown University, and Pathologist-in-Chief, Miriam Hospital, Providence, Rhode Island

Steven E. Brooks, M.S. • Isaac Albert Research Institute of the Kingsbrook Jewish Medical Center, Brooklyn, New York

Linda Hoffman, Ph.D. • Isaac Albert Research Institute of the Kingsbrook Jewish Medical Center, Brooklyn, New York

Guta Perle, B.S. • Isaac Albert Research Institute of the Kingsbrook Jewish Medical Center, Brooklyn, New York

Abraham Saifer, Ph.D. • Chief of Biochemistry, Isaac Albert Research Institute of the Kingsbrook Jewish Medical Center, and Professor of Biochemistry, Touro College, Brooklyn, New York

Larry Schneck, M.D. • Director of Neurology, Kingsbrook Jewish Medical Center, and Clinical Professor of Neurology, State University of New York, Downstate Medical Center, Brooklyn, New York

Bruno W. Volk, M.D. • Director, Isaac Albert Research Institute of the Kingsbrook Jewish Medical Center, and Clinical Professor of Pathology, State University of New York, Downstate Medical Center, Brooklyn, New York

PREFACE

The history of so-called storage diseases goes back to the end of the 19th and to the beginning of the 20th century when Fabry, Tay, Sachs, Gaucher, Niemann, Hunter, and Hurler first described the disorders which up to now are called by their eponym. The clinical descriptions soon were followed by pathologic studies, and within a short time the hereditary characters of these rare afflictions came to be recognized.

Although sporadic reports during the early part of this century dealt with biochemical analysis of the "stored" materials in these disorders, it was actually in the late 1930s that the abnormal deposits started to attract the increasing attention of chemists. S. H. Thannhauser brought the broad concept of lipidoses as a group of related disorders to the attention of the medical profession for the first time, and in 1939 Klenk observed that the brain of a patient with Tay–Sachs disease contained greatly increased amounts of a glycolipid for which he proposed the name "ganglioside." Work carried out in the past 20 years has thrown new light on these afflictions and has pinpointed the enzymatic and lipid abnormalities associated with the various "storage" diseases. Moreover, electron microscopic studies have permitted detailed investigations of the fine structure of the various organs of afflicted patients. Thus, the multiphasic approach to the study of these disorders has brought about a remarkable cross-fertilization within related fields and has led to discoveries of new diseases, which include the group of gangliosidoses. As of now, the enzyme deficiencies underlying most of the afflictions have been elucidated. This knowledge became the indispensible basis for the detection of heterozygotes and for the prenatal diagnosis of homozygotes.

Quite often, results obtained with newly refined techniques have made obsolete the contributions of the pioneering early workers who, with comparatively primitive methods, were able to make significant contributions to the understanding of these disorders. Until the early 1960s, Tay–Sachs disease was considered to be the only known gangliosidosis. However, with

the use of newer methods in biochemistry and enzyme chemistry, it became
possible to recognize additional variants and subdivisions of ganglioside
diseases.

At the same time it became necessary to abandon old concepts of
classification which were based primarily on clinical observations. Thus, the
designation of the late infantile form of Jansky–Bielschowsky, the juvenile
form of Spielmeyer–Vogt, and the adult form described by Kuf, all previously considered as variants of Tay–Sachs disease, has become untenable
on the basis of extensive electron microscopic, biochemical, and enzymatic
chemical studies.

At present there is no single, clearly defined, clinical, chemical, or morphological criterion that will distinguish and identify the various types of
ganglioside "storage" diseases. For example, the clinical features of
Sandhoff's and Tay–Sachs disease are almost identical, and the diagnosis of
each is based upon essentially chemical criteria such as the absence of the
isoenzyme hexosaminidase A in Tay–Sachs disease and the absence of the
isoenzymes A and B in Sandhoff's disease. However, it has been reported
that an apparently normal adult was identified with complete absence of the
isoenzyme hexosaminidase A. Thus, if one used only enzymatic criteria, this
patient would have to be considered to have a variant of Tay–Sachs disease.
The authors, therefore, recommend the retention of well-established, widely
recognized eponyms such as Tay–Sachs disease, Sandhoff's disease,
Norman–Landing disease, etc. to be followed by the accumulated substrate
and isoenzyme that is present. Zero indicates complete absence of all
isoenzymes. Thus Tay–Sachs disease would be designated as Tay–Sachs
disease [G_{M2} (B)], Sandhoff's disease [G_{M2} (0)], Bernheimer–Seitelberger
disease [G_{M2} (A,B)], Norman–Landing disease [G_{M1} (0)], and Derry's disease
[G_{M1} (A)].

Although the vast number of newer contributions in this rapidly
expanding field in the study of gangliosidoses have been reviewed by several
authors, there seems to be a need for work by clinicians, biochemists,
pathologists, and geneticists of a more elaborate composite background for
the better understanding of these disorders. To the best of our knowledge,
there are few places where, between the covers of a single volume, an in-
tegrated concept of the gangliosidoses has been attempted, to include
various avenues of approach to correlate this relatively new information.
Although therapeutic efforts have so far been unsuccessful, the prenatal
diagnosis of some of these disorders, particularly of Tay–Sachs disease, has
become an important tool for the intrauterine detection of these afflictions.
Thus, since replacement therapy with enzyme has not been successful so far,
for the foreseeable future, the pragmatic approach to some of the gangliosidoses, notably Tay–Sachs disease, involves the identification of the high-risk

pregnancies and prenatal diagnosis of the homozygotes. Ideally this approach may lead to complete eradication of some of the gangliosidoses.

By necessity, it is unavoidable that there will be overlaps of certain observations and ideas in the various chapters. However, it appears to us that the incorporation of some similar material in different parts of this volume would help to elucidate the presented facts. The selected illustrations depict some of the more characteristic features of the clinical aspects and the pathology of these diseases. Moreover, it is hoped that tables and figures pertaining particularly to biochemical and genetic areas will contribute to a better understanding of certain concepts.

The work of the authors has been aided by the existence at the Kingsbrook Jewish Medical Center of a 16-bed clinical unit that is entirely dedicated to the care and study of children afflicted with ganglioside diseases and related storage disorders. This has permitted the correlation of biochemical and pathologic studies with genetic observations during the period of hospitalization.

This multiphasic approach was successfully carried out through the benevolent cooperation of the administration of the Kingsbrook Jewish Medical Center, as well as through the enthusiastic and active support of the National Tay–Sachs and Allied Diseases Association, Inc. The important role this organization played in the progress of this study is gratefully acknowledged.

The authors are indebted to Mr. Herbert A. Fischler, Chief Medical Photographer, who prepared the microphotographs and other illustrations of this monograph. We, furthermore, wish to acknowledge the many contributions of various members of the professional, technical, and secretarial staff of the Isaac Albert Research Institute.

Lastly, the authors are grateful to Plenum Publishing Corporation for their excellent cooperation in making this monograph possible.

B. W. V.
L. S.

CONTENTS

Chapter 4

Masazumi Adachi and Bruno W. Volk

Chapter 5

Stanley M. Aronson

Chapter 6

Daniel Amsterdam

Chapter 7

SPONTANEOUS GANGLIOSIDOSES IN ANIMALS 215

Masazumi Adachi

Appendix A

METHODOLOGY: SPHINGOLIPID ANALYSIS 223

Linda M. Hoffman and Larry Schneck

Appendix E
METHODOLOGY: CELL CULTURE 265
Daniel Amsterdam and Steven E. Brooks

THE
GANGLIOSIDOSES

Chapter 1

HISTORICAL REVIEW

BRUNO W. VOLK

The term amaurotic family idiocy (AFI) is a clinical description which refers to a group of hereditary disorders characterized by progressive psychomotor and visual deterioration. The term ganglioside was introduced by Klenk[1] in 1939 for neuraminic-acid-containing glycolipids which he found in the brains of subjects with the infantile form of AFI which is now known as Tay–Sachs disease (TSD). The gangliosidoses are due to an inborn error of ganglioside metabolism resulting in an absolute increase in the tissue concentration of gangliosides. The terms Tay–Sachs disease and amaurotic family idiocy have often been used interchangeably. However, only three major classes of AFI are biochemically proven gangliosidoses:

1. G_{M2}-gangliosidosis. This group includes the most common type, Tay–Sachs disease (variant B), as well as Sandhoff's disease (variant O) and Bernheimer–Seitelberger disease (variant AB).
2. G_{M1}-gangliosidosis. This group includes Norman–Landing disease (type O) and Derry's disease (type A).
3. G_{M3}-gangliosidosis. This group has so far been reported in only two patients.

While the infantile form of AFI was first described by Tay[2] in 1881 and independently by Sachs[3] in 1887, for historical reasons it should be recorded

BRUNO W. VOLK. Isaac Albert Research Institute of the Kingsbrook Jewish Medical Center and State University of New York, Downstate Medical Center, Brooklyn, New York.

that after the turn of the century several investigators described familial disorders which occurred in young children, juveniles, or adults, which they considered to be variants of what is now known by the eponym TSD. Thus, Batten[4] in 1903 described cerebral degeneration with symmetrical changes in the macula of two members of a family, and he thought that this condition might be related to TSD; Mayou[5] in 1904 described first cousins with three children who had eyesight failure at six years of age, and he considered this condition identical with that described by Batten.[4] In 1905, Vogt,[6] in a clinical study, and, about a year later Spielmeyer,[7] independently, by means of pathologic observations established a juvenile form as a separate disease entity which they considered distinct from the infantile form of TSD. Jansky[8] in 1909, and Bielschowsky,[9] subsequently in 1913, described a disorder which they considered as a late infantile variety that first becomes apparent in the third or fourth year of life and that lasts for an additional three to four years. In 1925, Kufs[10] described the first patient with the late form of AFI which he considered as the adult variety of infantile TSD; the pertinent symptoms started at the age of 26 years and death occurred at age 38.

The contributions of Batten, Mayou, Jansky, Bielschowsky, Vogt, and Spielmeyer to the knowledge of the various forms of AFI with later onset has been recognized in the form of eponymic designations. More recently, Zeman and co-workers[11,12] coined the term "neuronal ceroid lipofuscinosis," based primarily on histochemical and electron microscopic studies. However, since their original description of the ultrastructural features of the cytoplasmic inclusions in the juvenile and adult forms of AFI, a variety of inclusion bodies have been observed by several authors.[13-32] Several investigators[18,33] failed to observe lipofuscin in so-called juvenile and adult forms of AFI and concluded that in most of these cases the cytoplasmic inclusions were different from lipofuscin and exhibited a variety of ultrastructural features showing morphologic variations, which are reflected by descriptive names such as multilocular, multilamellar, crescentic, curvilinear, pleomorphic "fingerprint," lipofuscin–lipid compound bodies, etc. Most biochemical studies of these disorders failed to identify a consistent lipid.[19,34-36] However, Bartsch,[36] who examined one of the brains studied by Seitelberger et al.,[14] observed that an increased concentration of all four major gangliosides and of ceramide lactoside and ceramide trihexoside is the expression of a specific metabolic disturbance of ganglioside metabolism and, therefore, the cause of the myoclonic variant of cerebral lipidosis because he found abnormalities in the sequence of hexoses. Andrews et al.[37] observed that in one of two cases 12% of the total gangliosides were represented by ganglioside G_{A3}, a breakdown product of ganglioside G_{M1}.

TSD, which was originally classified as the infantile form of AFI, is now generally accepted to designate a gangliosidosis where the "stored" material is G_{M2}-ganglioside. Warren Tay[2] in 1881 was the first to describe eyeground changes in a 12-month-old child who showed pronounced weakness and who had difficulty in holding up its head and moving its limbs. Tay observed "in the region of the yellow spot in each eye a conspicuous tolerably defined large white patch, and showing in its center a brownish red, fairly circular spot, contrasting strongly with the white patch surrounding it." He considered this a congenital disease, but could not offer any explanation as to its evolution. However, he observed a few months later that the optic disks had become atrophied. Subsequently, Tay[38] saw two additional cases in the same family and later[39] reported a case in another family in which a baby had previously died under similar conditions. Shortly after Tay's original report, a number of authors[40-44] published cases in which similar eyeground changes had been observed. Furthermore, the clinical description of the disease was identical with that reported by Tay. It became increasingly obvious that there was a disease entity occurring in young children in which definite symptoms appeared at about six months of age and which was inevitably fatal. The credit of providing the first clinical and pathologic description of this illness belongs to Bernard Sachs, who, not being aware of the ophthalmologic observations of Tay, gave a detailed report of the disease which is still valid. In his first publication[3] in 1887, he left open the question whether the lack of development is due to a previous inflammation. In a subsequent study[45] he maintained his original viewpoint with respect to the pathogenesis of this disease. However, in 1896, he became aware of the familiar character of this malady after having observed it in a sister of his earlier patient.[46] In that year alone he collected 19 cases, all of them children of Jewish families, and proposed the name of "amaurotic family idiocy." By 1898 he came to the conclusion[47] that TSD is a "heredo-degenerative form of disease occurring in infancy and characterized by a triad of manifestations; an arrest of all mental processes; a progressive weakness of all muscles of the body terminating in generalized paralysis; and by rapidly developing blindness associated with changes in the macula lutea, the cherry-red spot and optic atrophy."

While Sachs thus continued and expanded his studies of TSD, other authors observed similar cases which concurred with his clinical and pathological descriptions. Thus, Peterson[48] noted that the alterations of this illness were restricted to the sulci of the cortex and medulla and also believed that the condition was due to defective development. At the same time, Hirsch[49] also observed several such cases and corroborated, in general, the original report of Sachs. He furthermore noted that the disease was more disseminated than originally thought, and he observed typical alterations in the nerve cells of the gray matter of the spinal cord and, to a somewhat lesser degree, of the cerebellar cortex. He also described degenerative changes in the optic chiasm and optic tracts. Peculiarly enough, no alterations of the glial elements were observed, possibly due to the limitations of the staining techniques which were then available. In contrast to the original theory concerning the pathogenesis of this disease, as proposed by Sachs, Hirsch believed that it possibly resulted from acquired toxic degeneration, with the causative agent being transmitted through the mother's milk. At the same time, Kingdon and Russell,[50] corroborating the observations of various other authors, expressed the opinion that the underlying pathology of TSD results from a degenerative process of undetermined character.

Sachs[51,52] in the ensuing years continued to enlarge his original observations. This was followed by detailed clinical and pathologic descriptions of the disease by several other investigators.[53-57] Schaffer,[53-55] in a series of publications, emphasized the swelling of the cell body and dendrites of the neurons and focused attention upon the ubiquity of the disease process which involved, in addition to the ganglion cells, also the glial cells. He considered the disease a systemic illness restricted to the neuroectodermal derivatives. He furthermore suggested the concept that the disease involves the so-called hyaloplasm of the affected cells and hypothesized that this structural material of the cytoplasm first undergoes swelling and then evolves into coarse granules, which fill or replace the cytoplasmic matrix. He called this material "prelipoid granules," and theorized that these granules are converted into a simple fatty substance as the degenerative process progresses. Eventually degenerative products are taken up by the glial cells which act as macrophages, and then, during the evolution of the disease, these are transferred to the granular cells. Schaffer also believed that an arrest of myelination constitutes a part of the disease process.

During the first decade of this century the number of reported cases increased considerably.[58-61] In 1908, Apert[61] collected 82 indisputable cases. By 1933, Slome[62] was able to collate a total of 200 individuals with TSD from the world literature. The observations of the earlier authors were substantiated and expanded by many investigators.[63-79]

The first pathologic description of the retina in TSD was given in 1897 by Treacher Collins,[80] who observed gross degeneration of the ganglion cell layer associated with thinning and edema at the macula and thought that the latter findings were responsible for the typical eyeground changes. In the following year, Holden[81] confirmed the alterations in the ganglion cells and nerve fiber layers and emphasized, in particular, the degenerative changes in the ganglion cells, while noting that the other retinal layers were practically intact. He believed that the cause for the ophthalmoscopic picture was coagulative necrosis in the ganglion cells. In 1905, Shumway and Buchanan[82] confirmed the degenerative changes in the ganglion cells, many of which had disappeared so that even at the edge of the macula the cells were only one row thick. There was also some degeneration of the nerve-fiber layer and of the optic nerve, but no edema. Poynton, Parsons, and Holmes[83] observed typical changes of the macula. They believed that the cherry-red spot was due to the choroid shining through the degenerating ganglion cells and that the surrounding white area was the result of edema. In the following years a number of other authors[84-86] gave additional descriptions of the characteristic eyeground changes in TSD and, in general, confirmed the original observations.

Several cases have been reported in whom symptoms of TSD occurred either at birth or during the immediate neonatal period, and, therefore, were considered as a congenital form of the disorder. Thus, in 1917, Epstein[87] and, in 1941, Schick[88] reported cases with TSD in whom the clinical picture of the disorder appeared already during the second week after birth. Similarly, Norman and Wood[89] in 1941 reported another patient who they considered to have the congenital form of the disease, an 18-day-old girl with extreme microencephaly and who showed deposition of large amounts of lipid material in ganglion cells. Brown, Corner, and Dodgson[90] in 1954 reported that the younger sister of the patient of Norman and Wood also displayed extreme microencephaly and lived for six weeks. Jorgensen et al.[91] in 1964 reported a case of Niemann–Pick disease in a non-Jewish boy who died at the age of 29 months after a history of hepatosplenomegaly as well as progressive motor and mental retardation which started at the age of six months. There were characteristic foam cells in liver, spleen, bone marrow, thymus, several glands, and in connective tissue of small vessels. The neurons of the central nervous system were markedly swollen and several axons displayed local swelling. Histochemically, the foam cells contained a material that stained distinctly with Baker's acid hematin and Sudan black B. These observations, together with negative reactions with Sudan IV and PAS stains and the absence of metachromasia, appeared consistent with the accumulation of sphingomyelin. However, in addition, the neurons and some glial cells contained a material that was Alcian blue- and PAS-positive and showed metachromasia with thiazine, had a low isoelectric point, and could easily be extracted by chloroform–methanol and particularly by ethanol. These reactions suggested the presence of an acid glycolipid, e.g., gangliosides or related compounds. In 1965, Hagberg et al.[92] reported a 19-month-old non-Jewish boy who died from a progressive neurologic disorder which started before or at two weeks of age and presented a picture of TSD. At autopsy no recognizable neurons were seen in the brain. Many organs showed markedly enlarged reticuloendothelial cells. Biochemically, the ganglioside pattern was composed of ordinary brain gangliosides and gangliosides of an extracellular type. Studies of isolated gangliosides suggested that the major component was a disialoganglioside with a carbohydrate moiety with two hexoses. The authors believed that this disorder was a congenital form of AFI which belonged to a different type from that described earlier. In contrast to TSD, it was believed that this case could not be classified as a "true lipidosis." In 1968, Sandbank[93] reported two siblings who died shortly after delivery and showed severe generalized neurological symptoms. The brains displayed severe neuronal loss in the cortex accompanied by extensive gliosis. A few enlarged neurons showed accumulation of a PAS-positive lipid and the astrocytes contained Sudan-positive material. There were also severe atrophy of the cerebellum and extensive absence of myelin. Moreover, the reticuloendothelial cells in the liver, spleen, and lymph nodes contained the same material as the large neurons. Since biochemical studies were not performed, the author felt that a classification of this case will remain obscure until this is done.

Our present knowledge of the material stored in TSD is based primarily on the fundamental work of Klenk,[1] who, in 1939, observed that the brain in this disease contains greatly increased amounts of glycolipids, which include a substance later identified as N-acetylneuraminic acid or sialic acid. At first Klenk called this lipid "Substance X." However, he soon recognized[94-97] that this material contains ceramide and hexose but is distinguished from cerebroside primarily by the additional presence of a Bial-reactive substance, i.e., neuraminic acid or its derivatives. Klenk proposed the name "ganglioside" for this lipid and found it to be present in the cerebral cortex of TSD patients in concentrations 10–12 times that of normal.[98] Subsequently, Blix[99] observed that the gangliosides also contain hexosamine. In 1951 Folch et al.[100] isolated a ganglioside-like substance from the cerebral cortex which they called *strandin* and from which neuraminic acid was supposedly absent. Their observations, however, were not confirmed by other investigators,[101-104] and it appears now that peptidefree strandin is structurally identical with gangliosides. Subsequently, Rosenberg, Howe, and Chargoff[105] reported a high-molecular-weight neuraminic-acid-containing glycosphingolipid, called a *mucolipid*, which also contained amino acids. However, it seems very likely that these authors were also dealing with a ganglioside fraction containing a peptide chain.

The better understanding of the chemical pathology underlying TSD became possible only after the advent of improved chromatographic techniques. It was consequently found that there are differences in solubility properties of various gangliosides[106,107] It was also observed by the use of column or thin-layer chromatography that a definitive heterogeneity of ganglioside preparations exists.[108-116] It was moreover observed that in TSD a monosialoganglioside accumulates. It has been proven that the Tay–Sachs ganglioside (G_{M2}) is identical with the normal minor monosialoganglioside. Unlike the major monosialoganglioside, however, it lacks the terminal galactose.[108,114-116]

In view of the doubtful increase of gangliosides in what has been called the late infantile, juvenile, and adult forms of AFI, Suzuki and Chen[117] proposed a nomenclature for the two chemically well-delineated gangliosidoses. According to this classification, it was suggested that TSD be called G_{M2}-gangliosidosis and that generalized gangliosidosis be termed G_{M1}-gangliosidosis.

Svennerholm[109] noted an increase of ganglioside also in the livers of Tay–Sachs patients, evidence which seemed to indicate that this disorder represents a generalized disease of ganglioside metabolism. These findings appeared to be confirmed by electron microscopic studies by Volk and Wallace,[118] who also observed lipid cytosomes in livers of Tay–Sachs patients, and by Schneck, Kleinberg, and Volk,[119] who observed an increase of ganglioside in the heart muscle of patients with TSD.

In the past decade various authors[120-135] carried out histochemical and electron microscopic studies of the brains of Tay–Sachs patients and, thereby, contributed considerably to the understanding of the pathogenetic mechanisms of the disease. Landing and Freiman,[121] using various fat stains and histochemical procedures, came to the conclusion that the ganglion cells contain a lipoprotein complex, probably a glycolipid. Diezel,[123-127] in a series of histochemical studies, was able to demonstrate the accumulation of gangliosides in the cerebral cortex of patients with TSD. In detailed studies, he observed that the material found in the ganglion cells of the cerebral and cerebellar cortex was PAS-positive, sudanophilic, metachromatic with thiazin stains, and colored blue-green with Alcian blue. This tinctorial behavior, he concluded, indicated the presence of a protein-bound glycolipid which seemed identical with the gangliosides. Diezel pointed out that different degrees of lipid-to-protein linkages exist in various types of TSD, but that, as a rule, with the advancing age of the patient, more stored lipid is found as a protein and that a decreased solubility in fat solvents can be noted.

Terry, Korey, and co-workers,[131-135] in electron microscopic studies, observed membranous bodies in the cytoplasm of neurons and glial cells of patients with TSD, and they called them "membranous cytoplasmic bodies." Isolated fractions of these membranous cytoplasmic bodies obtained from Tay–Sachs brain tissue have shown that they consist of 90% lipid and 10% protein.[133] They contain large amounts of G_{M2}-ganglioside with an asialic acid–cholesterol–lipid ratio of 1:4:1. In light microscopic studies, Wallace, Lazarus, and Volk[136,137] observed an increase of acid phosphatase in neurons and glial cells of Tay–Sachs patients. They suggested that the increase in acid phosphatase activity is associated with the membranous cytoplasmic bodies described by Terry and Korey.[131] Furthermore, since acid phosphatase has been interpreted as being associated with lysosomes, the authors hypothesized that these bodies are the lysosomes in which gangliosides constitute the main structural component.

The light microscopic observations were confirmed in electron micro-

scopic studies by Wallace and colleagues,[136-138] who identified the localization of acid phosphatase and thiolacetate esterase activity in the cerebellum
of children with TSD. Enzymatic activity occurred in the membranous cytoplasmic bodies, in Purkinje, stellate, and astrocytic cells, and also in
hepatocytes[137,138] and Kupffer cells.[118] In keeping with the results obtained
by light microscopy, the authors concluded that the lipid structures are
lysosomes of the digestive or residual body type, reflecting the cellular efforts to eliminate the accumulated material.

Aronson, Saifer, Volk, and co-workers[139-142] reported serial biochemical
studies of serum and spinal fluid of patients with TSD. There was a
decrease of total serum protein and albumin together with a markedly
depressed amount of gamma globulin present, while, on the other hand, an
elevation of the alpha-2-globulin fraction was found. Furthermore,
decreases in neutral fats and phospholipids as well as of free cholesterol
levels were observed. These authors noted a significant elevation of total
fructoaldolase and glutamic oxaloacetic transaminase in serum and spinal
fluid during the first nine months of illness followed by a decline to normal
values during the protracted phase of the disease. This transient enzyme elevation in serum was interpreted as paralleling the process of ganglionic
destruction within the central nervous system. Aronson, Volk, and co-
workers[140,143-145] in a series of studies correlated the clinical and pathologic
data of over 50 cases of TSD during the evolution of the disease process and
noted that many of the children exhibited a significant increase in brain
weight and head circumference when their life expectancy was extended past
the age of 30 months. The paradoxic increase in the brain weight occurring
in the presence of neuronal disintegration was believed to be the result of an
excessive reactive gliosis.

While, in general, TSD in the vast majority of cases presents a rather
stereotyped pathologic and clinical picture, there are occasional atypical
cases on record. The first of these seems to be a report by Globus,[56] who
presented a case in which the stored intraneuronal material was stainable
only by the technique of Marchi for degenerating myelin. Bielschowsky[146]
reported a patient who at the time of death was two years and seven months
old and in whom demyelinating plaques unlike those of multiple sclerosis
were observed together with intraneuronal deposited lipids. The demyelination differed to some degree from the demyelinated areas which can be
frequently seen in the white matter of Tay–Sachs patients. Furthermore, the
staining properties of the intraneuronal deposits of this case differed also
inasmuch as they resembled more closely those of the juvenile or adult variety. Norman[147] recorded a one-year-old infant with tuberous sclerosis in
whom the ganglion cells contained a substance which histochemically had
some similarity to that observed in juvenile cases. Furthermore, the his-

tologic appearance of the neurons was more similar to that of juvenile cases than to the ganglion cells seen in the infantile form. Jervis[148] reported a family with a disorder that simulated TSD and gargoylism. The material deposited within the neurons stained faintly with both Sudan dyes and iron hematoxylin. Biochemical studies showed a high protagon (cerebrosides and sphingomyelin) concentration and the presence of neuraminic acid. Jervis[149] subsequently also reported a case with considerable accumulation of an iron-containing pigment within ganglion cells which were similar to those found in Hallervorden–Spatz disease.

Several authors[14,78,150-152] reported cases of TSD in whom inclusion bodies of Lafora (myoclonus bodies) were observed in some of the neurons, but particularly in the optic thalamus, substantia nigra, and dentate nucleus. Descamps and van Bogaert[76] reported a patient with TSD in a non-Jewish Walloon family who showed intracytoplasmic deposits simultaneously with demyelination, the latter being either primary or secondary in character. The catabolism progressed to the Sudanophilic state and there were systematized atrophies which recalled the olivopontocerebellar atrophies. Wildi[153] and Favarger and Wildi[154] reported histochemical and chemical observations in a patient with atypical TSD in whom a high concentration of cerebrosides was found and in whom the intraneuronal material was strongly acidic, although it gave a negative Bial reaction. Seitelberger[13,155] observed a case in whom the ganglion cells contained a "hyaline" material while the glial cells were filled with a Sudanophilic substance and some of the cells stained with iron hematoxylin. Bérard-Badier et al.[122] recorded a Tay–Sachs child with demyelination which resembled that observed in leukodystrophy. Mossakowski et al.[156,157] reported three siblings with a progressive neurological disease, in each of whom evidence of both TSD and metachromatic leukodystrophy was found on histologic examination. Histochemically, the material within the neurons was believed to be primarily ganglioside or some glycolipid intermediate between gangliosides and cerebrosides. The accumulated material was believed to be a cerebroside and/or cerebroside sulfuric acid or ester. Biochemical studies of the brain of two of these cases revealed in the white matter an augmentation in hexosamine in both and an increase in sulfatides, absolute in one patient and relative to the total lipids in the other case. The neuraminic acid content of the cortex was not increased.

Wolman[158] reported a 2½-year-old Tay–Sachs patient in whom the deposited material was composed of a mixture of a neutral glycolipid and cholesterol and, while there was no evidence for the presence of strongly acidophilic glycolipids, the deposited material stained intensely with the PAS method and was moderately Sudanophilic. Other authors[148,154,159] reported accumulation of extraneuronal pigment in TSD. Seitelberger's patients[13] exhibited the typical histochemical reaction of chromolipids including a bright yellow fluorescent acid fastness, performic acid Schiff staining, and a positive PAS reaction. In addition, the pigment granules were argentaffin.

De Vries and Amir[160] reported two patients with AFI. In one the disease started at the age of 6 months and death occurred at 2½ years. The other patient was four years old when observed, and had developed neurological symptoms and optic atrophy without the cherry-red spot and retinitis pigmentosa at the age of six months. Both patients showed extensive loss of ganglion cells with marked ballooning of the remaining neurons. There was also extensive demyelination. The brain weights were 430 and 400 g, respectively. The second patient also showed very extensive atrophy of the granular layer of the cerebellum, some of which contained PAS-positive material. The authors considered the first patient an atypical Tay–Sachs case, while they conjectured that the second patient represented the late infantile form of the disorder.

During the past years several attempts have been made to identify the homozygous and heterozygous cases of TSD. Thus, in 1962 Aronson and co-workers[161-162] reported a decrease of fructose-1-phosphate aldolase in the sera of children with TSD as well as in 95% of their parents. However, others[163] were unable to confirm these findings. In 1967 Balint et al.[164] noted that in TSD children and their presumably heterozygous parents a significant reduction of sphingomyelin occurred in the red blood cells both in terms of absolute concentration and as a percentage of total phospholipid. These authors thought that this decline in sphingomyelin represents a possibly useful method for the detection of heterozygous carriers in the Tay–Sachs trait. In 1968, Robinson and Stirling[165] reported that N-acetyl-β-D-hexosaminidase, which was the most likely enzyme to be implicated in the metabolic defect of TSD, could be separated into two isoenzymes, A and B (Hex A and Hex B). On the basis of this observation, Okada and O'Brien[166] observed that component A, which normally comprises over 50% of the total hexosaminidase activity in various tissues, was absent in brain and viscera from patients with TSD. Independently, Sandhoff[167] found a similar enzyme pattern in patients with TSD. O'Brien and co-workers[168] subsequently developed an assay of serum Hex A activity for the purpose of heterozygote detection. It was observed that obligate heterozygotes had a somewhat lower enzyme activity than control subjects and much higher than affected children, and Friedland et al.[169] reported that it was possible to distinguish heterozygotes by assay of Hex A in white blood cells. The specific enzymatic defect has also been demonstrated in various tissues, including extracts from frozen organs, plasma and serum, and cultured fibroblasts.[170,171]

A short time after Sachs expressed his opinion that AFI invariably occurs in Jews, it became obvious that this disease can also be found in children from non-Jewish backgrounds. The first case was recorded by Magnus[40] in an 18-month-old girl of non-Jewish extraction who exhibited clinical symptoms and eyeground changes apparently typical of TSD. Falkenheim,[59] in reviewing this subject, observed that in a series of 36 families, four non-Jewish children afflicted with this disorder were observed. Haveroch[172] observed 86 patients with TSD, seven of whom were non-Jewish. In the following years an increasing number of reports[173-180] recorded the occurrence of TSD in non-Jewish children, although the occurrence of this disease outside the Jewish religion was comparatively rare. Cockayne and Attlee[181] reported a typical case in a one-year-old English infant, the parents of whom were first cousins. The members of the Royal Society of Medicine who heard this report considered it to be a typical case of Tay–Sachs of the "Jewish type," the condition being identical with that originally recorded by Tay. Grear[182] confirmed the existence of TSD in an infant of non-Jewish extraction for the first time by postmortem examination. Throughout the years, a larger number of cases of TSD occurring in non-Jewish children has been recorded, including babies of Asiatic and Levantine origin as well as in Blacks.[183-187] Slome,[62] in a review of the 200 cases in the literature available at that time, found 18 reports of Tay–Sachs patients occurring in non-Jewish infants and calculated that in 20% of the cases the disease occurred in non-Jewish children. Aronson and Volk[188] observed a percentage of 10% of non-Jewish patients in their material of 219 children. Franceschetti et al.[189] noted an increase in nonconsanguineous infants with TSD in gentile families, and they considered this as possibly being due to an increased frequency of the pathogenetic gene or of latent heterozygotes in the population during the previous 20 years.

The ethnic preponderance of TSD in Jewish children has been confirmed by several formal surveys of death certificate registries in Israel and the United States.[190-192] Furthermore, Goldschmidt et al,[190] and others[188,192,193] noted that TSD occurs comparatively rarely in Oriental and African Jews, as compared with those of European extraction. They further observed that the abnormal gene seems to be concentrated primarily in Jews of eastern-European rather than western-European ancestry. These observations have been corroborated by Aronson and Volk,[188] who found that the majority of children with TSD derive primarily from the areas of the pre-World War I Russian–Polish border zone. It has been estimated that in the United States the disease occurs once in about 4000–6000 Jews and only once in approximately 300,000–500,000 non-Jewish births.[194] The gene frequency corresponded to 158 births of infants with TSD per million among the Ashkenazic Jews and 1.7 per million among non-Jews.[195] Based on esti-

mates of gene frequencies, population figures, and birth rates, it was calculated that about 50–60 children with TSD are born yearly in the United
States and that the world figure is probably 5–7 times this number.[196]

TSD is transmitted as an autosomal recessive trait and is found pre-
dominantly, but not exclusively, in descendants of Ashkenazic Jews.[184,192,197]
The carrier rate in this ethnic group is estimated to be 1 in 30, whereas in
Sephardic Jews the carrier rate is 1 in 100, and in Yemenite Jews and non-
Jews it is 1 in 300. In the United States an estimation of the studies of
mortality records give a heterozygote frequency of 0.026 for Ashkenazic
Jews and 0.0029 for non-Jews.[191,192,198] Demographic studies indicate the
epicenters occurred in northeastern Europe, and it has been speculated that
the augmented gene frequency of TSD in Ashkenazic Jews indicates that the
heterozygotes enjoy a small but distinctive survival advantage during their
reproductive period.[194]

There is general agreement that the inheritance of TSD is the result of
an autosomal recessive trait. Slome,[62] in an extensive study of 200 patients
reported up to 1933, observed a frequency of cases of approximately 25% in
69 sibships, half of which had four or more members, the fraction predicted
on the assumption that each parent carried a single recessive gene with
expression of the disease only in the homozygous stage. Slome[62] also observed a high rate of consanguinity in all racial groups, which was approximately 25% in Jewish and 50% in non-Jewish parents. Van Bogaert
and Klein[193] recorded their observations of 11 families in whom infantile, juvenile, and adult cases of AFI occurred. They observed that consanguinity
was common in the involved families. Their studies included a case of
consanguinity within a large Jewish pedigree, the disease occurring only in
the progeny of these doubly related matings. In the non-Jewish pedigrees
consanguinity was present in most cases.

In 1968, Sandhoff and co-workers[199,200] reported an "exceptional case
of Tay–Sachs disease" in which not only the cerebral levels of G_{M2}-ganglio-
sides were significantly increased, but where the asialo-G_{M2} also accumulated to a much greater extent than usual in TSD. In addition, there was a
marked increase of the neutral glycosphingolipid globoside in visceral
tissues, with a total Hex A and Hex B deficiency. Thus far, no ethnic predilection of this condition has been observed and none of the reported patients
were of Jewish descent.[196] Other authors[201-209] have confirmed Sandhoff's
original observation in additional patients, all of whom were non-Jewish.
There were alterations in neurons of the cerebral cortex, cerebellum, spinal
cord, and autonomic nervous system. There were also vacuolated histiocytes
present in various viscera, including the bone marrow, but the degree of
histiocytosis was not as prominent as that seen in Gaucher's disease or
Niemann–Pick disease. Also, Sandhoff[210] observed another variant of TSD

in which both Hex A and Hex B were present in the patient's biological fluids and tissues at above-normal activities, although there was still a marked accumulation of G_{M2}-ganglioside in brain tissue present.

Several authors[211-218] reported a late form of G_{M2}-gangliosidosis in which the patient developed ataxia and progressive psychomotor retardation in the second to sixth year of life and died at about five to fifteen years of age. All patients were of non-Jewish origin. The cherry-red spot and megalencephaly did not occur in these patients, although retinitis pigmentosa and/or optic atrophy could be observed. Both G_{M2}-ganglioside and asialo-G_{M2} accumulate in the brain,[219] as does G_{M2}-ganglioside in the liver and spleen.[212] Although there is less lipid stored in these organs than in typical cases of TSD, electron microscopic observations show that both membranous cytoplasmic bodies as well as less-well-defined lamellated structures are present. Various authors[220-222] demonstrated partial deficiency of Hex A in serum, various tissues, and fibroblasts of these cases.

In 1959 Norman et al.[223] described a patient with a specific form of AFI which they called "Tay–Sachs disease with visceral involvement." The clinical and pathological picture resembled TSD, however, in addition, there was accumulation of lipid-laden histiocytes in liver, spleen, and other organs. Also, in 1959, Craig et al.[224] described an infant with "foam cell" histiocytosis of the viscera, involvement of renal glomerular epithelium, and clinical radiological features suggestive of Hurler's disease. Since the foam cells did not contain acid mucopolysaccharides, their patient was described as "a metabolic neurovisceral disorder with accumulation of an unidentified substance; a variant of Hurler's disease?" In 1962, Landing and Rubinstein[225] reported this disorder under the name of "pseudo-Hurler's disease." Subsequently, Landing and co-workers[226] described eight patients with this disease from the clinical, radiological, and histochemical standpoints and concluded that the material stored in these patients was a relatively soluble, weakly acidic glycolipid, probably a ganglioside, and described this condition as a "familial neurovisceral lipidosis." This disorder has subsequently been reported variously as "a biochemically special form of infantile amaurotic idiocy,"[227] "generalized gangliosidosis,"[228] "late infantile systemic lipidosis,"[229] "Landing's disease,"[230] and "G_{M1}-gangliosidosis."[231] There are two clinical types: one with features similar to those of Hunter–Hurler disease, and the other with cerebral changes but absence of hepatosplenomegaly and skeletal deformities. Clinically the former, and more common, form shows many features of typical mucopolysaccharide disorders type 1, 2, and 3. The patients exhibit hepatosplenomegaly, skeletal changes, and progressive neurologic symptoms. The first manifestations usually appear within the first few months of life, and death in general occurs at the end of the second year. About half of the patients show a cherry-red spot in the macula.[226,228,230] In the second, and numerically smaller, group of patients, the late infantile form, the onset of the disease occurs between the third and sixth years of life, although some patients have reportedly lived longer.[221,230-239] It appears that in the late form only cerebral symptoms are present and that hepatosplenomegaly and skeletal deformities are absent.[235-239] Pathologic alterations include neuronal lipidosis, cytoplasmic ballooning of the glomerular epithelial cells, and visceral histiocytosis.[221,226,230] Electron microscopically, the neuronal cytoplasm is densely filled with lipid bodies which show considerable pleomorphism. The majority of them consist of concentrically arranged lamellae, while others display stacked concentric lamellae similar to the "zebra bodies."[240]

The infantile as well as the late infantile forms of G_{M1}-gangliosidosis show accumulation in brain or viscera of G_{M1}-ganglioside.[241-244] In the viscera there is, in addition, an increase of mucopolysaccharides which is similar to keratin sulfate.[234,245,246] Both forms are transmitted as an autosomal recessive trait.[247] G_{M1}-gangliosidosis is due to a marked deficiency of β-galactosidase in tissues,[248] skin fibroblasts,[249] and leukocytes.[242,250,251] In contrast to TSD, no ethnic predilections have appeared.

In 1966 Pilz and co-workers[252] reported a patient who had nonspecific symptoms suggestive of degeneration of the central nervous system and who died in the third year of life. There were abnormally high concentrations of G_{M3}-ganglioside and asialo-G_{M3}-ganglioside (galactosylglucosylceramide). The brain of this patient, however, had been stored in formalin so that it was impossible to perform enzyme studies.

At the annual meeting of the American Association of Neuropathologists held in June 1974, Max et al.[253] presented another case of G_{M3}-gangliosidosis who died at the age of 3½ months. Since the activities of the various enzymes were normal, the authors concluded that this disease was not due to a defective catabolic reaction, but was the result of a deficiency of ganglioside biosynthesis. Electron microscopically, the picture resembled more that of spongy degeneration of the central nervous system (van Bogaert-Bertrand) than that of any of the so-far-known "storage" diseases.

The advent of prenatal diagnosis through amniocentesis represents the most important step in the prevention of the birth of infants with incurable genetic mental defects and fatal genetic diseases. The utilization of biochemical and enzyme techniques permits identification of high-risk couples and the potential to detect homozygous affected fetuses in utero which makes it selectively possible for at-risk couples to have unaffected babies. In 1970, Schneck et al.[254] observed a case of TSD diagnosed during the second trimester of pregnancy. They demonstrated but trace amounts of Hex A in the amniotic fluid and in the uncultured amniotic fluid cells and subsequently confirmed the prenatal diagnosis by observing a deficiency of this enzyme in the liver and brain of the abortus. These biochemical observations were confirmed by the electron microscopic studies of Adachi *et al.*,[255,256] who found lipid cytosomes in neuronal cells of the central and autosomal nervous systems. Earlier observations by Schneck *et al.*[254] on cultured tissue of a 12-week-old embryo from a mother heterozygous for TSD indicated that the fetal deficiency of Hex A in conjunction with G_{M2} accumulation is detectable during an early stage of pregnancy. The prenatal diagnosis of TSD from amniotic fluid and uncultured and cultured amniotic cells has subsequently been confirmed by other investigators.[221,257,258]

The antenatal diagnosis of a fetus afflicted with G_{M1}-gangliosidosis and the postabortion confirmation of the diagnosis of the tissue obtained at hysterotomy was reported by several observers.[259,260]

During the past two decades several instances of lipid "storage" diseases in animals have been observed. The clinical, pathologic or, in some instances, also the biochemical observations suggested either the juvenile form of AFI[261-266] or human spontaneous leukodystrophy similar to Krabbe's disease.[267-269] In these reports the diagnosis was made primarily on the basis of histochemical criteria.

There are also, however, several reports which deal with diseases considered to be the counterpart of human gangliosidoses.[270-272] In 1968, Read and Bridges[270] reported a spontaneous lipidosis in two Yorkshire swine where membranous cytoplasmic bodies in the central nervous system similar to those in human TSD were present. Biochemical studies, however, were not performed. In 1970, Bernheimer and Karbe[271] and, in 1971, Karbe[272] reported morphologic and biochemical findings in dogs with two types of gangliosidosis. In a German shorthair pointer the disease was characterized by swollen neurons which contained "soluble," PAS-positive material in the form of membranous cytoplasmic bodies. Biochemically, the ganglioside content of the cortex was five times as high as that in the controls. The accumulated material had the properties of G_{M2}-gangliosidosis. In addition, an accumulation of G_{M3}-ganglioside was observed. It was believed that the disease in these animals resembled the late infantile form of G_{M2}-gangliosidosis. In an English setter the disease picture was pathologically characterized by neuronal storage of granules containing mainly insoluble, PAS-positive material and a slight enlargement of some of the neurons. There was a 1.5-times-higher accumulation of the ganglioside content, which could be only assigned to an increase of G_{M2}-ganglioside. In the spinal cord, the ganglioside content was twice as high as that in the controls, but no accumulation of any one particular ganglioside was observed. The authors concluded that the disease in this animal resembled the myoclonic variant of AFI. McGrath *et al.*[273] reported a morphologic study and Gambetti and associates[274] published biochemical observations of a cerebral lipidosis in dogs with similarities to TSD.

Baker and co-workers[275,276] reported biochemical and ultrastructural findings in a Siamese cat with G_{M1}-gangliosidosis which showed progressive motor disability associated with extensive neuronal degeneration due to accumulation of G_{M1}-ganglioside. Tissues from the brain and kidney showed a marked deficiency in β-galactosidase activity. The authors concluded that the disease was similar to the juvenile type of G_{M1}-gangliosidosis. Blakemore[277] observed a case of G_{M1}-gangliosidosis in a three-month-old cat in which the clinical, chemical, and pathologic features resembled those in man, and Handa and Yamakawa[278] performed biochemical analysis of the central nervous system of a family of Siamese cats afflicted with a hereditary neurological disease in which the accumulation of G_{M1}-ganglioside associated with a defect of β-galactosidase activity was observed. Donnelly and co-workers[279, 280] in structural, histochemical and chemical studies observed in Friesian calves a storage disease which was similar to the juvenile form of G_{M1}-gangliosidosis. The presence of gangliosidoses in various animal species, it is believed, will introduce a useful tool in the study of these diseases.

References

1. Klenk, E., Beiträge zur Chemie der Lipoidosen, Niemann–Picksche Krankheit und amaurotische Idiotie, *Z. Physiol. Chem.* **262**:128 (1939–1940).
2. Tay, W., Symmetrical changes in the region of the yellow spot in each eye of an infant, *Trans. Ophthalmol. Soc. U. K.* **1**:155 (1881).
3. Sachs, B., On arrested cerebral development with special reference to its cortical pathology, *J. Nerv. Ment. Dis.* **14**:541 (1887).
4. Batten, F. E., Cerebral degeneration with symmetrical changes in the maculae in two members of a family, *Trans. Ophthalmol. Soc. U. K.* **23**:386 (1902–1903).
5. Mayou, M. S., Cerebral degeneration with symmetrical changes in the maculae in three members of a family, *Trans. Ophthalmol. Soc. U. K.* **24**:142 (1904).
6. Vogt, H., Über familiäre amaurotische Idiotie und verwandte Krankheitsbilder, *Monatsschr. Psychiatr. Neurol.* **18**:161 (1905).
7. Spielmeyer, W., Über familiäre amaurotische Idiotien, *Neurol. Centralbl.* **24**:620 (1905).
8. Jansky, J., Über einen noch nicht beschriebenen Fall der familiären amaurotischen Idiotie mit Hypoplasie des Kleinhirns, *Z. Erforsch. Behandl. jugendl. Schwachsinns.* **3**:86 (1909–1910).
9. Bielschowsky, M., Über spätinfantile familiäre amaurotische Idiotie mit Kleinhirnsymptomen, *Dtsch. Z. Nervenheilkd.* **50**: 7 (1913–1914).
10. Kufs, H., Über eine Spätform und ihre heredo-familiären Grundlagen, *Z. Neurol. Psychiatr.* **95**:169 (1925).

11. Zeman, W. and Dyken, P., Neuronal ceroidlipofuscinosis (Batten's disease): Relationship to amaurotic family idiocy? *Pediatrics* **44**:570 (1969).

12. Zeman, W., Donahue, S., Dyken, P., and Green, J., The neuronal ceroidlipofuscinosis (Batten-Vogt syndrome), in: *Handbook of Clinical Neurology,* P. J. Vinken and G. W. Bruyn, eds., North-Holland, Amsterdam pp. 588-679 (1970).

13. Seitelberger, F., Sonderformen zerebraler Lipoidosen, *Fourth Int. Congr. Neuropathol.* **1**:3 (1962).

14. Seitelberger, F., Jacob, J., and Schnabel, R., The myoclonic variant of cerebral lipidosis, in: *Inborn Disorders of Sphingolipid Metabolism,* S. M. Aronson and B. W. Volk, eds., Pergamon Press, New York, pp. 43-74 (1967).

15. Sluga, E. and Majdetzki, T., Zur Ultrastruktur des Speichermaterials von spätinfantiler amaurotischer Idiotie, *Acta Neuropathol.* **9**:254 (1967).

16. Diezel, P. B., Rossner, J. A., Koppang, N., Ritzhaupt, P., and Bartling, D., Juvenile form of amaurotic family idiocy: A contribution to the morphological, histochemical and electron microscopic aspects, in, *Inborn Disorders of Sphingolipid Metabolism,* S. M. Aronson and B. W. Volk, eds., Pergamon Press, New York, pp. 23-42 (1967).

17. Escola-Pico, J., Über die Ultrastruktur der Speichersubstanzen bei Spätfällen von familiärer amaurotischer Idiotie, *Acta Neuropathol.* **3**:309 (1964).

18. Towfighi, J., Baird, H. W., Gambetti, P., and Gonatas, N. K., The significance of cytoplasmic inclusions in late infantile and juvenile amaurotic idiocy. An ultrastructural study, *Acta Neuropathol.* **23**:32 (1973).

19. Duffy, P. E., Kornfield, M., and Suzuki, K., Neurovisceral storage disease with curvilinear bodies, *J. Neuropathol. Exp. Neurol.* **27**:351 (1968).

20. Haltia, M., Rapola, J., and Santavuori, P., Infantile type of so-called neuronal ceroidlipofuscinosis. Histological and electron microscopic studies, *Acta Neuropathol.* **26**:157 (1973).

21. Benz, U.-U., Peiffer, J., and Schlote, W., Morphologische und biochemische Untersuchungen über einen Fall von juveniler amaurotischer Idiotie (neuronale Ceroid-Lipofuszinosis), in, *Aktuelle Probleme der Kinderpathologie,* H. Bredt and G. Seifert, eds., G. Fischer, Stuttgart pp. 427-432 (1972).

22. Carpenter, S., Karpati, G., and Andermann, F., Specific involvement of muscle, nerve and skin in late infantile and juvenile amaurotic idiocy, *Neurology* **22**:170 (1972).

23. Dolman, C. L. and Chang, E., Visceral lesions in amaurotic familial idiocy with curvilinear bodies, *Arch. Pathol.* **94**:425 (1972).

24. Elfenbein, I. B. and Cantor, H. E., Late infantile amaurotic idiocy with multilamellar cytosomes: An electron microscopic study, *J. Pediatr.* **75**:253 (1969).

25. Gambetti, P., The multilamellar cytosome in late infantile amaurotic idiocy, *J. Neuropathol. Exp. Neurol.* **29**:138 (1970).

26. Gonatas, N. K., Gambetti, P., and Baird, H., A second type of late infantile amaurotic idiocy with multilamellar cytosomes, *J. Neuropathol. Exp. Neurol.* **27**:371 (1968).

27. van Haelst, U. J. G. M. and Gabreëls, F. J. M., The electron microscopic study of the appendix as early diagnostic means in Batten-Spielmeyer-Vogt disease, *Acta Neuropathol.* **21**:169 (1972).

28. Ishii, T. and Gonatas, N. K., The multilamellar cytosome in late infantile amaurotic idiocy, *Acta Neuropathol.* **19**:265 (1971).

29. Richardson, M. E. and Bornhofen, J. H., Early childhood cerebral lipidosis with prominent myoclonus. Ultrastructural and histochemical studies of a cerebral biopsy, *Arch. Neurol.* **18**:34 (1968).

30. Schröder, J. M., Thomas, E., and Kollmann, F., Formvarianten kurvilineärer Zytosomen in Gehirn-, Leber- und Knochenmarksbiopsien bei neuroviszeralen Lipidosen, in: *Aktuelle*

Probleme der Kinderpathologie, H. Bredt and G. Seifert, eds., G. Fischer, Stuttgart, pp. 432–437 (1972).

31. Jakob, H. and Kolkmann, F.-W., Zur Pigmentvariante der adulten Form der amaurotischen Idiotie (Kufs), *Acta Neuropathol.* **26**:225 (1973).

32. Herman, M. H., Rubinstein, L. J., and McKhann, G. M., Additional electron microscopic observations on two cases of Batten-Spielmeyer-Vogt disease (neuronal ceroid lipofuscinosis), *Acta Neuropathol.* **17**:265 (1971).

33. Pallis, C. A., Duckett, S., and Pearse, A. G. E., Diffuse lipofuscinosis of the central nervous system, *Neurology* **17**:381 (1967).

34. Borri, P. F., Hooghwinkel, G. J. M., and Edgar, G. W. F., Brain ganglioside pattern in three forms of amaurotic idiocy and gargoylism, *J. Neurochem.* **13**:1249 (1966).

35. Bronstein, G., Elian, M., Sandbank, U., and Klibansky, C., Juvenile amaurotic idiocy. Clinical, histochemical and brain lipids investigation, *Confin. Neurol.* **24**:62 (1964).

36. Bartsch, G. G., Glycolipid abnormalities in a myoclonic variant of late infantile amaurotic idiocy, *J. Lipid Res.* **11**241 (1970).

37. Andrews, J. M., Sorenson, V., Cancilla, P. A., Price, H. M., and Menkes, N. J., Late infantile neurovisceral storage disease with curvilinear bodies, *Neurology* **21**:207 (1971).

38. Tay, W., A third instance in same family of symmetrical changes in the region of the yellow spot in each eye of an infant closely resembling those of embolism, *Trans. Ophthalmol. Soc. U. K.* **4**:158 (1884).

39. Tay, W., A fourth instance of symmetrical changes in the yellow-spot region of an infant closely resembling those of embolism, *Trans. Ophthalmol. Soc. U. K.* **7**:125 (1892).

40. Magnus, H., Eigentümliche congenitale Bildung der Macula lutea auf beiden Augen, *Klin. Monatsbl. Augenheilkd.* **23**:42 (1885).

41. Goldzieher, W., Ein eigentümlicher Spiegelbefund, *Centralbl. Prakt. Augenheilkd.* **11**:336 (1885).

42. Wadsworth, A., A case of congenital, zonular grayish-white opacity around the fovea, *Trans. Am. Ophthalmol. Soc.* **4**:572 (1887).

43. Hirschberg, J., Der graublaue Hof um den gelben Fleck, *Centralbl. Prakt. Augenheilkd.* **12**:14 (1888).

44. Knapp, H., Über angeborene, hofartige, weissgraue Trübung um die Netzhautgrube, Bericht über die 17, *Verh. Ophthalmol. Ges. Heidelberg* **17**:217 (1942).

45. Sachs, B., A further contribution to the pathology of arrested cerebral development, *J. Nerv. Ment. Dis.* **19**:663 (1892).

46. Sachs, B., A family form of idiocy, generally fatal associated with early blindness, *J. Nerv. Ment. Dis.* **21**:475 (1896).

47. Sachs, B., A family form of idiocy. *N. Y. State J. Med.* **63**:697 (1898).

48. Peterson, F., A case of amaurotic family idiocy with autopsy, *J. Nerv. Ment. Dis.* **25**:529 (1898).

49. Hirsch, W., The pathological anatomy of a fatal disease of infancy with symmetrical changes in the region of the yellow spot, *J. Nerv. Ment. Dis.* **25**:538 (1898).

50. Kingdon, E. C. and Russell, J. S. R., Infantile cerebral degeneration with symmetrical changes in the macula, *Proc. Roy. M. & Chir. Soc.* **9**:34 (1896–1897).

51. Sachs, B., On amaurotic family idiocy, *J. Nerv. Ment. Dis.* **30**:11 (1903).

52. Sachs, B., On amaurotic family idiocy, a disease chiefly of the gray matter, *J. Nerv. Ment. Dis.* **30**:1 (1905).

53. Schaffer, K., Zur Pathogenese der Tay-Sachs'schen Idiotie, *Neurol. Zentralbl.* **24**:386 (1905).

54. Schaffer, K., Tatsächliches und Hypothetisches an der Histopathologie der infantilamaurotischen Idiotie, *Arch. Psychiatr.* **64**:570 (1922).

55. Schaffer, K., General significance of Tay–Sachs disease, *Arch. Neurol. Psychiatr.* **14**:731 (1925).

56. Globus, J. H., Ein Beitrag zur Histopathologie der amaurotischen Idiotie (mit besonderer Berücksichtigung der Beziehungen zu den hereditären Kleinhirnerkrankungen und zur Merzbacher-Pelizaeusschen Krankheit), *Z. Ges. Neurol. Psychiatr.* **85**:424 (1923).

57. Hassin, G. B., A study of the histopathology of amaurotic family idiocy (infantile type of Tay–Sachs), *Arch. Neurol. Psychiatr.* **12**:640 (1924).

58. Mohr, M., Die Sachs'sche amaurotische Idiotie, *Arch. Augenheilkd.* **41**:285 (1900).

59. Falkenheim, K., Über familiäre amaurotische Idiotie, *Jahrb. Kinderheilkd.* **51**:2 (1901).

60. Provotelle, P., De l'idiotie amaurotique familiale (maladie de Warren Tay–Sachs); Étude monographique, Thèse de Paris, Univ. de Paris (1906).

61. Apert, L'idiotie amaurotique familiale (maladie de Tay–Sachs), *Sem. Med.* **3**:25 (1908).

62. Slome, D., The genetic basis of amaurotic family idiocy, *J. Genet.* **27**:24 (1933).

63. Bielschowsky, M., Zur Histopathologie und Pathogenese der amaurotischen Idiotie mit besonderer Berücksichtigung der zerebellaren Veränderungen, *J. Psychol. Neurol.* **26**:125 (1921).

64. Szymanski, J., Recherches anatomo-pathologiques des alterations de la rétine dans la maladie Tay–Sachs, *Bull. Mem. Soc. Fr. Ophthalmol.* **40**:449 (1927).

65. Westphal, A., Beitrag zur Lehre von der amaurotischen Idiotie, *Arch. Psychiatr.* **58**:248 (1917).

66. Globus, J. H., Amaurotic family idiocy, in: *Cytology and Cellular Pathology of the Nervous System*, W. Penfield, ed., Hoeber, New York, p. 1166 (1932).

67. Globus, J. H., Amaurotic family idiocy, *J. Mt. Sinai Hosp. N.Y.* **9**:451 (1942).

68. Ostertag, B., Entwicklungsstörungen des Gehirns und zur Histologie und Pathogenese, bes. der degenerativen Markerkrankung bei amaurotischer Idiotie, *Arch. Psychiatr. Nervenkr.* **75**:355 (1925).

69. Grinker, R. R., The microscopic anatomy of infantile amaurotic idiocy with special reference to the early cell changes and the intracellular lipids, *Arch. Pathol. Lab. Med.* **3**:768 (1927).

70. Von Santha, K., Neuer Beitrag zur Histopathologie der Tay–Sachs-Schafferschen Krankheit, *Arch. Psychiatr. Nervenkr.* **86**:665 (1929).

71. Feyrter, F., Zur Frage der Tay–Sachs-Schafferschen amaurotischen Idiotie, *Virchows Arch. A.* **304**:481 (1939).

72. Scheidegger, S., Amaurotische Idiotie. Ihre Stellung zu den Lipoidosen und die Beziehung zu der Niemann-Pickschen Krankheit, *Schweiz. Z. Pathol. Bakteriol.* **4**:28 (1941).

73. Lubin, A. J., Marburg, O., and Tamaki, K., Familial type of paralysis in infants and its relationship to other heredofamilial disorders. A clinico-pathologic study, *Arch. Neurol. Psychiatr.* **49**:27 (1943).

74. Giampalmo, A., Le tesaurosi lipidiche, *Atti Soc. Ital. Pat.* **2**:35 (1951).

75. Clément, R., Grunner, J., Rameix, P., and Bretagne, J., Idiotie amaurotique de Tay–Sachs, *Presse Med.* **61**:253 (1953).

76. Descamps, L. and van Bogaert, L., Documents anatomo-cliniques sur les idioties amaurotiques. I. Sur une forme infantile précoce isolée dans une souche aryenne, *J. Genet. Hum.* **5**:54 (1956).

77. Baker, A. B. and Platou, E. S., Cerebral changes in amaurotic family idiocy (Tay–Sachs disease), *Arch. Pathol.* **25**:75 (1938).

78. Marburg, O., Inclusion bodies and late fate of ganglion cells in infantile amaurotic family idiocy, *Arch. Neurol. Psychiatr.* **49**:708 (1943).

79. Volk, B. W., Pathologic anatomy, in: *Tay-Sachs Disease*, B. W. Volk, ed., Grune & Stratton, New York, pp. 36–67 (1964).

80. Collins, T., Sciatic nerves; occular changes, *Med. Chir. Trans.* **80**:101 (1897).

81. Holden, W. A., Pathological report on the eyes of Dr. Hirsch's patient with amaurotic family idiocy, *J. Nerv. Ment. Dis.* **25**:550 (1898).

82. Shumway, E. W. and Buchanan, M., Histological examination of the eyes in a case of amaurotic idiocy. *Am. J. Med. Sci.* **129**:35 (1905).

83. Poynton, F. J., Parsons, J. H., and Holmes, G., A contribution to the study of amaurotic family idiocy, *Brain* **29**:180 (1906).

84. Cohen, M., Report of a case of amaurotic family idiocy with histologic report on the eyes, *J. Am. Med. Assoc.* **48**:1751 (1907).

85. Verhoeff, F. H., Amaurotic family idiocy: Histological examination of a case in which the eyes were removed immediately after death, *Arch. Ophthalmol.* **38**:107 (1909).

86. Hancock, W. I. and Coats, G., Pathological examination of the freshly fixed eyes from a case of amaurotic family idiocy, *Brain* **35**:514 (1911).

87. Epstein, T., Amaurotic family idiocy, *N. Y. State J. Med.* **106**:887 (1917).

88. Schick, B., Personal communication to Rothstein, J. L. and Welt, S.: Infantile amaurotic idiocy, *Am. J. Dis. Child.* **62**:801 (1941).

89. Norman, M. and Wood, N., A congenital form of amaurotic family idiocy, *J. Neurol. Psychiatr.* **4**:175 (1941).

90. Brown, N. J., Corner, B. D., and Dodgson, M. C., A second case in the same family of congenital family cerebral lipidosis resembling amaurotic idiocy, *Arch. Dis. Child.* **29**:48 (1954).

91. Jorgensen, L., Blackstad, T. W., Harkmark, W., and Steen, J. A., Niemann–Pick disease: Report of a case with histochemical evidence of neural storage of acid glycolipids, *Acta Neuropathol.* **4**:90 (1964).

92. Hagberg, B., Hultquist, G., Öhman, R., and Svennerholm, L., Congenital amaurotic idiocy, *Acta Paediatr. Scand.* **54**:116 (1965).

93. Sandbank, U., Congenital amaurotic idiocy, *Pathol. Eur.* **3**:228 (1968).

94. Klenk, E., Beiträge zur Chemie der Lipoidosen, *Z. Physiol. Chem.* **267**:128 (1940).

95. Klenk, E., Neuraminsäure, das Spaltprodukt eines neuen Gehirnlipoids, *Z. Physiol. Chem.* **268**:50 (1941).

96. Klenk, E., Über die Ganglioside, eine neue Gruppe von zuckerhältigen Gehirnlipoiden, *Z. Physiol. Chem.* **273**:76 (1942).

97. Klenk, E., Über die Ganglioside des Gehirns bei der infantilen amaurotischen Idiotie vom Typus Tay-Sachs, *Ber. Dtsch. Chem. Ges.* **75**:1632 (1942).

98. Klenk, E., Die Chemie der Lipoidosen und der Entmarkungskrankheiten, *Wien. Z. Nervenheilkd.* **13**:309 (1957).

99. Blix, G., Einige Beobachtungen über eine hexosaminehältinge Substanz in Protagon Fraktion des Gehirns, *Skand. Arch. Physiol.* **80**:46 (1938).

100. Folch, J., Arsove, S., and Meath, J. A., Isolation of brain strandin, a new type of large molecule tissue component, *J. Biol. Chem.* **191**:819 (1951).

101. Bogoch, S., Studies on the structure of brain ganglioside, *Biochem. J.* **68**:319 (1958).

102. Chatagnon, C. and Chatagnon, P., Propriétés chemiques du strandin de Folch. Strandin et acide neuraminique, *Bull. Soc. Chim. Biol.* **36**:373 (1954).

103. Rosenberg, A. and Chargaff, E., Nitrogenous constituents of an ox brain mucolipid, *Biochim. Biophys. Acta* **21**:588 (1956).

104. Sperry, W. M., *Biochemistry of Developing Nervous System*, Academic Press, New York, p. 261 (1951).

105. Rosenberg, A., Howe, C., and Chargaff, E., Inhibition of influenza virus haemagglutination by brain lipid fraction, *Nature (London)* **177**:234 (1956).

106. Svennerholm, L., Chromatographic separation of human brain gangliosides, *J. Neurochem.* **10**:613 (1963).

107. Jatzkewitz, H., Pilz, H., and Sandhoff, K., Quantitative Bestimmungen von Gangliosiden und ihren neuramin-säurefreien Derivaten bei infantilen, juvenilen und adulten Formen der amaurotischen Idiotie und einer spätinfantilen biochemischen Sonderform, *J. Neurochem.* **12**:135 (1965).

108. Svennerholm, L., The chemical structure of normal human brain and Tay–Sachs gangliosides, *Biochem. Biophys. Res. Commun.* **9**:436 (1962).

109. Svennerholm, L., The metabolism of gangliosides in cerebral lipidoses, in: *Inborn Disorders of Sphingolipid Metabolism*, S. M. Aronson and B. W. Volk, eds., Pergamon Press, New York, pp. 169–186 (1967).

110. Svennerholm, L., The nature of the gangliosides in Tay–Sachs disease, in: *Cerebral Lipidoses. A Symposium*, L. van Bogaert, J. N. Cumings, and A. Lowenthal, Blackwell Oxford, pp. 139–145 (1957).

111. Svennerholm, L. and Raal, A., Composition of brain gangliosides, *Biochim. Biophys. Acta* **53**:422 (1961).

112. Gatt, S. and Berman, E. R., A new glycolipid in Tay–Sachs brain, *Biochem. Biophys. Res. Commum.* **4**:9 (1961).

113. Gatt, S. and Berman, E. R., Studies on brain lipids in Tay–Sachs disease. I. Isolation of two sialic acid-free glycolipids, *J. Neurochem.* **10**:43 (1963).

114. Klenk, E., Liedtke, U., and Gielen, W., Das Gangliosid des Gehirns bei der infantilen amaurotischen Idiotie vom Typ Tay–Sachs, *Z. Physiol. Chem.* **334**:186 (1963).

115. Kuhn, R. and Wiegandt, H., Die Konstitution der Ganglio-*N*-tetraose und des Gangliosids G_1, *Chem. Ber.* **96**:866 (1963).

116. Ledeen, R. and Salsman, K., Structure of the Tay–Sachs ganglioside, *Biochemistry* **4**:2225 (1965).

117. Suzuki, K. and Chen, G. C., Brain ceramide hexosides in Tay–Sachs disease and generalized gangliosidosis (G_{M1}-gangliosidosis), *J. Lipid Res.* **8**:105 (1967).

118. Volk, B. W. and Wallace, B. J., The liver in lipidosis. An electron microscopic and histochemical study, *Am. J. Pathol.* **49**:203 (1966).

119. Schneck, L., Kleinberg, W., and Volk, B. W., Cardiac gangliosides in sphingolipidoses, *Proc. Soc. Exp. Biol. Med.* **130**:404 (1969).

120. Allegranza, A., Studio istologico ed istochimico di un caso idiozia amaurotica dell'adulto (tipo Kufs), *Acta Neurol. Napoli* **11**:596 (1956).

121. Landing, B. H. and Freiman, D. G., Histochemical studies on the cerebral lipidoses and other cellular metabolic disorders, *Am. J. Pathol.* **33**:1 (1957).

122. Bérard-Badier, M., Pailas, J. E., Gastaut, H., and Edgar, G. W. F., Essai sur la signification des démyélinisations dans l'idiotie amaurotique infantile. Recherches électro-encéphalographiques, histochimiques et biochimiques, *Psychiatr. Neurol.* **132**:50 1958.

123. Diezel, P. B., Histochemische Untersuchungen an primären Lipoidosen. Amaurotische Idiotie, Gargoylismus, Niemann–Picksche Krankheit, Gauchersche Krankheit, mit besonderer Berücksichtigung des Zentralnervensystems, *Virchows Arch. A* **326**:89 (1954).

124. Diezel, P. B., Histochemischer Nachweis des Gangliosids in Ganglien und Gliazellen bei amaurotischer Idiotie und Isolierung der Lipoidspeichernden Zellen nach der Methode von M. Behrens, *Dtsch. Z. Nervenheilkd.* **171**:344 (1954).

125. Diezel, P. B., Bestimmung der Neuraminsäure im histologischen Schnittpräprat, *Naturwissenschaften* **42**:487 (1955).

126. Diezel, P. B., Histochemical study of primary lipidoses, in: *Cerebral Lipidoses. A Symposium*, L. van Bogaert, J. N. Cumings, and A. Lowenthal, eds., Blackwell Oxford, pp. 11–31 (1957).

127. Diezel, P. B., *Die Stoffwechselstörungen der Sphingolipoide*, Springer-Verlag, Berlin (1957).

128. Franceschetti, A., Wildi, E., and Klein, D., Examen anatomoclinique d'un cas d'idiotie amaurotique infantile (Tay–Sachs), *Acta Genet. et Stat. Med.* **5**:343 (1955).

129. Lazarus, S. S., Wallace, B. J., and Volk, B. W., Neuronal enzyme alterations in Tay–Sachs disease, *Am. J. Pathol.* **41**:579 (1962).

130. Wallace, B. J., Volk, B. W., and Lazarus, S. S., Glial cell enzyme alterations in infantile amaurotic idiocy (Tay–Sachs disease), *J. Neurochem.* **10**:439 (1963).

131. Terry, R. D. and Korey, S. R., Membranous cytoplasmic granules in infantile amaurotic idiocy, *Nature (London)* **188**:1000 (1960).

132. Terry, R. D., Korey, S. R., and Weiss, M., Electron microscopy of the cerebrum in Tay–Sachs disease, in: *Cerebral Sphingolipidoses: A Symposium on Tay–Sachs Disease and Allied Disorders*, S. M. Aronson and B. W. Volk, eds., Academic Press, New York, pp. 49–56 (1962).

133. Samuels, S., Korey, S. R., Gonatas, J., Terry, R. D., and Weiss, M., The membranous granules in Tay–Sachs disease, in, *Cerebral Sphingolipidoses: A Symposium on Tay–Sachs Disease and Allied Disorders*, S. M. Aronson and B. W. Volk, eds., Academic Press, New York, pp. 309–316 (1962).

134. Terry, R. D. and Weiss, M., Studies in Tay–Sachs disease. II. Ultrastructure of the cerebrum, *J. Neuropathol. Exp. Neurol.* **22**:18 (1963).

135. Terry, R. D. Korey, S. R., Studies in Tay–Sachs disease. V. The membrane of the membranous cytoplasmic body, *J. Neuropathol. Exp. Neurol.* **22**:98 (1963).

136. Wallace, B. J., Lazarus, S. S., and Volk, B. W., Electron microscopic and histochemical studies of viscera in lipidoses, in: *Inborn Disorders of Sphingolipid Metabolism*, S. M. Aronson and B. W. Volk, eds., Pergamon Press, New York, pp. 107–120 (1967).

137. Wallace, B. J., Volk, B. W., and Lazarus, S. S., Fine structural localization of acid phosphatase activity in neurons of Tay–Sachs disease, *J. Neuropathol. Exp. Neurol.* **53**:676 (1964).

138. Wallace, B. J., Volk, B. W., Schneck, L., and Kaplan, H., Fine structural localization of two hydrolytic enzymes in the cerebellum of children with lipidoses, *J. Neuropathol. Exp. Neurol.* **25**:76 (1966).

139. Aronson, S. M., Saifer, A., Perle, G., and Volk, B. W., Cerebrospinal fluid enzymes in central nervous system lipidoses (with particular reference to amaurotic family idiocy), *Proc. Soc. Exp. Biol. Med.* **97**:331 (1958).

140. Aronson, S. M., Saifer, A., Kanof, A., and Volk, B. W., Progression of amaurotic family idiocy as reflected by serum and cerebrospinal fluid changes, *Am. J. Med.* **24**:390 (1958).

141. Saifer, A., Aronson, S. M., Zymaris, M. C., and Volk, B. W., Serial biochemistry of serum and cerebrospinal fluid in amaurotic family idiocy (Tay–Sachs disease), *Proc. Soc. Exp. Biol. Med.* **91**:394 (1956).

142. Volk, B. W., Aronson, S. M., and Saifer, A., The serum neuraminic acid distribution. II. Clinical studies with special reference to amaurotic family idiocy (Tay–Sachs disease), *J. Lab. Clin. Med.* **50**:26 (1957).

143. Aronson, S. M., Lewitan, A., Rabiner, A. M., Epstein, N., and Volk, B. W., The megalencephalic phase of infantile amaurotic familial idiocy, *Am. Med. Assoc. Arch. Neurol. Psych.* **79**:151 (1958).

144. Aronson, S. M., Volk, B. W., and Epstein, N., Morphologic evolution of amaurotic family idiocy, *Am. J. Pathol.* **31**:609 (1955).

145. Kanof, A., Aronson, S. M., and Volk, B. W., Clinical progression of amaurotic family idiocy, *Am. Med. Assoc. J. Dis. Child.* **97**:656 (1959).

146. Bielschowsky, M., Über eine bisher unbekannte Form von infantiler amaurotischer Idiotie, *Z. Ges. Neurol. Psychiatr.* **155**:321 (1936).

147. Norman, R. M., Nerve-cell swelling of the juvenile amaurotic idiocy type, *Arch. Dis. Child.* **15**:244 (1940).

148. Jervis, G. A., Familial mental deficiency akin to amaurotic idiocy and gargoylism. An apparently new type, *Arch. Neurol. Psychiatr.* **47**:943 (1942).

149. Jervis, G. A., Hallervorden-Spatz Disease associated with amaurotic idiocy, *J. Neuropathol. Exp. Neurol.* **11**:4 (1952).

150. Liebers, M., Zur Histopathologie der amaurotischen Idiotie und Myoklonusepilepsie, *Z. Ges. Neurol. Psychiatr.* **111**:465 (1927).

151. Von Santha, K., Über drei reine von Niemann-Pickscher Krankheit verschonte Fälle der infantil-amaurotischen Idiotie, *Arch. Psychiatr. Nervenkr.* **93**:675 (1931).

152. Marchand, L., Borel, J., Laroche, J., and Ganry, C.; Idiote infantile de Tay-Sachs. Forme myoclono-épileptique chez deux frères (considérations cliniques, anatomo-pathologiques et héréditaires), *Encéphale* **45**:1 (1956).

153. Wildi, E., Contribution à l'étude anatomo-pathologique et chimique de la maladie de Tay-Sachs, Thèse Médecine, Genève, No. 1978, Imprimerie Centrale (1950).

154. Favarger, P. and Wildi, E., Chemical analysis and histochemical examination of an atypical case of Tay-Sachs disease, in: *Cerebral Lipidoses. A Symposium,* L. van Bogaert, J. N. Cumings, and A. Lowenthal, eds., Blackwell Oxford, pp. 146–158 (1957).

155. Seitelberger, F., Eine unbekannte Form von infantiler Lipoid-speicher-Krankheit des Gehirns, *Proc. 1st Int. Congr. Neuropathol.* **3**:323 (1952).

156. Mossakowski, M. J., Mathieson, G., and Cumings, J. N.; On the relationship of metachromatic leucodystrophy and amaurotic idiocy, *Brain,* **84**:585 (1961).

157. Mossakowski, M. J., Mathieson, G., and Cumings, J. N., The association of amaurotic idiocy and metachromatic leucodystrophy: A histochemical and biochemical study, *Proc. 4th Int. Congr. Neuropathol.* **1**:205 (1962).

158. Wolman, M., Histochemical study of the brain in an atypical case of amaurotic idiocy, *Acta Neuropathol.* **1**:73 (1961).

159. Seitelberger, F. and Simma, K., On the pigment variant of amaurotic idiocy, in: *Cerebral Sphingolipidoses: A Symposium on Tay-Sachs Disease and Allied Disorders,* S. M. Aronson and B. W. Volk, eds. Academic Press, New York, pp. 29–48 (1962).

160. De Vries, E. and Amir, A. P., An atrophic type of amaurotic idiocy. Report of two cases, *Psychiatr. Neurol. Neurochir.* **67**:231 (1964).

161. Aronson, S. M., Saifer, A., Perle, G., and Volk, B. W., The biochemical identification of the carrier state of Tay-Sachs disease, *Proc. Soc. Exp. Biol. Med.* **111**:664 (1962).

162. Volk, B. W., Aronson, S. M., and Saifer, A., Editorial. Fructose-1-phosphate aldolase deficiency in Tay-Sachs disease, *Am. J. Med.* **36**:481 (1964).

163. Hue, L., Van Hoof, F., and Hers, H. G., Serum aldolase in Tay-Sachs disease and in fructose intolerance, *Am. J. Med.* **51**:758 (1971).

164. Balint, J. A., Kyriakides, E. C., and Spitzer, H. L., On the chemical changes in the red cell stroma in Tay-Sachs disease: Their value as genetic tracers, in, *Inborn Disorders of Sphingolipid Metabolism,* S. M. Aronson and B. W. Volk, eds., Pergamon Press, New York, pp. 423–430 (1967).

165. Robinson, D. and Stirling, J. L., N-Acetyl-β-glucosaminidase in human spleen, *Biochem. J.* **107**:321 (1968).

166. Okada, S. and O'Brien, J. S., Tay-Sachs disease. Generalized absence of β-D-N-acetyl-hexosaminidase components, *Science* **165**:698 (1969).

167. Sandhoff, K., Variation of β-N-acetylhexosaminidase-pattern in Tay-Sachs disease, *FEBS Lett.* **4**:351 (1969).

168. O'Brien, J. S., Okada, S., Chen, A., and Fillerup, D. L., Tay-Sachs disease: Detection of heterozygotes and homozygotes by serum hexosaminidase assay, *New Engl. J. Med.* **283**:15 (1970).

169. Friedland, J., Schneck, L., Saifer, A., Pourfar, M., and Volk, B. W., Identification of Tay-Sachs disease carriers by acrylamide gel electrophoresis, *Clin. Chim. Acta* **28**:397 (1970).

170. Kolodny, E. H., Brady, R. O., and Volk, B. W., Demonstration of an alteration of ganglioside metabolism in Tay-Sachs disease, *Biochem. Biophys. Res. Commun.* **37**:526 (1969).

171. Okada, S., Veath, M. L., Leroy, J., and O'Brien, J. S., Ganglioside G_{M2} storage disease: Hexosaminidase deficiencies in cultured fibroblasts. *Am. J. Hum. Genet.* **23**:55 (1971).

172. Haveroch, A., Störung des Gedächtnisses. Unmöglichkeit der Zeitbestimmung bei den Erinnerungen, *Neurol. Zentralbl.* **23**:375 (1904).

173. Tarr, E. M., A case of amaurotic family idiocy of non-Jewish parentage, *Louisville Month. J. Med. Surg.* **22**:353 (1914–1915).

174. Van Starck, M. P., Amaurotic family idiocy, *Mbl. Kinderheilkd.* **18**:39 (1920).

175. Levy, A., Amaurotic family idiocy, *Am. J. Ophthaolmol.* **6**:408 (1923).

176. Hoppe, L. O. and Clay, G. E., Amaurotic family idiocy with report of a case in a gentile, *Arch. Pediatr.* **41**:389 (1924).

177. Finnoff, W. E., Amaurotic family idiocy, *Am. J. Ophthalmol.* **8**:570 (1925).

178. Lebbetter, T., A case of amaurotic family idiocy in an infant of nonsemitic parentage, *Can. Med. Assoc. J.* **14**:367 (1925).

179. Zannoni, C., Amaurotic idiocy, *Rev. Gen. Ophthalmol.* **39**:299 (1925).

180. Duran, J., Amaurotic family idiocy, *Arch. Oftalmol. Hisp. Am.* **26**:232 (1926).

181. Cockayne, E. A. and Attlee, J., Amaurotic family idiocy in an English child. *Proc. R. Soc. Med.* **8**:414 (1959).

182. Grear, J. N., Jr., Infantile amaurotic family idiocy with report of a case in a child of non-Jewish parentage, *South. Med. J.* **23**:324 (1951).

183. Cordes, F. C. and Horner, W. D., Infantile amaurotic family idiocy in two Japanese families, *Am. J. Ophthalmol.* **12**:558 (1929).

184. Aronson, S. M., Valsamis, M. P., and Volk, B. W., Infantile amaurotic idiocy. Occurrence, genetic considerations and pathophysiology in the non-Jewish infant, *Pediatrics* **26**:229 (1960).

185. Maruyama, Y., Takeuchi, S., Tajiri, R., Hayano, S., and Makita, A., A case of infantile amaurotic family idiocy (Tay-Sachs disease). A clinical and pathological study with biochemical analysis, *Med. J. Shinshi Univ.* **5**:237 (1960).

186. Duke, J. R. and Clark, D. B., Infantile amaurotic family idiocy (Tay-Sachs disease) in the Negro race, *Am. J. Ophthalmol.* **53**:232 (1926).

187. Ghai, O. P. and Kheterpal, S., Amaurotic family idiocy. Report of a case of Tay-Sachs disease with a brief review, *Indian J. Child Health* **12**:107 (1963).

188. Aronson, S. M. and Volk, B. W., Genetic and demographic considerations concerning Tay-Sachs disease, in: *Cerebral Sphingolipidosis: A Symposium on Tay-Sachs Disease and Allied Disorders,* S. M. Aronson and B. W. Volk, eds., Academic Press, New York, pp. 375–395 (1962).

189. Franceschetti, A., Klein, D., and Babel, J., Les manifestations oculaires des troubles primitifs du métabolisme des lipides. Étude clinique, génétique et anatomo-pathologique, *Arch. Neuropsiquiat.* **13**:68 (1955).

190. Goldschmidt, E., Lenz, R., Marin, S., Ronen, A., and Ronen, I., Frequency of the Tay-Sachs gene in the Jewish communities of Israel, *Proc. 25th Annu. Meet. Genet. Soc. Am.* 27 (1956).

191. Kozinn, P. J., Wiener, H., and Cohen, P., Infantile amaurotic family idiocy, *J. Pediatr.* 51:58 (1957).

192. Myrianthopoulos, N. C., Some epidemiologic and genetic aspects of Tay-Sachs disease, in: *Cerebral Sphingolipidoses: A Symposium on Tay-Sachs Disease and Allied Disorders,* S. M. Aronson and B. W. Volk, eds., Academic Press, New York, pp. 359–374 (1962).

193. van Bogaert, L. and Klein, D., Observations sur l'hérédité des idioties amaurotiques et de la spléno-hépato-mégalie lipidiènne (11 familles), *J. Genet. Hum.* 4:23 (1955).

194. Myrianthopoulos, N. C. and Aronson, S. M., Reproductive fitness and selection in Tay-Sachs disease, in: *Inborn Disorders of Sphingolipid Metabolism,* S. M. Aronson and B. W. Volk, eds., Pergamon Press, New York, pp. 431–444 (1967).

195. Shaw, R. F. and Smith, A. P., Is Tay-Sachs disease increasing? *Nature (London)* 224:1213 (1969).

196. O'Brien, J. S., Okada, S., Ho, M. W., Fillerup, D. L., Veath, M. L., and Adams, K., Ganglioside-storage diseases, *Fed. Proc. Fed. Am. Soc. Exp. Biol.* 30:956 (1971).

197. Fuhrmann, W., Genetic aspects of lipidoses, in: *Lipids and Lipidoses,* G. Schettler, ed., Springer-Verlag, New York, pp. 490–528 (1967).

198. Aronson, S. M., Epidemiology, in: *Tay-Sachs Disease,* B. W. Volk, ed., Grune & Stratton, New York, pp. 118–153 (1964).

199. Sandhoff, K., Andreae, W., and Jatzkewitz, H., Deficient hexosaminidase activity in an exceptional case of Tay-Sachs disease with additional storage of kidney globoside in visceral organs, *Life Sci.* 7:283 (1968).

200. Pilz, H., Müller, D., Sandhoff, K., and ter Meulen, V., Tay-Sachssche Krankheit mit Hexosaminidase-Defekt. Klinische, morphologische und biochemische Befunde bei einem Fall mit viszeraler Speicherung von Nierenglobosid, *Dtsch. Med. Woclenschr.* 93:1833 (1968).

201. Sandhoff, K., Jatzkewitz, H., and Peters, G., Die infantile amaurotische Idiotie und verwandte Formen also Gangliosid-Speicherkrankheiten, *Naturwissenschaften* 56:356 (1969).

202. Suzuki, Y., Jacob, J. C., Suzuki, K., Kutty, K. M., and Suzuki, K., G_{M2}-gangliosidosis with total hexosaminidase deficiency, *Neurology* 21:313 (1971).

203. O'Brien, J. S., Okada, S., Ho, M. W., Fillerup, D. L., Veath, M. L., and Adams, K., Ganglioside storage diseases, in: *Lipid Storage Diseases. Enzymatic Defects and Implications,* J. Bernsohn and H. J. Grossman, eds., Academic Press, New York, pp. 225–274 (1971).

204. Krivit, W., Desnick, R. J., Lee, J., Moller, J., Wright, F., Sweeley, C. C., Snyder, P. D., and Sharp, H. L., Generalized accumulation of neutral glycosphingolipids with G_{M2} ganglioside accumulation in the brain. Sandhoff's disease (variant of Tay-Sachs disease), *Am. J. Med.* 52:763 (1972).

205. O'Brien, J. S., Five gangliosidoses, *Lancet* 2:805 (1969).

206. Harzer, K., Sandhoff, K., Schall, M., and Kollmann, F., Enzymatische Untersuchungen im Blut von Überträgern einer Variante der Tay-Sachsschen Erkrankung (Variante O.), *Klin. Wochenschr.* 49:1189 (1971).

207. Strecker, G. and Montreuill, J., Description d'une oligosaccharodosurie accompagant une ganglioside G_{M2} à deficit total en *N*-acetyl-hexosaminidases, *Clin. Chim. Acta* 33:395 (1971).

208. Snyder, P. D., Krivit, W., and Sweeley, C. C., Generalized accumulation of neutral gly-

cosphingolipids with G_{M2} ganglioside accumulation in the brain, *J. Lipid Res.* **13**:128 (1972).

209. Résibois, A. and Tondeur, M., Ultrastructure of Sandhoff's disease. *Proc. 6th Int. Congr. Neuropathol.* 1047 (1970).
210. Sandhoff, K., Harzer, K., Wässle, W., and Jatzkewitz, H., Enzyme alterations and lipid storage in three variants of Tay–Sachs disease, *J. Neurochem.* **18**:2469 (1971).
211. Suzuki, Y. and Suzuki, K., Partial deficiency of hexosaminidase A in juvenile G_{M2}-gangliosidosis, *Neurology* **20**:848 (1970).
212. Suzuki, K., Suzuki, K., Rapin, I., Suzuki, Y., and Ishii, N., Juvenile G_{M2}-gangliosidosis, *Neurology* **20**:190 (1970).
213. Young, P., Ellis, R. B., Lake, B. D., and Patrick, A. D., Tay–Sachs disease and related disorders: Fractionation of brain N-acetyl-β-hexosaminidase on DEAE-cellulose, *FEBS Lett.* **9**:1 (1970).
214. Menkes, J. H., O'Brien, J. S., Okada, S., Grippo, J., Andrews, N. J., and Cancilla, P. A., Juvenile G_{M2}-gangliosidosis: Biochemical and ultrastructural studies on a rare variant of Tay–Sachs disease, *Arch. Neurol.* **25**:14 (1971).
215. Bernheimer, H. and Seitelberger, F., Über das Verhalten der Ganglioside im Gehirn bei 2 Fällen von spätinfantiler amaurotischer Idiotie, *Wien. Klin. Wochenschr.* **80**:163 (1968).
216. Volk, B. W., Adachi, M., Schneck, L., and Saifer, A., Systemic late infantile amaurotic idiocy-monosialogangliosidosis, *J. Neuropathol. Exp. Neurol.* **28**:171 (1969).
217. Klibansky, C., Saifer, A., Feldman, N. I. Schneck, L., and Volk, B. W., Cerebral lipids in a case of systemic G_{M2}-gangliosidosis of a late infantile type, *J. Neurochem.* **17**:339 (1970).
218. Volk, B. W., Adachi, M., Schneck, L., Saifer, A., and Kleinberg, W., G_5-ganglioside variant of systemic late infantile lipidosis, *Arch. Pathol.* **87**:393 (1969).
219. Seitelberger, F., Sluga, E., and Bernheimer, H., Studies on neuronal lipid dystrophies, in: *Cerebral Lipidoses,* A. N., Vincente P. Dustin, and A. Lowenthal, eds., Presses Académiques Européennes, Brussels, 116–127 (1968).
220. Schneck, L., Friedland, J., Pourfar, M., Saifer, A., and Volk, B. W., Hexosaminidase activities in a case of systemic G_{M2}-gangliosidosis of late infantile type, *Proc. Soc. Exp. Biol. Med.* **133**:997 (1970).
221. O'Brien, J. S., Ganglioside storage diseases, in: *Advances in Human Genetics,* H. Harris and K. Hirschhorn, eds., Plenum Press, New York, pp. 39–98 (1972).
222. Brett, E. M., Ellis, R. B., Haas, L., Ikonne, J. U., Lake, B. D., Patrick, A. D., and Stephens, R., Late onset G_{M2}-gangliosidosis. Clinical, pathological and biochemical studies, *Arch. Dis. Child.* **48**:775 (1973).
223. Norman, R. M., Urich, H., Tingey, A. H., and Goodbody, R. A., Tay–Sachs disease with visceral involvement and its relationship to Niemann–Pick disease, *J. Pathol. Bacteriol.* **78**:409 (1959).
224. Craig, J. M., Clarke, J. T., and Banker, B. Q., Metabolic neurovisceral disorder with accumulation of unidentified substance: Variant of Hurler's syndrome? *Am. J. Dis. Child.* **98**:577 (1959).
225. Landing, B. H. and Rubinstein, J. H., Biopsy diagnosis of neurologic diseases in children with emphasis on the lipidoses, in: *Cerebral Sphingolipidoses: A Symposium on Tay–Sachs Disease and Allied Disorders,* S. M. Aronson and B. W. Volk, eds., Academic Press, New York, pp. 1–14 (1962).
226. Landing, B. H., Silverman, F. N., Craig, J. M., Jacoby, M. D., Lahey, M. E., and Chadwick, D. L., Familial neurovisceral lipidosis: Analysis of eight cases of syndrome previously reported as "Hurler-variant," "pseudo-Hurler disease," and "Tay–Sachs disease with visceral involvement," *Am. J. Dis. Child.* **108**:503 (1964).

227. Jatzkewitz, H. and Sandhoff, K., On a biochemically special form of infantile amaurotic idiocy, *Biochim. Biophys. Acta* **70**:354 (1963).

228. O'Brien, J. S., Stern, M. B. Landing, B. H., O'Brien, J. K., and Donnell, G. N., Generalized gangliosidosis. Another inborn error of ganglioside metabolism? *Am. J. Dis. Child.* **109**:338 (1965).

229. Gonatas, N. K. and Gonatas, J., Ultrastructural and biochemical observations on a case of systemic late infantile lipidosis and its relationship to Tay–Sachs disease and gargoylism, *J. Neuropathol. Exp. Neurol.* **24**:318 (1965).

230. Sacrez, R., Juif, J. G., Gigonnet, J. M., and Gruner, J. E., La maladie de Landing. Ou Idiotie amaurotique infantile precoce avec gangliosidose generalisée de type G_{M1}, *Pediatrie* **22**:143 (1967).

231. Suzuki, K., Suzuki, K., and Chen, G. C., G_{M1}-gangliosidosis (generalized gangliosidosis). Morphology and chemical pathology, *Pathol. Eur.* **3**:389 (1968).

232. Hooft, C., Vlietinck, R. F., Dacremont, G., and Kint, A., G_{M1}-gangliosidosis type II, *Eur. Neurol.* **4**:(1970).

233. Patton, V. M. and Dekaban, A. S., G_{M1}-gangliosidosis and juvenile cerebral lipidosis. Clinical, histochemical and chemical study, *Arch. Neurol.* **24**:529 (1971).

234. Suzuki, K., Suzuki, K., and Kamoshita, S., Chemical pathology of G_{M1}-gangliosidosis (generalized gangliosidosis), *J. Neuropathol. Exp. Neurol.* **28**:25 (1969).

235. Derry, D. M., Fawcett, J. S., Andermann, F., and Wolfe, L. S., Late infantile systemic lipidosis. Major monosialogangliosidosis delineation of two types, *Neurology* **18**:340 (1968).

236. Hubain, P., Adam, E., Dewelle, A., Druez, G., Farriaux, J.-P., and Dupont, A., Étude d'une observation de gangliosidose G_{M1}, *Helv. Paediatr. Acta* **24**:337 (1969).

237. Kint, J. A., Dacremont, G., and Vlietinck, R., Type II G_{M1}-gangliosidosis? *Lancet* **2**:108 (1969).

238. Schettler, G. and Kahlke, W., Gangliosidosis, in: *Lipids and Lipidoses*, G. Schettler, ed., Springer-Verlag, Berlin, pp. 213–359 (1967).

239. Wolfe, L. S., Callahan, J., Fawcett, J. S., Andermann, F., and Schriver, C. G., G_{M1}-gangliosidosis without chondrodystrophy or visceromegaly, *Neurology* **20**:23 (1970).

240. Aleu, F. P., Terry, R. D., and Zellweger, H., Electron microscopy of two cerebral biopsies in gargoylism, *J. Neuropathol. Exp. Neurol.* **24**:456 (1967).

241. Hooft, C., Senesael, L., Delbeke, M. J., Kint, J. A., and Dacremont, G., The G_{M1}-gangliosidosis (Landing's disease), *Eur. Neurol.* **2**:225 (1969).

242. O'Brien, J. S., Generalized gangliosidosis, *J. Pediatr.* **75**:167 (1969).

243. Seringe, P., Plainfosse, B., Lautmann, F., Lorilout, J., Calamy, G., Berry, J. B., and Watchi, J. M., Gangliosidose generalizsée du type Norman–Landing. A G_{M1} étude a propose d'un cas diagnostique du vivant du malade, *Ann. Pediatr.* **15**:165 (1968).

244. Suzuki, K., Cerebral G_{M1}-gangliosidosis: Chemical pathology of the visceral organs, *Science* **159**:1471 (1968).

245. Callahan, J. W. and Wolfe, L. S., Isolation and characterization of keratan sulfates from the liver of a patient with G_{M1}-gangliosidosis type I, *Biochim. Biophys. Acta* **215**:527 (1970).

246. O'Brien, J. S., G_{M1}-gangliosidoses, in: *The Metabolic Basis of Inherited Disease*, J. B. Stanbury, J. B. Wyngaarden, and D. S. Fredrickson, eds., McGraw-Hill, New York, pp. 639–662 (1972).

247. O'Brien, J. S., Generalized gangliosidosis. The clinical delineation of birth defects, *Birth Defects Orig. Art. Ser.* **5**:190–206 (1969).

248. Okada, S. and O'Brien, J. S., Generalized gangliosidosis: Beta-galactosidase deficiency, *Science* **160**:1002 (1968).

249. Sloan, H. R., Uhlendorf, B. W., Jacobson, C. B., and Fredrickson, D. S., β-Galactosidase in tissue culture derived from human skin and bone marrow. Enzyme defect in G_{M1}-gangliosidosis, *Pediatr. Res.* **3**:532 (1969).

250. Singer, H. S. and Schafer, I. A., White cell beta-galactosidase activity, *New Engl. J. Med.* **282**:571 (1970).

251. Singer, H. S., Nankervis, G. A., and Schafer, I. A., Leukocyte beta-galactosidase activity in the diagnosis of generalized G_{M1}-gangliosidosis, *Pediatrics* **49**:352 (1972).

252. Pilz, H., Sandhoff, K., and Jatzkewitz, H., A disorder of ganglioside metabolism with storage of ceramide lactoside, monosialoceramide lactoside and Tay–Sachs ganglioside in brain, *J. Neurochem.* **13**:1273 (1966).

253. Max, S. R., Maclaren, N. K., Brady, R. P., Fishman, P., Tallman, J., Garcia, J. H., Cornblath, M., Tanaka, J., Viloria, J. E., and Kamijyo, Y., G_{M3} gangliosidosis: A new lipid storage disease with a defect in ganglioside biosynthesis, presented at the 50th Annual Meeting of the American Association of Neuropathologists, Boston, Mass. June. 1974.

254. Schneck, L., Friedland, J., Valenti, C., Adachi, M., Amsterdam, D., and Volk, B. W., Prenatal diagnosis, of Tay–Sachs disease, *Lancet* **1**:582 (1970).

255. Adechi, M., Schneck, L., and Volk, B. W., Ultrastructural studies of eight cases of fetal Tay–Sachs disease, *Lab. Invest.* **30**:102 (1974).

256. Adachi, M., Torii, J., Schneck, L., and Volk, B. W., The fine structure of fetal Tay–Sachs disease, *Arch. Pathol.* **91**:48 (1971).

257. O'Brien, J. S., Okada, S., Fillerup, D. L., Veath, M. L., Adornato, B., Brenner, P. H., and Leroy, J. G., Tay–Sachs disease: Prenatal diagnosis, *Science* **172**:61 (1971).

258. Padeh, B. and Navon, R., Diagnosis of Tay–Sachs disease by hexosaminidase activity in leukocytes and amniotic fluid cells, *Israel J. Med. Sci.* **7**:259 (1971).

259. Lowden, J. A., Cutz, E., Conen, P. E., Rudd, N., and Doran, T., Prenatal diagnosis of G_{M1}-gangliosidosis, *New Engl. J. Med.* **288**:225 (1973).

260. Kaback, M. M., Sloan, H. R., Sonneborn, M., Herndon, R. M., and Percy, A. K., G_{M1}-gangliosidosis type I. *In utero* detection and fetal manifestations, *J. Pediatr.* **82**:1037 (1973).

261. Hagen, L. O., Lipid dystrophic changes in the central nervous system in dogs, *Acta Pathol. Microbiol. Scand* **33**:22 (1953).

262. Ribelin, W. E. and Kintner, L. D., Lipodystrophy of the central nervous system in a dog. A disease with similarities to Tay–Sachs disease of man, *Cornell Vet.* **46**:532 (1956).

263. Fankhauser, R., Degenerative lipoid-idiotische Erkrankung des Zentralnervensystems bei zwei Hunden. *Schweiz. Arch. Tierheilkd.* **107**:73 (1965).

264. Read, W. K. and Bridges, C. H., Neuronal lipodystrophy. Occurrence in an inbred strain of cattle, *Pathol. Vet.* **6**:235 (1969).

265. Koppang, N., Neuronal ceroid-lipofuscinosis in English setters. Juvenile amaurotic familiar idiocy (AFI) in English setters. *J. Small Anim. Pract.* **10**:639 (1970).

266. Karbe, E. and Schiefer, B., Familiar amaurotic idiocy in male German shorthair pointers, *Pathol. Vet.* **4**:223 (1967).

267. Fankhauser, R., Luginbuhl, H., and Hartley, W. J., Leukodystrophie vom Typus Krabbe beim Hund. *Schweiz. Arch. Tierheilkd.* **105**:198 (1963).

268. Fletcher, T. F., Kurtz, H. J., and Low, D. G., Globoid cell leukodystrophy (Krabbe type) in the dog, *J. Am. Med. Assoc.* **149**:165 (1966).

269. Jortner, B. S. and Jonas, A. M., The neuropathology of globoid-cell leucodystrophy in the dog. A report of two cases, *Acta Neuropathol.* **10**:171 (1968).

270. Read, W. K. and Bridges, C. H., Cerebrospinal lipodystrophy in swine. A new disease model in comparative pathology, *Pathol. Vet.* **5**:67 (1968).

271. Bernheimer, H. and Karbe, E., Morphologische und neurochemische Untersuchungen von zwei Formen der amaurotischen Idiotie des Hundes: Nachweis einer G_{M2}-Gangliosidose, *Acta Neuropathol.* **16**:243 (1970).

272. Karbe, E., G_{M2}-Gangliosidose und andere neuronale Lipodystrophien mit Amaurose beim Hund. Eine vergleichende histopathologische, histochemische, elektronenmikroskopische und biochemische Studie, *Arch. Exp. Veterinaer med.* **25**:1 (1971).

273. McGrath, J. T., Kelly, A. M., and Steinberg, S. A., Cerebral lipidosis in the dog, *J. Neuropathol. Exp. Neurol.* **27**:141 (1968).

274. Gambetti, L. A., Kelly, A. M., and Steinberg, S. A., Biochemical studies in a canine gangliosidosis, *J. Neuropathol. Exp. Neurol.* **29**:137 (1970).

275. Baker, H. J., Lindsey, J. R. McKhann, G. M., and Farrell, D. F., Neuronal G_{M1}-gangliosidosis in a Siamese cat with beta-galactosidase deficiency, *Science* **174**:838 (1971).

276. Farrell, D. F., Baker, H. J., Herndon, R. M., Lindsey, J. R., and McKhann, G. M., Feline G_{M1}-gangliosidosis: Biochemical and ultrastructural comparisons with the disease in man, *J. Neuropathol. Exp. Neurol.* **32**:1 (1973).

277. Blakemore, W. F., G_{M1}-gangliosidosis in a cat, *J. Comp. Pathol.* **82**:179 (1972).

278. Handa, S. and Yamakawa, T., Biochemical studies in cat and human gangliosidosis, *J. Neurochem.* **18**:1275 (1971).

279. Donnelly, W. J. C., Sheahan, B. J., and Rogers, T. A., G_{M1}-gangliosidosis in Friesian calves, *J. Pathol.* **111**:173 (1973).

280. Donnelly, W. J. C., Sheahan, B. J., and Kelly, M., Beta-galactosidase deficiency in G_{M1}-gangliosidosis of Friesian calves, *Res. Vet. Sci.* **15**:139 (1973).

BIOCHEMICAL AND CLINICAL ASPECTS

LARRY SCHNECK

Lipids, with certain notable exceptions, may be operationally defined as organic-solvent-soluble, water-insoluble compounds. The three major classes of lipids in the central nervous system are cholesterol, glycerophospholipids, and sphingolipids. Sphingosines are 1,3-dihydroxy-2-amino-hydrocarbons that form a series of lipids by substitution on both the 1-hydroxyl and the amino groups. At present, more than 30 sphingosines and their hydroxy derivatives (phytosphingosines) have been recorded from natural lipids. The amino group of sphingosine is usually acylated with a long-chain (C_{14}–C_{26}) fatty acid. This amide, N-acylsphingosine, is generically known as ceramide. It is the backbone for the synthesis of sphingolipids. The different sphingolipids are formed when the terminal hydroxy group of ceramide is substituted with various compounds. In sphingomyelin, the primary hydroxy group of sphingosine is esterified with choline phosphate. The glycosphingolipids are sphingolipids with a sugar moiety attached through β-glycosidic linkage to the corresponding ceramide. Cerebroside is the generic term for a group of ceramide monohexosides. Ceramide glucose is known as glucocerebroside and ceramide galactose as galactocerebroside. The latter monohexoside is the major cerebroside in normal adult brain. Sulfatides are sulfuric acid esters of cerebrosides with the sulfate at the carbon atom 3 of the galactose moiety. Complex glycosphingolipids are ceramide glycosides

LARRY SCHNECK. Kingsbrook Jewish Medical Center and State University of New York, Downstate Medical Center, Brooklyn, New York.

containing more than one monosaccharide unit and are known as ceramide oligosaccharides. A ceramide dihexoside contains two sugar moieties; ceramide trihexoside, three sugars; ceramide tetrahexoside, four sugars; etc. The ceramide oligosaccharides may be partitioned into the neutral glycolipids and the gangliosides. The carbohydrate residues of the neutral glycolipids are important in various immunochemical reactions.[1-3]

Gangliosides are a class of complex lipids which, by definition, contain sialic acid, mostly as N-acetyl- or N-glycolylneuraminic acid. There is an obvious need for a simple, generally accepted designation for the different types of gangliosides. Since the R_f values of the gangliosides are dependent upon the solvent system used and different fractions may have very similar migratory rates,[4] a nomenclature based upon a structural analysis is preferred. Svennerholm's code system[5] based upon the composition of the carbohydrate chain is employed in this book. In this system, G stands for ganglioside; index M, D, and T for monosialosyl, disialosyl, and trisialosyl units, respectively; and subindex 1 for the major tetraglycosylceramide, index 2 for the trihexoside, and 3 for the diglycosylceramide (lactosylceramide). Figure 1 gives the chemical structure of the more common brain gangliosides and their designation according to Svennerholm.

Chemical Analysis

Once the biological tissue is disrupted by mechanical means, the extracting solvent must be capable of penetrating the tissue and rupturing both the hydrophobic as well as electrostatic bonds. Therefore, a mixture of solvents such as chloroform and methanol is employed to provide both nonpolar and polar properties. The extraction–partition–dialysis method of Folch-Pi, Lees, and Stanley[6] is widely used. The lipids are extracted with chloroform:methanol 2:1 (vol/vol). The addition of monovalent ions, e.g., Na^+ or K^+ up to 0.25 M concentration, facilitates phase separation by breaking up emulsions. The ions also increase the efficiency of ganglioside extraction from tissues. The chloroform–methanol-soluble extract is then partitioned into a lower, organic, and an upper, aqueous, phase. The aqueous phase contains gangliosides which are contaminated with nonlipid material. Almost all the other lipids are in the lower, organic, phase. The aqueous phase is then dialyzed against distilled water to remove nonlipid contaminants. The Folch-Pi procedure will extract over 90% of tissue gangliosides. However, it is only efficient for fairly small amounts of ganglioside and is severely limited when applied to sucrose-contaminated subcellular fractions prepared by gradient centrifugation. Furthermore, when the concentration of the mixed gangliosides in the aqueous phase is

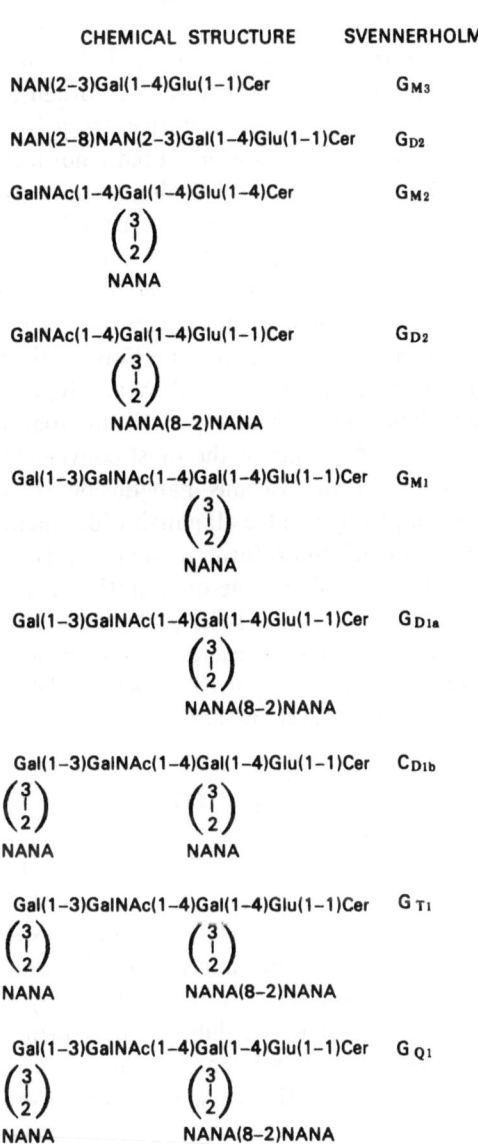

CHEMICAL STRUCTURE   SVENNERHOLM

NAN(2–3)Gal(1–4)Glu(1–1)Cer G_{M3}

NAN(2–8)NAN(2–3)Gal(1–4)Glu(1–1)Cer G_{D2}

GalNAc(1–4)Gal(1–4)Glu(1–4)Cer G_{M2}

$\begin{pmatrix} 3 \\ | \\ 2 \end{pmatrix}$

NANA

GalNAc(1–4)Gal(1–4)Glu(1–1)Cer G_{D2}

$\begin{pmatrix} 3 \\ | \\ 2 \end{pmatrix}$

NANA(8–2)NANA

Gal(1–3)GalNAc(1–4)Gal(1–4)Glu(1–1)Cer G_{M1}

$\begin{pmatrix} 3 \\ | \\ 2 \end{pmatrix}$

NANA

Gal(1–3)GalNAc(1–4)Gal(1–4)Glu(1–1)Cer G_{D1a}

$\begin{pmatrix} 3 \\ | \\ 2 \end{pmatrix}$

NANA(8–2)NANA

Gal(1–3)GalNAc(1–4)Gal(1–4)Glu(1–1)Cer C_{D1b}

$\begin{pmatrix} 3 \\ | \\ 2 \end{pmatrix}$ $\begin{pmatrix} 3 \\ | \\ 2 \end{pmatrix}$

NANA   NANA

Gal(1–3)GalNAc(1–4)Gal(1–4)Glu(1–1)Cer G_{T1}

$\begin{pmatrix} 3 \\ | \\ 2 \end{pmatrix}$ $\begin{pmatrix} 3 \\ | \\ 2 \end{pmatrix}$

NANA   NANA(8–2)NANA

Gal(1–3)GalNAc(1–4)Gal(1–4)Glu(1–1)Cer G_{Q1}

$\begin{pmatrix} 3 \\ | \\ 2 \end{pmatrix}$ $\begin{pmatrix} 3 \\ | \\ 2 \end{pmatrix}$

NANA   NANA(8–2)NANA

FIGURE 1. Cerebral gangliosides. Abbreviations: Cer, ceramide; Glu, glucose; Gal, galactose, GalNAC, Galactosamine; and NANA, *N*-acetylneuraminic acid.

less than 150 μg/ml (below the critical micelle concentration), there is loss of gangliosides through the dialysis membrane.[7] Therefore, under certain circumstances, column chromatography[8] may be preferable to partition dialysis. Formalin-fixed tissue should not be used since formalin can result in selective destruction of certain gangliosides.[9] Because gangliosides by definition contain sialic acid, their quantitative assay is often based upon the concentration of sialic acid. Two widely used colorimetric methods employ resorcinol[10] or thiobarbituric acid.[11] While the thiobarbituric acid is the more sensitive of the two (5 μg sialic acid vs. 10 μg), it is less reliable. A recently developed fluorometric method[12] can measure as little as 0.3 μg sialic acid. A serious limitation to both the colorimetric and fluorometric methods is their inability to distinguish between the various types of sialic acid. False chromagens may seriously interfere with the colorimetric analysis. Both these limitations are avoided by gas–liquid chromatography of the lipid-bound sialic acid.[13] Thin-layer chromatography (TLC) with silica gel is now established as one of the most convenient and rapid techniques for the analysis of the various ganglioside fractions. No single solvent system will completely resolve all ganglioside fractions, but for most purposes, a combination of chloroform:methanol:NH_4OH and n-propanol:H_2O is acceptable. Suzuki's simple quantitative method of analysis of ganglioside patterns directly from TLC plates has wide applicability.[14] However, before one can assign molecular homogeneity to a ganglioside fraction on TLC, one must have supportive structural data. See Appendix A for the general analytic scheme used in our laboratory.

Distribution and Development Patterns

While gangliosides were initially believed to be localized mainly in the neuronal cell body,[15] subsequent studies have shown that these lipids are constituents of myelin[16] and nerve-ending complexes (synaptosomes).[17] There is marked enrichment of the microsomal fraction.[18] Neuronal perikarya, glial cells, and peripheral nerve cells have only small amounts of ganglioside.[19,20] The bovine adrenal medulla, a component of the autonomic nervous system, is surprisingly rich in gangliosides of the hematoside (G_{M3}) type, and the sialic acid is of both the N-acetyl and N-glycolylneuraminic types.[21] Whereas bovine brain also contains N-glycolylneuraminic acid, none has been found in human brain.[21] Extraneuronal gangliosides, especially of the hematoside type, have been identified in plasma membranes of various nonneural tissues.[22-24] Gangliosides, particularly G_{M1}, are components of myelin.[20] Recently, Ledeen reported that a monosialoganglioside of the galactocerebroside type was also a myelin component and may be characteristic of oligodendroglial membranes.[25]

Myelin gangliosides are metabolically inactive when compared to gangliosides in nerve endings.[26] Nerve endings receive most, if not all, of their gangliosides via rapid axonal transport from the perikaryon.[25]

Ganglioside concentrations and patterns change markedly during human brain development.[27,28] In human brain, there is a true twofold increase in ganglioside from the third fetal month to birth and another twofold increase from birth to adulthood. Even greater increases have been found in neonatal rat brain[29] and embryonic chicken brain.[30] In the early stages of human fetal development, there is a high percentage of G_{M1}-ganglioside. With maturation there is a steady increase in the percentage of G_{D1a}, with a concomitant decrease in the relative percentage of G_{M1} and G_{T1}. Although no marked differences in ganglioside patterns of white and gray matter are seen at birth, there is a marked G_{M1} enrichment of white matter by one year of age. This coincides with the period of rapid myelination. The cerebellar cortex shows a later increase in total ganglioside concentration. By 18 months, G_{T1} comprises over a third of the total cerebellar gangliosides. Parallel ganglioside developmental patterns were noted in rat brain. Ganglioside ceramides also change with maturation.[29,31,32] The sphingosine of fetal and infant cerebral gangliosides changes from C_{18} at birth to equal concentrations of C_{18} and C_{20} sphingosine at maturity. The ceramide fatty acids have a very high percentage of C_{18} (stearic) acid but little, if any, of the α-hydroxy and longer-chain (C_{22}–C_{24}) fatty acids normally found in cerebrosides or sulfatides.[33,34] In contrast to all the brain gangliosides, except for the myelin monosialogalactocerebroside, extraneuronal gangliosides have longer-chain saturated and unsaturated fatty acids.[33-36]

Biosynthesis and Degradation

The biosynthesis and degradation of gangliosides occurs by the sequential addition or subtraction of sugars in the oligosaccharide moiety. The stepwise addition of activated monosaccharides is catalyzed by glycosyltransferases that are specific for each step.[37] The synthetic pathway for the formation of sialic acid via the condensation of phosphorylated N-acetylmannosamine with phosphoenolpyruvate is well established.[38,39] N-acetylneuraminic acid (NANA) is activated by linkage to cytosine monophosphate (CMP). The other sugars are activated by linkage to uridine diphosphate (UDP). The incorporation of CMP-NANA or CMP-N-glycolylneuraminic acid is catalyzed by sialyltransferase enzymes. These transferases differ from each other on the basis of their specificity toward the substrate. While most of the enzymatic reactions for the synthesis of gangliosides have been fairly well established, the pathway for the incorporation of the second sialic acid into the ganglioside molecule is still not resolved. It has been suggested that G_{D1b} and G_{T1} are synthesized from disialosyllactosylceramide.[40] It is also not known whether there is a specific sialyltransferase for the myelin ganglioside, monosialosylgalactocerebroside. During development, the rate of formation of a specific ganglioside is dependent on the relative activities of specific glycosyltransferases. Burton has written an excellent and comprehensive review on the enzymes involved in ganglioside biosynthesis.[41]

The degradation of gangliosides occurs via the stepwise removal of sugars by hydrolytic enzymes localized in the lysosomal fraction. Neuraminidase may exist in more than one form, as suggested by the data of Leibowitz and Gatt.[42] It had been claimed that because of steric hindrance, the sialic acid bound to the internal galactose is not liberated by bacterial neuraminidase.[43] However, the increased concentrations of asialotrihexosylceramide in fetal Tay–Sachs disease (TSD) brain[44] and infant G_{M2}-gangliosidosis[45] support Jatzkewitz's contention that the asialotrihexosylceramides in brain are formed from their corresponding gangliosides.[46] For a detailed discussion of the properties of the enzymes involved in the hydrolysis of G_{M1}- and G_{M2}-ganglioside, see Chapter 3.

One must be careful in attempting to extrapolate and correlate *in vitro* with *in vivo* data. The *in vitro* enzyme interaction with complex lipids may be a function of the physical state of the substrate (monomer *vs.* micelle) and a differential specificity of the purified enzyme to monomers and aggregated polymers.[47] The interpretation and comparison of the *in vivo* radioactive-tracer studies must take into account the radioactive precursor used, the route of injection, the age and species of the experimental animal, the size of the precursor pool, and the metabolic heterogeneity of the tissue being studied. It is, therefore, not surprising that there is conflicting interpretation of data on turnover times of various brain gangliosides, precursor pools, and synthetic pathways. The turnover time of "metabolically active" gangliosides is quite rapid. The half-time may be considerably less than 10 days.[48] The percent incorporation of the labeled precursor seems to be a function of the rate of accumulation of the ganglioside. Figure 2 summarizes the probable synthetic and degradative pathways of ganglioside biosynthesis.

Biological Function

Although the biological functions of gangliosides are not known, they probably play an important role in membrane structure and function. Their pattern is altered in virally transformed cells.[49-51] They may participate in cellular recognition and adhesion.[52] Gangliosides may also function as membrane receptor sites[53] and influence ion transport across membranes.[54]

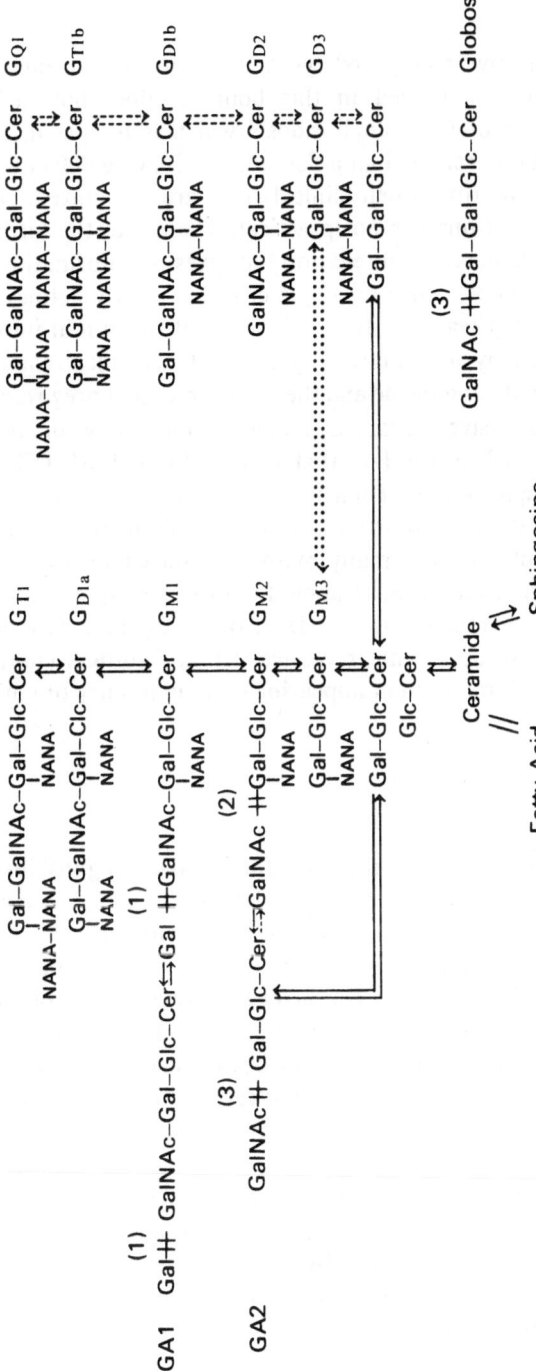

FIGURE 2. Metabolic pathways of glycolipids (lacto series), and enzymatic blocks (╫) in gangliosidoses. (1) β-Galactosidase, (2) Hex A, and (3) Hex B. Abbreviations: Cer, ceramide; Glc, glucose; Gal, galactose; GalNAC, galactosamine; NANA, N-acetylneuraminic acid; G_{A1}, asialoceramide tetrahexoside; and G_{A2}, asialoceramide trihexaside.

Clinical Aspects

Table 1 lists the five recognized types of ganglioside storage diseases and the nomenclature employed in this book. It does not include the recently reported case of G_{M3}-gangliosidosis which is unique in that it is caused by a biosynthetic rather than a degradative enzyme defect.[55] Because of the variability in the time when clinical signs are recognized, classification based upon time of onset is not practical. The use of the terms type 1 and type 2 implies phenotypic segregation but gives no information regarding the enzyme deficiency. Since no single criterion clearly defines and distinguishes the various disease entities, it is felt that maximum information can best be conveyed by a combined eponymic–biochemical classification that includes the stored ganglioside and the isoenzymes that are *present*.

The almost explosive advances made in the study of these rare disorders are illustrated by the fact that from 1881 to 1964 TSD was the only recognized gangliosidosis. Then in a period of five years, four other ganglioside storage diseases were clinically recognized and biochemically defined.[56-63] It is probable that many of the so-called non-Jewish cases of TSD (G_{M2} variant B) were in fact Sandhoff's disease (G_{M2} variant 0). This latter disorder may eventually rival TSD in frequency of case reports. All five gangliosidoses are autosomal recessive, lethal disorders characterized by severe neurological impairment appearing early in infancy or childhood.

G_{M2}-Gangliosidoses

Tay–Sachs disease is the prototype for all the gangliosidoses. Over several thousand cases have been reported. Its clinical course is based upon a typical and predictable evolution of signs and symptoms.[64-66] Over 90% have occurred in Jewish children, usually of Ashkenazic descent. Within the first six months of life, there is a characteristic clinical triad of cherry-red macula, exaggerated extension response to sound, and psychomotor arrest. The cherry-red spot may not be present at birth.[66] It results from degeneration of ganglion cells at the macula which is framed by a fluffy white border of lipid-laden ganglion cells. It is not pathognomonic of this disease and has been observed in other sphingolipidoses such as Sandhoff's disease, Niemann–Pick disease, Norman–Landing disease (G_{M1}, variant 0); metachromatic leukodystrophy, and Goldberg's syndrome.[67] The retinal receptor cells are preserved as proven by the electroretinographic studies of Pampiglione and co-workers.[68] The exaggerated extension response to sound has been erroneously called hyperacusis.[66] Tanaka *et al.,* using a variety of

TABLE 1. Cerebral Gangliosides in Ganglioside Storage Diseases[a]

	Normal	G_{M2}-Gangliosidosis			G_{M1}-Gangliosidosis	
		TSD (B)	Sandhoff (0)	Bernheimer–Seitelberger (AB)	Norman–Landing (0)	Derry (A)
Total gangliosides	3.0–5.0	13.0–18.0	16.6	7.0–9.6	11.0–19.0	10.7–14.2
Asialo-G_{M2} (G_{A2})	0.2	3.0–6.5	9.3–13.0	1.0–1.5	—	2.6–3.5
Asialo-G_{M1} (G_{A1})	0.2	Trace	Trace	Trace	1.0–4.0	2.6–3.5
Ganglioside distribution (% of total ganglioside SA)						
G_{M3}	0.5–1.0	1–2	2.0	2–3	1–2	1–2
G_{M2}	1–3	78–90	86	39–59	2–3	2–3
G_{M1}	17–25	1–5	6	10–12	70–80	70–80

[a] Values for total gangliosides, asialo-G_{M2}, and asialo-G_{M1} are expressed as mg/100 mg total lipid. Derived from O'Brien.[80]

audiological techniques, have shown that this auditory response is probably related to involvement of the supranuclear auditory pathways.[69]

These infants, during the first year of life, have a doll-like facial appearance, with pale, translucent skin, long eyelashes, fine hair, and pink coloring.[66] Under six months they are often apathetic, hypotonic, and fail to sit or turn over. A rare case may sit, stand, or even crawl. After age one, they are hypotonic, paretic, and have exaggerated tendon reflexes. By eighteen months of age, there is an obvious macrocephaly which is caused by cerebral gliosis. At this age, the child appears blind and no longer shows appropriate cognitive or affective responses to visual stimuli. However, the pupils continue to respond to light even though optic atrophy may be obvious. At this stage, the visual-evoked cortical response is usually absent.[68] A detailed clinical description of the evolution of eye signs in TSD was reported by Jampel and Quaglio.[70]

Generalized convulsions are not common during the first two years of life. Even in the terminal stages, opisthotonic posturing and clonus are more common than generalized convulsions. Abnormal laughter (gelastic seizures) is often noted around one year of age. This sign is usually associated with or precedes abnormal changes in the electroencephalogram.[71] Before one year of age, the waking EEG is usually normal. After one year, the EEG shows high-voltage slow wave activity with single and multiple spikes. In the early stages, the sleep EEG may show a change in the frequency of sleep spindles. In the later stages of the disorder, it is difficult to electroencephalographically distinguish the sleep from the waking record.[68] Between three and five years of age, the children are in a vegetative state and usually die from intercurrent infections. There are no abnormal lymphocytes, visceromegaly, or foam cells. The spinal fluid may show increased concentrations of G_{M2}-ganglioside.[72]

The clinical picture of Sandhoff's disease is similar to that of TSD.[60] Sandhoff's disease has not yet been reported in children of Jewish descent. Both TSD and Sandhoff's disease may have electrocardiographic abnormalities.[73,74] The urinary sediment in Sandhoff's disease may contain increased concentrations of globoside,[74] and foam cells have been noted in the bone marrow.[75]

The clinical picture of Bernheimer–Seitelberger disease [G_{M2} (A,B)] is distinctly different from Tay–Sachs and Sandhoff's diseases.[61,62,76,77] Until the end of the first year, the children appear normal. The most common initial sign is locomotor ataxia which becomes manifest between two and six years of age. This is followed by dyskinesia, progressive loss of speech, blindness, decerebrate rigidity, and minor motor seizures. Whereas optic atrophy and retinitis pigmentosa may be present, the cherry-red spot is not seen.

G_{M1}-Gangliosidoses

The G_{M1}-gangliosidoses were first defined as a clinical pathological entity by Landing et al. in 1964.[56] They have been identified in various ethnic groups in Europe, Asia, and North America,[56-58,78,79] and have been recorded under various names, e.g., Norman–Landing disease,[56] Derry's disease,[59] generalized gangliosidosis,[58] and late infantile systemic lipidosis (type 1 and 2).[59] The division into two types, 1 and 2, was based upon clinical criteria, and these types are genotypically as well as phenotypically distinct. The clinical features of 25 cases of Norman–Landing disease [G_{M1} (0)] and 11 patients with Derry's disease [G_{M1} (A)] have been summarized by O'Brien.[80]

In Norman–Landing disease [G_{M1} (0)], the clinical signs and symptoms are apparent shortly after birth: Appetite is poor, the cry is weak, sucking is impaired, and the extremities are edematous. The infant cannot sit and does not smile. By one year of age he becomes decerebrate, blind, deaf, and requires tube feeding. The child seldom survives beyond two years. Although tonic–clonic fits are said to be common, the only EEG abnormalities are nonspecific, 3- to 4-Hz high-voltage waves. The infant has a dull, apathetic look, coarse facial features, prominent frontal bossing, gum hypertrophy, hirsutism, macroglossia, dorsolumbar kyphosis, enlargement at the epiphyseal joints, and deformities of hands and feet. Hepatosplenomegaly is prominent within a few months after birth. Corneal opacities have not been noted, but cherry-red spots have been observed in about half the cases. Radiological abnormalities similar to those of Hurler's disease are recorded in a great majority of the infants that survive beyond six months of age. The undermining of the anterior clinoids produces a J-shaped sella. The vertebral bodies are beaked; the ribs are spatulate and there are marked skeletal deformities in the feet, pelvis, and hands. The long bones show early periosteal thickening and rarefaction. The disorder has been called pseudo-Hurler's disease because of the facial features, bony abnormalities, and prominent visceromegaly. Foam cells in bone marrow and other organs, and vacuolated lymphocytes have been found in many cases. The patients usually die from bronchopneumonia before age two. Many do not survive the first six months of life.

Derry's disease [G_{M1} (A)] is often referred to as juvenile G_{M1}-gangliosidosis because of the later onset of clinical signs and symptoms, and the longer survival time. In contrast to Norman–Landing disease, clinical signs are not apparent before six months of age. The facies appears normal. Visceromegaly is not prominent. There are no gross skeletal abnormalities and radiographic changes are minimal. Appendicular ataxia, a common early clinical sign, usually appears after the first year. It is rapidly followed by psychomotor deterioration. Progressive weakness and spasticity in the extremities eventually culminates in decerebrate rigidity. Seizures are common. They appear as any combination of *grand mal* fits, staring spells, myoclonic convulsions, and opisthotonic posturing. The EEG is grossly abnormal. Electromyography in both types is normal.[79] Cherry-red maculae have not been observed. Vacuolated lymphocytes and foam cells are usually present. In the terminal stages, the children are blind, deaf, and decerebrate. Death usually occurs between five and fifteen years of age.

Certain clinical features common to both G_{M1}- and G_{M2}-gangliosidoses seem to be related to the age of onset. In the "infantile" forms of both G_{M1}- and G_{M2}-gangliosidoses, cherry-red spots are observed, whereas in the "juvenile" types they are absent. It would appear that with maturity, the retinal ganglion cells become more resistant to degeneration. In contrast, true seizures and associated EEG abnormalities are more prevalent in the late-onset varieties.

Since antenatal diagnosis is now practical, the clinician must have a high index of suspicion that any patient with progressive psychomotor deterioration starting early in infancy or childhood may have a sphingolipid disorder. This is true even with a negative family history. Spongy degeneration of white matter, the mucopolysaccharidoses, and the ceroid-lipofuscinoses are some of the nonsphingolipidoses that should be considered in the differential diagnosis. At present, the neuronal sphingolipidoses are not amenable to enzyme-replacement therapy.[81] Therefore, for the foreseeable future, the pragmatic approach involves identification of the high-risk pregnancy and antenatal diagnosis. Amniocentesis has been performed in all five types,[75,79,82-86] and homozygote fetuses have been aborted in TSD and G_{M1}-gangliosidosis (0) cases.[84-86]

Storage Compounds

For the sake of clarity and brevity, the chemical pathology of all five types will be considered simultaneously rather than sequentially. They are all generalized or systemic gangliosidoses.[87-89] The gray matter of the central nervous system has the highest concentration of the stored ganglioside. The increased storage of the ganglioside in the neuronal tissue results in a secondary dysmyelination with associated alteration of myelin lipids. The inclusion bodies contain the stored ganglioside, and their chemical composition reflects the alterations in the brain lipids. The amount of cerebral ganglioside in the "juvenile" types is approximately equal to or less than that found in the "infantile" types. The degradative enzyme, a lysosomal enzyme whose defective activity results in accumulation of the corresponding ganglioside, is also required for the degradation of related oligosaccharides, mucopolysaccharides, and glycoproteins. Figure 2 illustrates the presumed metabolic pathways of the gangliosides and derived glycolipids and the assumed enzymatic block. Tables 1, 2, and 3 compare the chemical pathology of the five types of gangliosidoses.

As seen in Table 1, the levels of increased cerebral G_{M2}-ganglioside in TSD and Sandhoff's disease are similar,[74,75,88,90] but the level of asialoceramide trihexoside in Sandhoff's disease is two- to threefold that of TSD.[88] Except for the case reported by Sandhoff,[88] the levels of cerebral G_{M2}- and asialoceramide trihexoside in Bernheimer–Seitelberger's disease are less than in Tay–Sachs and Sandhoff's diseases.[62,77] Even in the fetal state of TSD, there are increased levels of both G_{M2}-ganglioside and its asialoglycolipid.[44] Brunngraber and associates found that there was a fourfold increase in N-acetylglucosamine and mannose in the dialyzable glycopeptides in the brains of patients with Tay–Sachs and Sandhoff's diseases.[91] In Sandhoff's disease, globoside, a ceramide tetrahexoside with a terminal galactosamine, is stored in various viscera including spleen, liver, and kidney.[61,74,75,90,92] (Table 2) Increased concentrations of this compound can be detected in plasma and urinary sediment.[74]

In G_{M1}-gangliosidosis there are increased levels of G_{M1}-ganglioside and its asialoceramide tetrahexoside in brain and viscera.[58,89,93] Both types of G_{M1}-gangliosidosis contain increased amounts of a keratin sulfate species of mucopolysaccharide and sialomucopolysaccharide in the viscera.[89,94,96] There is an increased excretion of urinary glycopeptide.[97] Suzuki noted higher levels of visceral G_{M1} and keratin sulfate-like mucopolysaccharides in the cases with skeletal deformities,[98] but there were notable exceptions. (See Tables 1, 3.)

The chemical composition of the membranous cytoplasmic bodies in

TABLE 2. G_{M2}-Gangliosidoses Liver Glycolipids[a]

Glycolipid	Control	TSD	Sandhoff
Total gangliosides[b]	0.06	0.10	0.18
G_{M2} [c]	29	152	915
Ceramide trihexoside[c]	68	40	188
Globoside[c]	85	62	9790

[a] Derived from data of Kolodny.[75]
[b] Expressed as % dry weight.
[c] μmol/g dry weight.

TABLE 3. Visceral Storage in G_{M1}-Gangliosidoses[a]

	Liver			Spleen		
	Normal	Norman–Landing (0)	Derry (A)	Normal	Norman–Landing (0)	Derry (A)
Total ganglioside[b]	36.7	73.9	29.9	42.6	68.8	68.2
G_{M1}[b]	1.2	24.3	1.5	1.0	20.1	4.2
G_{M3}[b]	30.8	32.8	18.8	26.4	27.2	51.3
Glycoprotein[c]	171	679	545	212	713	689
Mucopolysaccharide[c]	207	2260	1070	254	702	656

[a] Derived from Suzuki et al.[89]
[b] Values are expressed as μg of NANA/100 mg of chloroform–methanol-insoluble residue.
[c] Values are expressed as μg of hexosamine/100 mg of chloroform–methanol-insoluble residue.

both G_{M1}- and G_{M2}-gangliosidoses are similar except for the type of ganglioside and its asialoglycolipid.[89] Ganglioside comprised one third of the dry weight. There were large amounts of proteolipid present, and over 95% of the cerebroside was glucocerebroside.

The chemical abnormalities in white matter are consistent with a nonspecific myelin breakdown. In the white matter and myelin there are low concentrations of proteolipid protein and glycolipids, and significant amounts of esterified cholesterol.[89] Eto and Suzuki also noted similar fatty acid patterns of the esterified cholesterol in G_{M1}-gangliosidosis, TSD, and Schilder's demyelination disease.[99]

Enzyme Defects

Can the differences in the stored glycolipids be correlated with their respective isoenzyme patterns? What is the structural and genetic relationship between hexosaminidase A and B? Numerous publications have confirmed the fact that the storage of G_{M2}-ganglioside is associated with absent or deficient activity of Hex A.[88,100-103] Since both Hex A and Hex B can hydrolyze the terminal amino sugar of globoside, the absence of both Hex A and Hex B in Sandhoff's disease explains the accumulation of this glycolipid in Sandhoff's disease. However, there is no ready explanation for the increase storage of the asialo derivative of G_{M2} in the fetal[44] and infant[87] brains of variants B and AB gangliosidoses cases. The fact that this ceramide trihexoside has the same sphingosine, fatty acid, and sugar patterns of G_{M2}-ganglioside indicates that it is derived from or metabolically linked to G_{M2}.[31,32] Since Hex B can (in vitro) degrade this ceramide trihexoside to ceramide lactoside,[88] this glycolipid ought not to be stored in either Tay Sachs [G_{M2} (B)] or Bernheimer–Seitelberger [G_{M2} (A,B)] diseases. It has been suggested that this asialoceramide trihexoside becomes entrapped in the membranous cytoplasmic bodies and is thus protected from enzymatic degradation.[88] The amorphous nature of the lipid cytosome in the fetus would vitiate this hypothesis.[104] In vitro studies have indicated that $G_{\overline{M2}}$-ganglioside inhibits Hex B, and this inhibition could produce the increase in the asialo-G_{M2} derivative.[105] Another less likely possibility is that G_{M2} inhibits a sialyltransferase reaction[106] that converts G_{A2} to G_{M2}. Tallman et al. hypothesized that Hex A and Hex B are different conformational states of the same enzyme.[107] Wenger reported that both Hex A and Hex B could hydrolyze G_{M2} by a complex between brain neuraminidase and hexosaminidase.[105] However, both hypotheses lack experimental confirmation (see Chapter 3 in this book). Brunngraber suggests that the combined action of both Hex A and Hex B are required to affect the catabolic breakdown of the heteropolysaccharide chain of the glycoproteins.[91] A similar combined action on sphingoglycolipids may be necessary *in vivo* but not *in vitro*.

Okada and O'Brien, using radioactive $G_{\overline{M1}}$-ganglioside and synthetic substrates, found a deficiency of β-galactosidase in $G_{\overline{M1}}$-gangliosidosis.[94] MacBrinn and co-workers demonstrated that the undersulfated mucopolysaccharides and glycoprotein in the visceral organs of $G_{\overline{M1}}$-gangliosidosis patients were not degraded by use of a purified preparation of galactosidase from the liver of a case with Norman–Landing disease.[108] It can be concluded that the missing β-galactosidase has a high specificity for the terminal galactose of G_{M1}-ganglioside and of the above-mentioned mucopolysaccharides and glycoproteins. Ho and O'Brien separated the galactosidases by starch gel electrophoresis into a fast-moving component A and slower-moving components B and C.[109] In Norman–Landing disease, all β-galactosidase isoenzymes were deficient, whereas in one case of Derry's disease, only B and C were absent.[109] If this characteristic isoenzyme pattern proves true, then other variants, e.g., types B and C, may be uncovered.

Fetal TSD and Norman–Landing disease brains have elevated levels of G_{M2}- and G_{M1}-ganglioside, respectively,[82-86] and abnormal lipid cytosomes.[85,86,104] Hex A is absent in fetal TSD tissues.[82-84] Lowden *et al.* reported reduced, but nevertheless significant, β-galactosidase activity in fetal Norman–Landing-disease tissue.[85] However, Kaback *et al.*, using acetate gel electrophoresis, found that while α- and β-galactosidase isoenzymes were absent, the C isoenzyme was present in the brain of a saline-aborted [G_{M1} (0)] fetus.[86]

Somatic-cell hybrids tested for Hex A and Hex B showed discordant segregation of these two isoenzymes.[110] This segregation suggested that the genes coding for their expression were not linked. The discordant segregation was not complete. Hex A was never present in the absence of Hex B, although Hex B was present in the absence of Hex A. This supports a structural relationship between Hex A and Hex B. Hex B may be converted to Hex A by a sialosyltransferase, and the defect in TSD may be due to an absence of this transferase. This is unlikely since Srivastava *et al.* found differences in the amino acid composition of Hex A and Hex B.[111] Furthermore, this hypothesis does not explain the G_{M2}-gangliosidosis AB subtype. The proposal of Tallman *et al.* that the two different isoenzymes are conformational states of the same enzyme[107] runs counter to the observed partial discordant segregation of Hex A and Hex B.[111] The discordant segregation of Hex A and Hex B can occur if the two isoenzymes share a common structural subunit and if each have one other different subunit.[73,74,112] This hypothesis offers the simplest explanation for the observed subtypes in G_{M2}-gangliosidoses. It would also explain the subtype of other sphingolipidoses such as G_{M1}-gangliosidoses and metachromatic leukodystrophy. Galjaard *et al.* were able to experimentally confirm this hypothesis when Tay–Sachs cells [G_{M2} (B)] and Sandhoff cells [G_{M2} (0)] were hybridized, and Hex A activity was detected in the hybrid-cell preparation.[113] Navon *et al.* suggested that the apparent absence of Hex A in healthy adults may be due to compound heterozygosity for the common TSD allele and a rare variant allele.[114] Further immunochemical and physical chemical studies should resolve some of these perplexing problems.

References

1. Rapport, M. M., Graf, L., Skipski, P., and Alonzo, N. F., Immunochemical studies of organ and tumor lipids. VI. Isolation and properties of cytolipin, *Cancer* **12**:438 (1959).
2. Hakomori, S. J. and Jeanloz, R. W., Glycolipids as membrane antigens, in: *Blood and Tissue Antigens*, D. Aminoff, ed., Academic Press, New York, pp. 149–161 (1970).
3. Siddiqui, B. and Hakomori, S. J., A revised structure for the Forsmann glycolipid hapten, *J. Biol. Chem.* **246**:5766 (1971).
4. Penick, R. J., Meisler, M. H., and McCluer, R. H., Thin-layer chromatographic studies of human brain gangliosides, *Biochim. Biophys. Acta* **116**:279 (1966).
5. Svennerholm, L., Chromatographic separation of human brain gangliosides, *J. Neurochem.* **10**:613 (1963).
6. Folch-Pi, J., Lees, M., and Sloane-Stanley, G. H., A simple method for the isolation and purification of total lipides from animal tissue, *J. Biol. Chem.* **226**:497 (1957).
7. Kanfer, J. M. and Spielvogel, C., On the loss of gangliosides by dialysis, *J. Neurochem.* **20**:1483 (1973).
8. Rouser, G., Kritchevsky, G., and Yamamoto, A., Column chromatographic and associated procedures for separation and determination of phosphatides and glycolipids, in: *Lipid Chromatographic Analysis*, G. V. Marinetti, ed., Marcel Decker, New York, Vol. 1, pp. 99–161 (1967).
9. Suzuki, K., The pattern of mammalian brain gangliosides. II. Evaluation of the extraction procedures, post-mortem changes and the effect of formalin preservation, *J. Neurochem.* **12**:629 (1965).
10. Svennerholm, L., Quantitative estimation of sialic acids. II. A colorimetric resorcinol–hydrochloric acid method, *Biochim. Biophys. Acta* **24**:604 (1957).
11. Warren, L., The thiobarbituric acid assay of sialic acids, *J. Biol. Chem.* **234**:197 (1959).
12. Hess, H. H. and Rolde, E., Flurometric assay of sialic acid in brain gangliosides, *J. Biol. Chem.* **239**:3215 (1964).
13. Yu, R. K. and Ledeen, R. W., Gas–liquid chromatographic assay of lipid-bound sialic acids: Measurement of gangliosides in brain of several species, *J. Lipid Res.* **11**:506 (1970).
14. Suzuki, K., A simple and accurate micromethod for quantitative determination of ganglioside patterns, *Life Sci.* **3**:1227 (1964).

15. Klenk, E., Über die Ganglioside, eine neue Gruppe von zuckerhältigen Gehirnlipoiden, *Hoppe-Seyler's Z. Physiol. Chem.* **273**:76 (1942).

16. Suzuki, K., Poduslo, S. E., and Norton, W. T., Gangliosides in the myelin fraction of developing rats, *Biochim. Biophys. Acta* **144**:375 (1967).

17. Burton, R. M., Howard, R. E., Baer, S., and Balfour, Y. M., Gangliosides and acetylcholine of the central nervous system, *Biochim. Biophys. Acta* **84**:441 (1964).

18. Eichberg, J., Whittaker, V. P., and Dawson, R. M., Distribution of lipids in subcellular particles of guinea-pig brain, *Biochim. J.* **92**:91 (1964).

19. Derry, D. M. and Wolfe, L. S., Gangliosides in isolated nervous and glial cells, *Science* **158**:1450 (1967).

20. Norton, W. T. and Poduslo, S. E., Isolation and some properties of whole neuroglia and neuronal perikarya from rat brain, *Fed. Proc. Fed. Am. Soc. Exp. Biol.* **28**:734 1969.

21. Ledeen, R., Salsman, K., and Cabrera, M., Gangliosides of bovine adrenal medulla, *Biochemistry* **7**:2287 (1968).

22. Yamakawa, T. and Suzuki, S., The chemistry of the lipids of posthemolytic residue or stroma of erythrocytes. I. Concerning the ether-insoluble lipids of hyophilized horse blood stroma, *J. Biochem. (Tokyo)* **38**:199 (1951).

23. Klenk, H. D. and Choppin, P. W., Glycosphingolipids of plasma membranes of cultured cells and an enveloped virus (SV$_5$) grown in these cells, *Proc. Natl. Acad. Sci. U.S.A.* **66**:57 (1970).

24. Renkonen, O., Gahmberg, C. G., Simons, K., and Kääriäinen, L., Enrichment of gangliosides in plasma membranes of hamster kidney fibroblasts, *Acta Chem. Scand.* **24**:733 (1970).

25. Ledeen, R. and Yu, R. K., Gangliosides as constituents of nervous system membranes, in: *Biological Diagnosis of Brain Disorders,* S. Bogoch, ed., Spectrum, New York, pp. 247–257 (1973).

26. Suzuki, K., Formation and turnover of myelin gangliosides, *J. Neurochem.* **17**:209 (1970).

27. Suzuki, K., The pattern of mammalian brain gangliosides. III. Regional and developmental differences, *J. Neurochem.* **12**:969 (1965).

28. Vanier, M. T., Holm, M., Öhman, R., and Svennerholm, L., Developmental profiles of gangliosides in human and rat brain, *J. Neurochem.* **18**:581 (1971).

29. Rosenberg, A. and Stern, N., Changes in sphingosine and fatty acid components of the gangliosides in developing rat and human brain, *J. Lipid Res.* **7**:122 (1966).

30. Garrigan, O. W. and Chargaff, E., Studies on the mucolipids and the cerebrosides of chicken brain during embryonic development, *Biochim. Biophys. Acta* **70**:452 (1963).

31. Schneck, L., Adachi, M., and Volk, B. W., The fetal aspects of Tay–Sachs disease, *Pediatrics* **49**:342 (1972).

32. Naoi, M. and Klenk, E., The sphingosine bases of the gangliosides from developing human brain and from brains of amaurotic idiots, *Hoppe-Seyler's Z. Physiol. Chem.* **353**:1677 (1972).

33. Avrova, N. F. and Zabelinskiï, S. A., Fatty acids and long chain bases of vertebrate brain gangliosides, *J. Neurochem.* **18**:675 (1971).

34. Kishimoto, Y., Agranoff, B. W., Radin, N. S., and Burton, R. M., Comparisons of the fatty acids of lipids of subcellular brain fractions, *J. Neurochem.* **16**:397 (1969).

35. Feldman, G. L., Feldman, L. S., and Rouser, G. P., The isolation and partial characterization of ganglioside and ceramide polyhexosides from the lens of the human eye, *Lipids* **1**:4 (1966).

36. Svennerholm, L., Gangliosides and other glycolipids of human placenta, *Acta Chem. Scand.* **19**:1506 (1965).

37. Kaufman, B., Basu, S., and Roseman, S., Studies on the biosynthesis of gangliosides, in: *Inborn Disorders of Sphingolipid Metabolism*, B. W. Volk and S. M. Aronson, eds., Pergamon Press, New York, pp. 193–213 (1967).

38. Jourdian, G. W. and Roseman, S., Intermediary metabolism of sialic acid, *Ann. N. Y. Acad. Sci.* **106**:202 (1963).

39. Warren, L., Blacklow, R. S., and Spearing, C. W., Biosynthesis and metabolism of sialic acids, *Ann. N. Y. Acad. Sci.* **106**:191 (1963).

40. Svennerholm, L., Gangliosidoses, in: *Handbook of Neurochemistry. III. Metabolic Reactions in the Nervous System*, A. Lajtha, ed., Plenum Press, New York, pp. 425–452 (1970).

41. Burton, R. M., Glycolipid metabolism, in: *Fundamentals of Lipid Chemistry*, R. M. Burton and F. C. Guerra, eds., BI-Science, Webster-Groves, Mo., pp. 373–403 (1972).

42. Leibowitz, Z. and Gatt, S., Enzymatic hydrolyses of sphingolipids. VII. Hydrolysis of gangliosides by a neuraminidase from calf brain, *Biochim. Biophys. Acta* **152**:136 (1968).

43. Kuhn, R. and Wiegandt, H., Die Konstitution der Ganglio-*N*-tetraose und Gangliosids G_1, *Chem. Ber.* **96**:866 (1963).

44. Schneck, L., Pinkett, B., and Volk, B. W., Asialo-GM_2 ganglioside in fetal brain Tay-Sachs disease, *J. Neurochem.* **24**:183 (1974).

45. Sandhoff, K. and Jatzkewitz, H., The chemical pathology of Tay-Sachs disease, in: *Sphingolipids, Sphingolipidoses and Allied Disorders*, B. W. Volk and S. M. Aronson, eds. Plenum Press, New York, pp. 305–319 (1972).

46. Jatzkewitz, H., Pilz, H., and Sandhoff, K., The quantitative determination of gangliosides and their derivatives in different forms of amaurotic idiocy, *J. Neurochem.* **12**:135 (1965).

47. Gatt, S., Barenholz, Y., Borkovski-Kubiler, I., and Liebovitz, B. G., Interaction of enzymes with lipid substrates, in: *Sphingolipids, Sphingolipidoses and Allied Disorders*, B. W. Volk and S. M. Aronson. eds., Plenum Press, New York, pp. 237–256 (1972).

48. Burton, R. M., Biochemistry of sphingosine containing lipids, in: *Lipids and Lipidoses*, G. Schettler, ed., Springer-Verlag, Berlin, pp. 122–167 (1967).

49. Brady, R. O. and Mora, P. T., Alterations in ganglioside pattern and synthesis in SV_{40}- and polyoma virus-transformed mouse cell lines, *Biochim. Biophys. Acta* **218**:308 (1970).

50. Dawson, G., Kemp, S. F., Stoolmiller, A. C., and Dorfman, A., Biosynthesis of glycosphingolipids by mouse neuroblastoma (NB41A), rat glia (RGC-6) and human glia (CHB-4) in cell culture, *Biochem. Biophys. Res. Commun.* **44**:687 (1971).

51. Hakomori, S. I., Teather, C., and Andrews, H., Organizational difference of cell surface "hematoside" in normal and virally transformed cells, *Biochem. Biophys. Res. Commun.* **33**:563 (1968).

52. Roseman, S., The synthesis of complex carbohydrates by multiglycosyltransferase systems and their potential function in intercellular adhesion, *Chem. Phys. Lipids* **5**:270 (1970).

53. Van Heyningen, W. E., The fixation of tetanus toxin, strychnine, serotonin, and other substances by ganglioside, *J. Gen. Microbiol.* **31**:375 (1963).

54. McIlwain, H., Polybasic and polyacidic substances as aggregates and the excitability of cerebral tissues electrically stimulated *in vitro*, *Biochem. J.* **90**:442 (1964).

55. Max, S. R., Maclaren, N. K., Brady, R. O., Fishman, P., Tallman, J., Garcia, J. H., Cornblath, M., Tanaka, J., Viloria, J. E., and Kamijyo, Y., G_{M3} gangliosidosis: A new

lipid storage disease with a defect in ganglioside biosynthesis, presented at the 50th Annual Meeting of the American Association of Neuropathology, Boston, Mass., June 1974.

56. Landing, B. H., Silverman, F. N., Craig, M. M., Jacoby, M. D., Lahey, M. E., and Chadwick, D. L., Familial neurovisceral lipidosis, *Am. J. Dis. Child.* **108**:503 (1964).

57. Gonatas, N. K. and Gonatas, J., Ultrastructural and biochemical observations on a case of systemic late infantile lipidosis and its relationship to Tay–Sachs disease and gargoylism. *J. Neuropathol. Exp. Neurol.* **24**:318 (1965).

58. O'Brien, J. S., Stern, M. B., Landing, B. H., O'Brien, J. K., and Donnell, N. G., Generalized gangliosidosis. Another inborn error of ganglioside metabolism, *Am. J. Dis. Child.* **109**:338 (1965).

59. Derry, D. M., Fawcett, J. S., Andermann, F., and Wolfe, L. S., Late infantile systemic lipidosis. Major monosialogangliosidosis, delineation of two types, *Neurology* **18**:340 (1968).

60. Bernheimer, H. and Seitelberger, F., Über das Verhalten der Glioside im Gehirn bei 2 Fällen von spätinfantiler amaurotischer Idiotie, *Wein Klin. Wochenschr.* **80**:163 (1968).

61. Sandhoff, K., Andreae, U., and Jatzkewitz, H., Deficient hexosaminidase activity in an exceptional case of Tay–Sachs disease with additional storage of kidney globoside in visceral organs, *Life Sci.* **7**:283 (1968).

62. Suzuki, K., Suzuki, K., Rapin, I., Suzuki, Y., and Ishii, N., Juvenile G_{M2}-gangliosidosis, *Neurology* **20**:190 (1970).

63. Schneck, L., Friedland, J., Pourfar, M., Saifer, A., and Volk, B. W., Hexosaminidase activities in a case of systemic G_{M2}-gangliosidosis, *Proc. Soc. Exp. Biol. Med.* **133**:997 (1970).

64. Tay, W., Symmetrical changes in the region of the yellow spot in each eye of an infant, *Trans. Ophthalmol. Soc. U. K.* **1**:155 (1881).

65. Sachs, B., A family form of idiocy, generally fatal associated with early blindness, *J. Nerv. Ment. Dis.* **21**:475 (1896).

66. Schneck, L., The clinical aspects of Tay–Sachs disease, in: Tay–Sachs Disease, B. W. Volk, ed., Grune & Stratton, New York, pp. 16–35 (1964).

67. Cotlier, E., Tay–Sachs disease and Fabry's disease: Clinical and chemical diagnosis of two metabolic eye diseases, *Bull. N.Y. Acad. Med.* **50**:777 (1974).

68. Pampiglione, G., Privett, G., and Harden, A., Tay–Sachs disease: Neurophysiological studies in 20 children, *Dev. Med. Child. Neurol.* **16**:201 (1974).

69. Tanaka, Y., Taguchi, K., and Arayama, T., Auditory responses in Tay–Sachs disease, *Pract. Oto-Rhino-Laryngol.* **31**:46 (1969).

70. Jampel, R. S. and Quaglio, N. D., Eye movements in Tay–Sachs disease, *Neurology* **14**:1013 (1964).

71. Schneck, L., The early electroencephalographic and seizure characteristics of Tay–Sachs disease, *Acta Neurol. Scand.* **41**:163 (1965).

72. Bernheimer, H., Ganglioside im Liquor cerebrospinalis und Tay–Sachssche Erkrankung, *Klin. Wochenschr.* **46**:258 (1968).

73. Rodriguez-Torres, R., Schneck, L., and Kleinberg, W., Electrocardiographic and biochemical abnormalities in Tay–Sachs disease, *Bull. N.Y. Acad. Med.* **47**:717 (1971).

74. Desnick, R. J., Snyder, P. D., Desnick, S. J., Krivit, W., and Sharp, H. L., Sandhoff's disease: Ultrastructural and biochemical studies, in: *Sphingolipids, Sphingolipidoses and Allied Disorders,* B. W. Volk and S. M. Aronson, eds., Plenum Press, New York, pp. 351–371 (1972).

75. Kolodny, E. H., Sandhoff's disease: Studies on the enzyme defect in homozygotes and detection of heterozygotes, in: *Sphingolipids, Sphingolipidoses and Allied Disorders,* B. W. Volk and S. M. Aronson, eds., Plenum Press, New York, pp. 321–341 (1972).

76. Volk, B. W., Adachi, M., Schneck, L., Saifer, A., and Kleinberg, W., G_5-ganglioside variant of systemic late infantile lipidosis. Generalized gangliosidosis, *Arch. Pathol.* **87**:393 (1969).

77. Menkes, J. H., O'Brien, J. S., Okada, S., Grippo, J., Andrews, J. M., and Cancilla, P. A., Juvenile G_{M2} gangliosidosis. Biochemical and ultrastructural studies on a new variant of Tay–Sachs disease, *Arch. Neurol. (Chicago)* **25**:14 (1971).

78. Dacremont, G. and Kint, J. A., G_{M1}-ganglioside accumulation and beta-galactoside deficiency in a case of G_{M1}-gangliosidosis (Landing disease), *Clin. Chim. Acta* **21**:421 (1968).

79. Taori, G. M., Basu, D. K., Chandi, S., Raman, P. T., Abraham, J., Leelavathy, R., and Job, C. K., G_{M1} Gangliosidosis, *J. Neurol. Sci.* **21**:77 (1974).

80. O'Brien, J. S., Ganglioside storage diseases, in: *Advances in Human Genetics*, H. Harris and K. Hirschhorn, eds., Plenum Press, New York, Vol. 3, pp. 39–98 (1972).

81. Schneck, L., Amsterdam, D., Brooks, S. E., Rosenthal, A., and Volk, B. W., The Tay–Sachs disease fibroblast model: Failure to respond to exogenous hexosaminidase A, *Pediatrics* **52**:221 (1973).

82. Schneck, L., Friedland, J., Valenti, C., Adachi, M., Amsterdam, D., and Volk, B. W., Prenatal diagnosis of Tay–Sachs disease, *Lancet* **1**:582 (1970).

83. O'Brien, J. S., Okada, S., Fillerup, D. L., Veath, B., Adornato, B., Brenner, P. H., and Leroy, J., Tay–Sachs disease: Prenatal diagnosis, *Science* **172**:61 (1971).

84. Yabuuchi, H., Sumi, K., Kurachi, K., and Hanai, J., Studies on cerebral lipidosis. Prenatal diagnosis of Tay–Sachs disease, *Acta Paediatr.* Jpn. Overseas Ed. **13**:13 (1971).

85. Lowden, J. A., Cutz, E., Conen, P. E., Rudd, N., and Doran, T. A., Prenatal diagnosis of G_{M1}-gangliosidosis, *New Engl. J. Med.* **288**:225 (1973).

86. Kaback, M. M., Sloan, H. R., Sonneborn, M., Herndon, R. M., and Percy, A. K., G_M-Gangliosidosis type I: *In utero* detection and fetal manifestations, *J. Pediatr.* **82**:1037 (1973).

87. Eeg-Olofsson, L., Kristensson, K., Sourander, P., and Svennerholm, L., Tay–Sachs disease: A generalized metabolic disorder, *Acta Paediatr. Scand.* **55**:546 (1966).

88. Sandhoff, K., Harzer, K., Wässle, W., and Jatzkewitz, H., Enzyme alterations and lipid storage in three variants of Tay–Sachs disease, *J. Neurochem.* **18**:2469 (1971).

89. Suzuki, K., Suzuki, K., and Kamoshita, S., Chemical pathology of G_{M1}-gangliosidosis (generalized gangliosidosis), *J. Neuropathol. Exp. Neurol.* **28**:25 (1969).

90. Suzuki, Y., Jacob, J. C., Suzuki, K., Kutty, K. M., and Suzuki, K., G_{M2}-Gangliosidosis with total hexosaminidase deficiency, *Neurology* **21**:313 (1971).

91. Brunngraber, E. G., Brown, B. D., and Aro, A., Glycoproteins in brain tissues of the O-variant of G_{M2}-gangliosidosis, *J. Neurochem.* **22**:125 (1974).

92. Snyder, P. D., Krivit, W., and Sweeley, C. C., Generalized accumulation of neutral glycosphingolipids with G_{M2} ganglioside accumulation in the brain, *J. Lipid Res.* **13**:128 (1972).

93. Patton, V. M. and Dekaban, A. S., G_{M1}-gangliosidosis and juvenile cerebral lipidosis, *Arch. Neurol. (Chicago)* **24**:529 (1971).

94. Okada, S. and O'Brien, J. S., Generalized gangliosidosis: Beta-galactosidase deficiency, *Science* **160**:1002 (1968).

95. Wolfe, L. S., Callahan, J., Fawcett, J. S., Andermann, F., and Scriver, C. R., G_{M1} gangliosidosis without chondrodystrophy or visceromegaly, *Neurology* **20**:23 (1970).

96. Dawson, G., Glycosphingolipid abnormalities in liver from patients with glycosphingolipid and mucopolysaccharide storage diseases, in: *Sphingolipids, Sphingolipidoses and Allied Disorders*, B. W. Volk and S. M. Aronson, eds., Plenum Press, New York, pp. 395–413 (1972).

97. Wolfe, L. S., Clarke, J. T. R., and Senior, R. G., Biochemical studies on G_{M1}-gangliosi-

dosis and ceramide trihexosidosis, in: *Sphingolipids, Sphingolipidoses and Allied Disorders*, B. W. Volk and S. M. Aronson, eds., Plenum Press, New York, pp. 373–384 (1972).

98. Suzuki, Y., Crocker, A. C., and Suzuki, K., G_{M1}-gangliosidosis: Correlation of clinical and biochemical data, *Arch. Neurol. (Chicago)* 24:58 (1971).

99. Eto, Y. and Suzuki, K., Fatty acid composition of cholesterol esters in brains of patients with Schilder's disease, G_{M1}-gangliosidosis and Tay–Sachs disease, and its possible relationship to the beta-position fatty acids of lecithin, *J. Neurochem.* 18:1007 (1971).

100. Kolodny, E. H., Brady, R. O., and Volk, B. W., Demonstration of an alteration of ganglioside metabolism in Tay–Sachs disease, *Biochem. Biophys. Res. Commun.* 37:526 (1969).

101. Okada, S. and O'Brien, J., Tay–Sachs disease: Generalized absence of a beta-D-N-acetylhexosaminidase component, *Science* 165:698 (1969).

102. Sandhoff, K., The hydrolysis of Tay–Sachs ganglioside (TSG) by human N-acetyl-beta-D-hexosaminidase A, *FEBS Lett.* 11:342 (1970).

103. Tallman, J. F., Johnson, W. G., and Brady, R. O., The metabolism of Tay–Sachs ganglioside: Catabolic studies with lysosomal enzymes from normal and Tay–Sachs brain tissue, *J. Clin. Invest.* 51:2339 (1972).

104. Adachi, M., Torii, J., Schneck, L., and Volk, B. W., The fine structure of fetal Tay–Sachs disease, *Arch. Pathol.* 91:48 (1971).

105. Wenger, D. A., Okada, S., and O'Brien, J. S., Studies on the substrate specificity of hexosaminidase A and B from liver, *Arch. Biochem. Biophys.* 153:116 (1972).

106. Goldstone, A., Konecny, P., and Koenig, H., Lysosomal hydrolases: Conversion of acidic to basic forms by neuraminidase, *FEBS Lett.* 13:68 (1971).

107. Tallman, J. F., Brady, R. P., Quirk, J. M., Villalba, M., and Gal, A. E., Isolation and relationship of human hexosaminidases, *J. Biol. Chem.* 249:3489 (1974).

108. MacBrinn, M. D., Okada, S., Ho, M. W., Hu, C. C., and O'Brien, J. S., Generalized gangliosidoses: Impaired cleavage of galactose from a mucopolysaccharide and a glycoprotein, *Science* 163:949 (1969).

109. Ho, M. W. and O'Brien, J. S., Differential effect of chloride ions on beta-galactosidase isoenzymes: A method for separate assay, *Clin. Chim. Acta* 32:443 (1971).

110. Talley, P. A., Rattazzi, M. C., and Shows, T. B., Human beta-D-N-acetyl-hexoaminidases A and B: Expression and linkage relationships in somatic cell hybrids, *Proc. Natl. Acad. Sci. U.S.A.* 71:1569 (1974).

111. Srivastava, S. K. and Beutler, E., Studies on human beta-D-N-acetyl-hexosaminidases. III. Biochemical genetics of Tay–Sachs and Sandhoff's diseases, *J. Biol. Chem.* 249:2054 (1974).

112. Murphy, J. V., Wolfe, H. J., Balazs, E. A., and Moser, H. W., A patient with deficiency of arylsulfatases A, B, C, and steroid sulfatase, associated with storage of sulfatide, cholesterol sulfate and glycosaminoglycans, in: *Lipid Storage Diseases*, J. Bernsohn and H. Grossman, eds., Academic Press, New York, pp. 67–109 (1971).

113. Galjaard, H., Hoogeveen, A., de Wit-Verbeek, H. A., Reuser, A. J. J., Keljzer, W., Westerveld, A., and Bootsma, D., Tay–Sachs and Sandhoff's disease: Intergenic complementation after somatic cell hybridization, *Expt. Cell Res.* 87:444 (1974).

114. Navon, R., Padeh, B., and Adam, A., Apparent deficiency of hexosaminidase A in healthy members of a family with Tay–Sachs disease, *Am. J. Hum. Genet.* 25:287 (1973).

ENZYMES

ABRAHAM SAIFER

Introduction

The "sphingolipidoses" constitute a group of heritable diseases involving storage of various glycosphingolipids mainly in the central nervous system.[1] There are two major types of neural glycosphingolipids; cerebroside and its sulfate ester, sulfatide, are characteristic of white matter, and gangliosides are characteristic of gray matter. Storage of cerebrosides are found in Gaucher's disease (glycosylceramide),[2] Fabry's disease (galactosylgalactosylglucosylceramide),[3] Krabbe's disease (galactosylceramide),[4] lactosylceramide lipidosis,[5] metachromatic leukodystrophy (galactosyl-3-sulfate ceramide),[6] Niemann–Pick disease (phosphorylcholine ester of ceramide),[7] and fucosidosis (tetra- and pentahexoside ceramide).[8] There are six known gangliosidoses. Three of these, Tay–Sachs disease (TSD),[9] late infantile lipidosis,[10,11] and Sandhoff's disease[12] involve mainly storage of the G_{M2}-ganglioside in brain tissue. Two others, Norman–Landing disease,[13] or general gangliosidosis,[14] and Derry's disease,[15] or juvenile gangliosidosis,[14] result in an accumulation of the G_{M1}-ganglioside in brain and other tissues. A disorder of ganglioside metabolism with storage of both G_{M2}- and G_{M3}-gangliosides has been reported in a single patient by Pilz et al.[16]

It is now generally accepted that gangliosides are the precursors of those sphingolipids which do not contain sialic acid, i.e., cerebrosides and sphingomyelin,[17,18] and that the marked increases of gangliosides found in

ABRAHAM SAIFER. Isaac Albert Research Institute of the Kingsbrook Medical Center and Touro College, Brooklyn, New York.

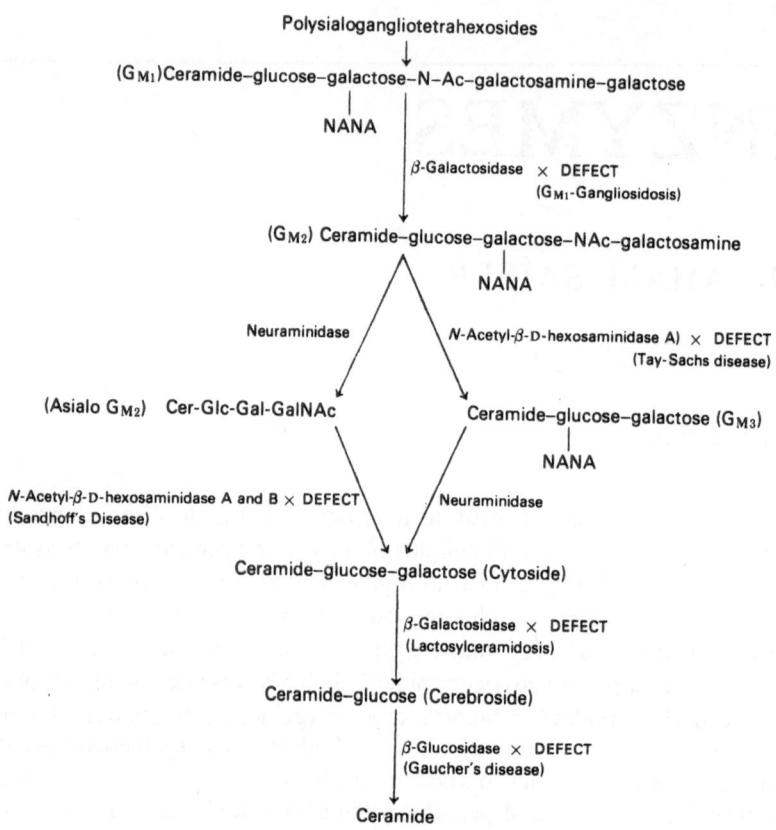

FIGURE 1. Enzymatic blocks in the degradative ganglioside metabolic pathway which would explain storage of complex lipids in various gangliosidoses and in Gaucher's disease.

the gangliosidoses are due to enzymatic blocks in the catabolic pathways from gangliosides to cerebrosides[19] as is illustrated in Figure 1.

Tay–Sachs Disease [G_{M2} (B)]

Since TSD, or infantile amaurotic idiocy, is the most common type of this group of sphingolipidoses and the prototype of the other gangliosidoses, it will be discussed first.

Early Studies of Enzymes in Tay–Sachs Disease

The utility of alterations in the enzyme and isoenzyme levels of biological fluids and tissues for the diagnosis and prognosis of disease has been widely explored over the last decade.[20] For the most part, enzyme studies of such material obtained from patients with TSD, prior to the establishment of the structure of the G_{M2}-ganglioside by Svennerholm,[21,22] involved determinations of the glycolytic and transaminating cytoplasmic enzymes such as those shown in Figure 2.[23] Enzyme determinations of the serum and cerebrospinal fluid (CSF) of 36 patients with TSD, 6 children with Niemann–Pick disease, and 1 with juvenile TSD were performed by Aronson et al.[24] at approximately monthly intervals over a period of up to four years. Tissue enzyme levels were determined in about 30 of these cases whose diagnoses were confirmed at postmortem examination. The various

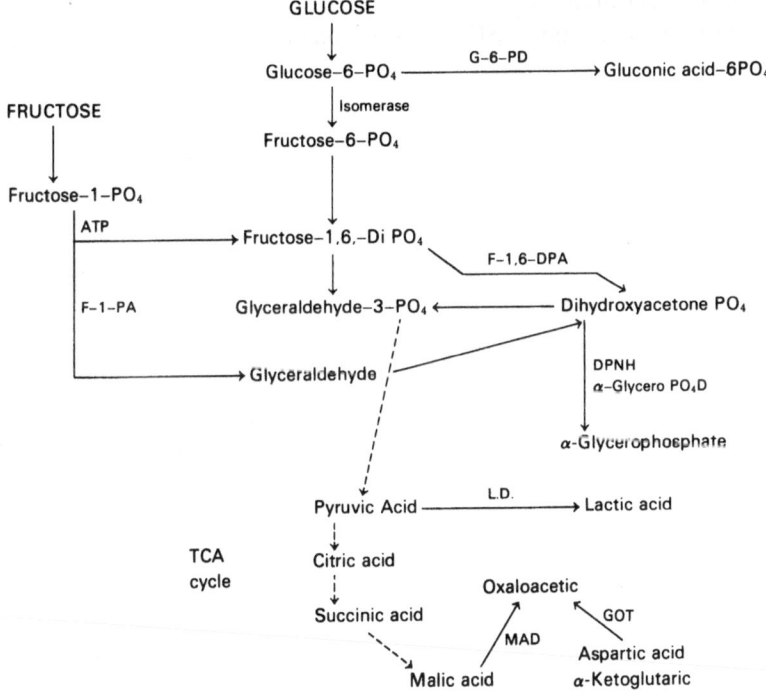

FIGURE 2. Glycolytic and transaminating enzymes which have been studied in relation to possible differences from normal levels in the biological fluids and tissues of patients with Tay-Sachs disease. From Saifer.[23]

phases of the disease, with respect to its progression, are based upon pathologic and clinical criteria which are discussed in detail by Aronson *et al*.[25] Early in the course of this investigation,[24] it was found that both serum and CSF lipase, alkaline phosphatase, and leucine aminopeptidase levels were within normal limits; the phosphohexose isomerase results paralleled those of aldolase; and the malic dehydrogenase values were similar to those obtained with lactic dehydrogenase. Further serial studies of these enzymes with respect to the progression of TSD were therefore discontinued. The mean serially determined serum and CSF aldolase levels of Tay–Sachs patients with progression of the disease are shown in Figure 3. The levels of serum aldolase were in the high normal range in the early phase, rising slightly toward the end of this phase, and gradually declining to normal limits as the protracted phase of the disease proceeded. In contrast, the aldolase activity in the CSF was distinctly abnormal, the change being most apparent in the earliest stages of the disease. The elevations persisted throughout the protracted phase but approached the upper levels of normal in patients older than 4 years.

Serial serum and CSF glutamic–oxaloacetic transaminase (GOT)

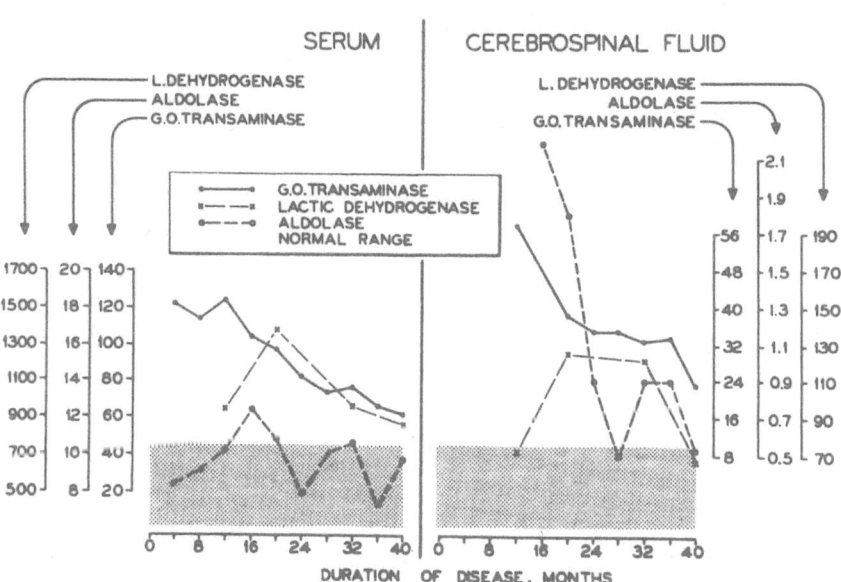

FIGURE 3. Mean serially determined serum and CSF glycolytic and transaminating enzyme levels during the progression of Tay–Sachs disease. From Aronson, S. M., Saifer, A., and Volk, B. W., Serial enzyme studies of serum and cerebrospinal fluid in amaurotic family idiocy, *A.M.A. J. Dis. Child.* **97**:684 (1959).

values obtained as TSD progresses are also shown in Figure 3. An approximately fivefold increase over normal serum levels is present during the early phase, with gradual regression toward normal values during the protracted phase of the disorder. The activity of this enzyme in the CSF closely conforms to that of the serum, with a return to normal values as the disease extends to the protracted phase. Serum and CSF lactic dehydrogenase (LDH) levels, as is illustrated in Figure 3, also exhibit marked elevations in the initial phases of the disease with a gradual return to normal values in the latter stages of the disease. In contrast to the results obtained for TSD, elevated LDH levels are not observed in patients with Niemann–Pick disease. No elevation of glycolytic or transaminating enzymes have been found in the single case of juvenile TSD investigated, reflecting the extremely low rate of brain-tissue destruction in this condition.

The GOT and LDH content of various regions of brain tissue from autopsies of Tay–Sachs children were determined (Table 1). In the early phase of the disease, reduction of GOT and aldolase levels in the cerebral white matter were the most pronounced changes, with little or no reduction in the LDH values. A profound decrease of tissue GOT and aldolase content characterize the protracted phase of TSD, with similar reduction of LDH only in the cerebral gray and white matter.

TABLE 1. Tissue Enzyme Levels in Tay–Sachs Disease[a]

		Phase of disease		
Region	Control	1 (0–14 months)	2 (15–29 months)	3 (over 30 months)
Glutamic oxaloacetic transaminase (GOT)[b]				
Cerebral gray matter	20,500	14,490	13,200	13,030
Cerebral white matter	16,000	8,330	6,810	7,700
Basal ganglia	20,200	15,600	16,320	12,850
Cerebellum	22,100	16,670	13,460	11,900
Brain stem	27,000	17,840	17,580	14,900
Lactic dehydrogenase (LDH)[b]				
Cerebral gray matter	78,800	72,640	59,980	65,800
Cerebral white matter	72,000	68,180	42,181	46,150
Basal ganglia	80,000	91,170	88,840	82,500
Cerebellum	85,000	118,530	127,280	137,700
Brain stem	132,000	124,490	131,440	135,000

[a] Data from Saifer.[23]
[b] Enzyme units/g of wet tissue.

The demonstration of abnormal variations in a number of enzymes in serum, CSF and tissues in TSD does not justify the designation of any one of these biochemical abnormalities as the basic anomaly of this disorder. The serum aldolase elevation has been previously equated with secondary muscle atrophy[26] and, therefore, probably reflects the nonspecific atrophy of the peripheral musculature in Tay–Sachs and Niemann–Pick patients. The elevated levels in some of the biologic fluids are associated with a parallel depression of tissue enzyme values, suggesting that the rise in enzymatic activity reflects a nonspecific neurocytolysis. This concept was confirmed in a later study of LDH isoenzyme distribution in the cerebral sphingolipidoses by Saifer et al.[27] They found distinctive serum isoenzyme LDH patterns with agar gel electrophoresis which resembled those found in normal brain tissue. The ratio of LDH-3: LDH-5 provided a useful statistical indicator for differentiating diseases involving brain ganglioside storage from those with storage of conjugated cerebroside compounds, e.g., Niemann–Pick disease, metachromatic leucodystrophy, etc. (Table 2). The reversion to normal enzyme levels in the terminal stages of the disease can be attributed to the stage of exhaustion resulting from complete cellular destruction. Since the highest levels were noted in CSF in the early phase of Tay–Sachs disease, it must be assumed that the increase of certain enzymes precedes the histologically observed neuronal disintegration and that the disturbance is already present in neonatal life and prior to the occurrence of clinical symptoms.

In the course of carrying out these enzyme determinations on the biologic fluids of Tay–Sachs children, similar determinations were performed on the sera of their parents. Normal values were obtained for these obligatory carriers except for fructose-1,6-diphosphate aldolase values, which were somewhat depressed. Since it had been suggested that the activity of this enzyme actually represents the combined action of two glycolytic enzymes, i.e., fructose-1,6-diphosphate aldolase and fructose-1-phosphate aldolase, it was thought that determinations of the latter enzyme, using fructose-1-phosphate as the substrate, might serve to identify carriers of TSD.[28] However, a subsequent publication by Schneck et al.,[29] in which liver fructose-1-phosphate aldolase activity in TSD was found to be reduced to only about 60% of normal levels, negated the possibility that determinations of this enzyme might turn out to be a useful test for carrier detection.

The important discovery that the brains of children with Tay–Sachs disease contain greatly increased amounts of a new type of water-soluble lipid, which he named "ganglioside," was made by Klenk.[30,31] Subsequent studies by Klenk and other investigators, extending over several decades, found that the ganglioside that accumulates in TSD, i.e., the "Tay–Sachs ganglioside" or G_{M2}-ganglioside (Figure 1), differs in solubility and

TABLE 2. LDH Isoenzyme Distribution in Normal Adults (25) and Normal Children (8) and in Patients with Storage Diseases of the Central Nervous System.[a]

Subjects[b]		Total LDH	LDH-1 units	LDH-2 units	LDH-3 units	LDH-4 units	LDH-5 units	LDH-3:LDH-5
Normal adults (25)	Mean	341	131	110	57	27	20	3.3
	± SD	158	73	73	46	33	15	1.6
Normal children (8)	Mean	398	149	127	74	33	15	5.1
	± SD	130	58	41	26	17	7	1.3
TSD (10)	Mean	1373	510	588	232	31	11	28
	± SD	579	204	271	111	27	6.0	23
SLIAI-1	5 years	400	146	163	78	5	8	9.7
SLIAI-2	6 years	660	226	279	123	20	12	10
JAI-1	—	544	134	175	103	68	64	1.6
JAI-2	—	520	127	212	81	38	62	1.3
JAI-3	9.5 years	235	102	79	38	11	6	6.4
IMLD	2.5 years	880	271	246	182	98	83	2.2
NPD-1	2.7 years	300	97	115	28	13	47	−0.6
NPD-2		620	254	283	27	11	45	−0.6
MPS-III	2.5 years	560	196	249	69	26	20	3.3

[a] Data from Saifer et. al.[27]
[b] TSD, Tay–Sachs disease; SLIAI, systemic late infantile amaurotic idiocy; JAI, juvenile amaurotic idiocy; IMLD, infantile metachromatic leukodystrophy; NPD, Niemann–Pick disease; MPS-III, mucopolysaccharidosis (type III)-Sanfilippo.

chromatographic properties from the major brain gangliosides[18,22,32] and is an elaboration of a minor ganglioside, and its asialo derivative,[32,33] which is present in normal brain to an extent of less than 5% of the total gangliosides.[34] After Svennerholm[21] and Klenk et al.[35] showed the Tay–Sachs ganglioside to possess the same structural formula as the major normal monosialoganglioside, cf. G_{M1}, Figure 1, except for the terminal galactose, its correct structure was elucidated by Makita and Yamakawa.[36]

The Search for the Enzyme Deficiency in Tay–Sachs Disease

Once the structure of the G_{M2}-ganglioside, and those of the other normal brain gangliosides, were known,[32,37,38] it became possible to speculate realistically with regard to the metabolic defect in TSD. TSD is an autosomal, recessive, inherited disorder with progressive mental and motor deterioration beginning in early childhood and with an invariably fatal outcome at about 4 years of age.[9,19,39] Based on the one-gene–one-enzyme hypothesis, it is assumed that such a disease results from a double dose of a mutant gene which gives rise to a deficient or inactive enzyme.[40] There is no experimental evidence that the accumulation of the G_{M2}-ganglioside is due to increased synthesis, and such a hypothesis would be contrary to the finding of catabolic defects in most other recessive genetic disorders. Several possibilities can be advanced for a deficient enzyme which would account for an increase of the G_{M2}-ganglioside in TSD.

1. The deficient enzyme catalyzes the reaction:

$$G_{M2}\text{-ganglioside} \xrightarrow[\text{transferase)}]{\text{(UDP-galactose}} G_{M1}\text{-ganglioside}$$

The absence of this enzyme could account for the increase in the G_{M2}-ganglioside in TSD if it were accompanied by a marked reduction in the G_{M1}-ganglioside (Figure 1). However, Suzuki et al.[41] found slightly increased amounts of the G_{M1}-ganglioside in TSD.

2. $G_{M2}\text{-ganglioside} \xrightarrow{\text{(neuraminidase)}} \text{asialo-}G_{M2}\text{-ganglioside}$

The possibility that this enzyme was deficient in TSD was negated by the report of Kolodny et al.,[42] who showed that G_{M2}-ganglioside neuraminidase was normal in muscle from patients with TSD.

Many investigators[18] had suggested that the enzymatic block in TSD is due to the inactivity of N-acetyl-β-D-hexosaminidase, that is, the hexosaminidase which serves to remove the N-acetylgalactose residue from the G_{M2}-ganglioside.

3. $G_{M2}\text{-ganglioside} \xrightarrow{\text{(hexosaminidase)}} G_{M3}\text{-ganglioside}$

This possibility also appeared to be eliminated when several investigators,[12,43] using artificial substrates, found markedly increased levels of total hexosaminidase activity in kidney and brain tissue of TSD children. This situation changed dramatically when Robinson and Stirling[44] reported that normal human spleen contains two isoenzymes of hexosaminidase, A and B. This important finding led several investigators[43,45,46] to reinvestigate this problem and to conclude that hexosaminidase A (Hex A) was the deficient enzyme in TSD.

Studies of the Assay of Total N-Acetyl-β-D-hexosaminidase

Prior to 1961, the preferred substrates for the quantitative assay of total N-acetyl-β-D-hexosaminidase activity in biological fluids or tissues was β-phenyl-2-acetylamino-2-deoxy-D-glucoside[47] or its p-nitro derivative,[48] in which the phenol released by the enzyme was measured colorimetrically. Furiya and Fukuda[49] applied this procedure to the determination of the total hexosaminidase activity of the various organs of the mouse and found the highest activity in kidney, testis, spleen, and liver, as is seen in Figure 4.

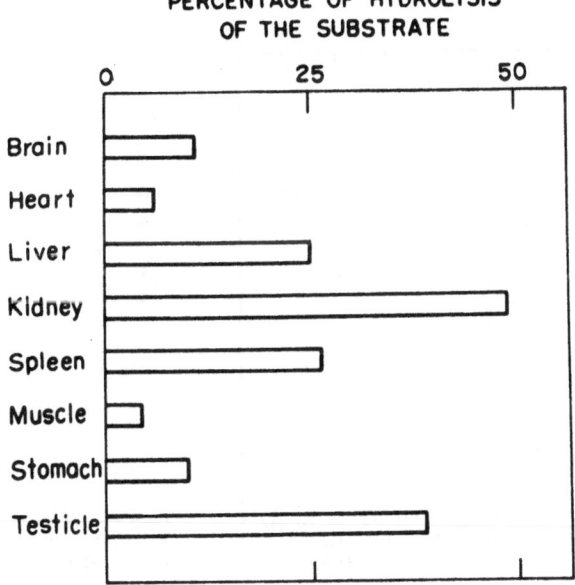

FIGURE 4. Total N-acetyl-β-D-hexosaminidase activity in tissues from various organs of the mouse. From Furiya and Fukada.[49]

These investigators also applied the method to serum from healthy individuals and from patients with various diseases. They found that elderly individuals (>60 years of age) exhibited higher activity (Figure 5), that elevated values were obtained in such diseases as nephritis, hepatitis, diabetes, and stomach cancer, and that especially high values were found during pregnancy which gradually increased toward term (Figure 6).

The use of the more sensitive and convenient fluorogenic substrate, 4-methylumbelliferyl-N-acetyl-β-D-glucosaminide, was introduced by Leaback and Walker.[50] The biological fluid containing the enzyme was incubated at 37°C for 30 min with 0.05 M sodium citrate buffer, pH 5.0, 0.01% albumin, and 0.264 mM 4-methylumbelliferyl-N-acetyl-β-D-glucosaminide; appropriate blanks were also incubated. The reaction was terminated and the liberated 4-methylumbelliferone converted into the anionic form by the addition of 0.2 M glycinate buffer, pH 10.65. The 4-methylumbelliferone was then estimated fluorometrically using an excitation wavelength of 365 nm and an emission wavelength of 405 nm. Their procedure for total hexosaminidase assay was applied by Woolen and Turner[51] to plasma from normal subjects and from patients with various diseases. Except for the fact that they reported normal values in most kidney conditions, their results confirmed those of Furiya and Fukuda.[49]

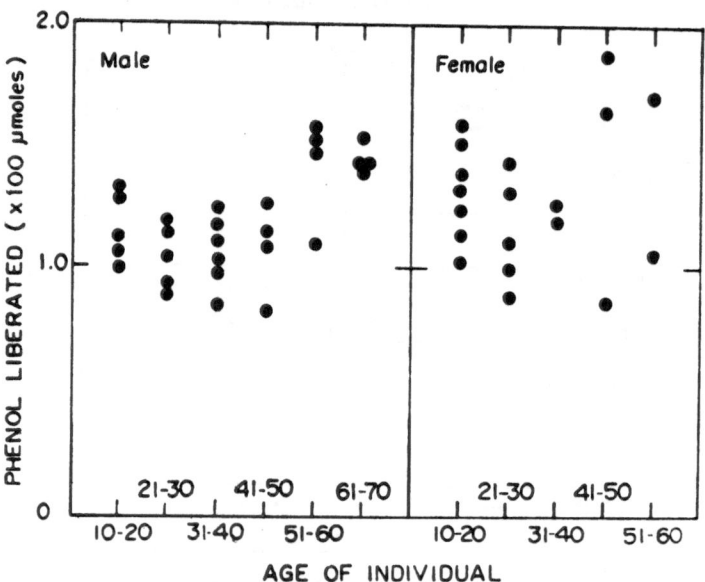

FIGURE 5. Variation of serum total N-acetyl-β-D-hexosaminidase with age. From Furiya and Fukada.[49]

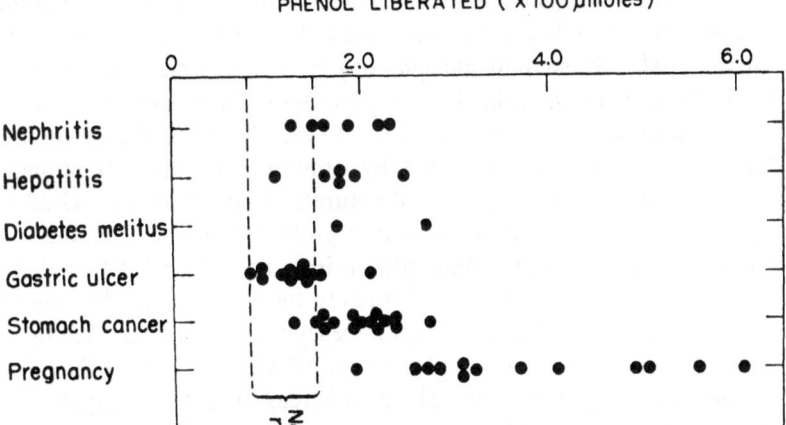

FIGURE 6. Serum total N-acetyl-β-D-hexosaminidase levels in healthy adults and in patients with various diseases. From Furiya and Fukada.[49]

However, Price et al.[52] reported increased urinary hexosaminidase activity in patients with surgical renal trauma; Sandman et al.[53] found the activity of this enzyme to reflect physiological changes in the kidney, and that its frequent measurement was useful in the diagnosis of renal damage caused by rejection and ischemia.

The assay of total hexosaminidase levels of various biological fluids and tissues is not only important for the diagnosis and detection of carriers of TSD as an integral part of the determination of the Hex A levels of such fluids, but also because many of the conditions which give rise to elevated enzyme values such as pregnancy, diabetes, cancer, kidney disease, etc., will generally yield Hex A results in the TSD-carrier range.

Studies of the Isoenzymes of N-Acetyl-β-D-hexosaminidases

As mentioned previously, the key study which led to the discovery of the enzymatic defect in TSD was that of Robinson and Stirling,[44] who reported that the N-acetyl-β-D-glucosaminidase of human spleen could be separated into two components, Hex A and Hex B, by starch gel electrophoresis at 4°C in 0.04 M phosphate buffer at pH 7.0. The Hex B component moved slightly toward the cathode while the Hex A migrated an appreciable distance toward the anode. The two isoenzymes present in splenic extracts were also separable by means of DEAE-cellulose column chromatography. Hex B was washed rapidly through the column by the buffer mixture (0.01 M sodium phosphate, pH 6.0) in which the tissue was originally homogenized; while Hex A was eluted by means of a 0–0.3 M NaCl gradient in the same buffer. If the DEAE-cellulose column-chromatography step was preceded by ammonium sulfate fractionation (precipitate between 40% and 70% of saturation) and Sephadex G-200 gel filtration, then Hex A was concentrated fiftyfold and Hex B sevenfold.

Both enzymes showed similar pH optima, i.e., pH 4.5–5.0 in 0.05 M sodium citrate or 0.05 M citrate–phosphate buffer and had the same K_m value (6.7×10^{-4} M). However, when the enzymes were maintained in solutions of varying pH (2.0–8.0) for 10 min at 37°C, it was found that Hex B was stable between pH 3.0 and pH 7.0, whereas Hex A was rapidly denatured if the pH was varied by more than one unit from the optimum of 4.5. Hex B was also found to be more stable with respect to denaturation by heat. At pH 5.0 and 50°C, it was completely stable for 30 min, while Hex A lost 65% of its initial activity under these conditions. As will be discussed later in this chapter, both of these differences in physical properties of the isoenzymes, and of their differences in electrophoretic mobility, were utilized in the development of procedures suitable for carrier testing based upon assays of the Hex A content of various biological fluids. All the inhibitors tested by these investigators showed the same degree of inhibition against both Hex A and Hex B, except for dithiothreitol, which inhibited Hex A to a maximum of 15% and Hex B to one of 30% inhibition. When p-nitrophenyl-N-acetyl-β-D-galactosaminide was used as a substrate in place of the corresponding glucosaminide, both Hex A and Hex B showed about 12% of their former activity under the same experimental conditions.[54] Treatment of purified Hex A with neuraminidase R.D.E. (glucosaminidase-free) produced a number of components of decreasing anodic mobility with starch gel electrophoresis which the authors attributed to the successive removal of 2, 3, 4, 5, 7, and 12 molecules of sialic acid, with the latter being equivalent in mobility to Hex B. Hex B was unaffected by similar neuraminidase treatment. Subcellular fractionation of human spleen tissue indicated that both Hex A and Hex B were present in the lysosomal fraction whereas the supernatant contained only the Hex A form of the enzyme.

Purification and Properties of Hex A and Hex B

Although there is substantial experimental evidence for the presence of a large number of different hexosaminidases which have been partially purified from plant,[55] bacterial,[56] and mammalian[57-58] sources, this review will be confined to a discussion of the purification and characterization of the two main hexosaminidase isoenzymes (Hex A and Hex B) present in human biological fluids and tissues. In general, all other investigators have followed the separation and purification scheme for Hex A and Hex B first proposed by Robinson and Stirling.[44] Sandhoff and Wässle[60] have extracted and purified Hex A and Hex B from human liver about 4000- and 2000-fold by column chromatography and isoelectric focusing, respectively. They found that both enzymes have an apparent molecular weight of about 130,000, that they both act upon p-nitrophenyl-N-acetyl-β-D-glucosaminide and -galactosaminide substrates, and that their close structural relationship is indicated by similarities in the effect of various inhibitors on their enzyme activity and the ready conversion of Hex A to a form with the same isoelectric point as Hex B. Li and co-workers[61] extracted and purified Hex A and Hex B from human liver (125- and 2.7-fold increases, respectively) and from human urine (113- and 12.2-fold increases, respectively) essentially employing the technique of Robinson and Stirling[44] except that CM-cellulose chromatography was used to further purify the partially purified Hex A obtained after DEAE-cellulose chromatography. Carroll and Robinson[62] improved upon their previously published procedure[44] for the separation and purification of Hex A and Hex B from human tissue by using both CM-cellulose chromatography and isoelectric focusing to obtain purified preparations from human liver of Hex A (87-fold increase) and of Hex B (61-fold increase). Verpoorte[63] purified Hex A from human citrated blood by protein precipitation with polyethylene glycol-6000 (3.0 to 25.0% fraction) at 4°C, dissolution in 0.01 M phosphate buffer (pH 6.0), precipitation with 25% Na_2SO_4, dissolution in cold water, removal of inactive protein by precipitation with 0.02 M $ZnSO_4$, concentration of the active fraction by DEAE-Sephadex column chromatography with 0.05 M citrate buffer (pH 4.5) elution, precipitation with 31% $(NH_4)_2SO_4$ at pH 7.0, chromatography of the precipitate dissolved in 0.01 M phosphate buffer (pH 7.0) on DEAE-cellulose, and rechromatography on Sephadex G-200; this yielded 14% of the original material but with approximately 195 times the Hex A activity of serum. A single peak was obtained by rechromatography on G-200, upon electrophoresis in gels containing 0.1% sodium dodecyl sulfate (SDS), after isoelectric focusing (maximum activity at pH 4.73) in the presence of Triton X-100, and with sedimentation velocity at pH 6.0 (coefficient about 4.0), indicating both the high degree of purity of the Hex A preparation and the absence of other proteins. Hex A from serum was found to have an apparent weight-average molecular weight of about 105,000 from sedimentation equilibrium and meniscus depletion data at pH 7.2, as did the carboxymethylated enzyme in 6 M guanidine hydrochloride. A molecular weight of 107,000 was estimated from Sephadex G-200 chromatography, significantly below the value of 140,000 obtained for bovine spleen Hex A using a somewhat different extraction and purification procedure.[59] When 4-methylumbelliferyl-N-acetyl-β-D-glucosaminide was employed as the substrate, Lineweaver–Burk plots of the initial reaction velocities at pH 4.5 and 37°C of serum Hex A gave a K_m value of 0.58 $\pm$ 0.037 mM and a V_{max} value of 0.078 $\pm$ 0.011 μmol/min/mg. The addition of 0.01% bovine or human serum albumin had little effect on the K_m value, but it increased the V_{max} to 0.098 and 0.094, respectively. Both Hg^{2+} and Ag^+ ions strongly inhibit the enzyme, and the inhibition can be completely prevented by cysteine. Although neither Cu^{2+} or ascorbate ions inhibit the enzyme significantly, the presence of both ions simultaneously inhibits the reaction to about 9% of its activity in 0.05 M citrate buffer alone. Verpoorte[63] also performed amino acid analyses on hydrolyzed samples of purified serum Hex A and the results are shown in Table 3. No free sulfhydryl groups could be detected and the glucosamine appeared to be a part of a covalently bound carbohydrate moiety.

Srivastava et al.[64] have described the purification and properties of human placental Hex A (4000-fold) and of Hex B (2000-fold), and a schematic representation of their purification procedure is presented in Figure 7. Their publication also details a second purification method for Hex A and Hex B in which the active fraction obtained after the first Sephadex G-200 gel filtration, cf. Figure 7, is subjected to separation by calcium phosphate gel chromatography and purification of each isoenzyme by DEAE-Sephadex, ECTEOLA-cellulose, CM-Sephadex, and CM-cellulose column chromatography and preparative polyacrylamide disk electrophoresis. Purified Hex A and Hex B obtained with these steps moved on polyacrylamide gel electrophoresis as single protein bands with virtually all of the enzyme activity. However, the placental hexosaminidases were found to differ electophoretically and immunochemically from the similar isoenzymes isolated from liver and fibroblasts. In contrast to the reports of other investigators,[44,65,66] neuraminidase failed to convert heat-labile Hex A to a heat-stable form with properties similar to Hex B.

In the second of three articles, Srivastava and co-workers[67] reported on the kinetic and structural properties of Hex A and Hex B purified to homogeneity from human placenta.[64] Both enzymes were found to have pH optima of 4.4 using 4-methylumbelliferyl-β-D-N-acetylglucosaminide in citrate–phosphate buffer, and similar K_m values (0.5 mM) and heats of activation (10,500 cal). The cupric ion was the only divalent cation to exert an appreciable inhibition of their enzyme activity, i.e., 25%, while acetate was the only anion which brought about a 75% inhibition of both enzymes. The p-hydroxymercuribenzoate (1 mM) almost completely inhibited both Hex A and Hex B activity. Using sedimentation equilibrium, the molecular weight of Hex A was found to be 100,000 $\pm$ 3000 while that of Hex B was 104,000

TABLE 3. Chemical Composition of N-Acetyl-β-D-hexosaminidases Purified from Human Fluids and Tissues

	Serum[a]	Placenta[b]	
	Hex A (mol %)	Hex A (mol %)	Hex B (mol %)
Amino acids[c]			
Lysine	9.0	6.70	6.64
Histidine	2.3	2.74	2.77
Arginine	3.5	7.14	6.86
Ammonia	10.3	—	—
Aspartic acid	9.5	9.56	9.18
Threonine	6.3	5.80	6.60
Serine	6.7	5.67	7.33
Glutamic acid	13.9	11.24	10.17
Proline	4.9	5.42	5.43
Glycine	5.2	3.16	3.13
Alanine	7.7	3.64	3.89
Half-cystine	2.1	2.25	1.62
Valine	6.3	6.27	6.24
Methionine	1.1	1.42	1.38
Isoleucine	2.4	4.15	4.60
Leucine	10.1	10.08	9.90
Tyrosine	2.8	7.45	7.57
Phenylalanine	4.4	7.30	6.60
Tryptophan	1.8	—	—
Carbohydrates			
Sialic acid	1.4[d]		
Neutral carbohydrate	30.0[d]		
Glucosamine	3.5[d]		
Galactosamine	Not detected	2.6[e]	1.5[e]

[a] Data from Verpoorte.[63]
[b] Data from Srivastava *et al.*[67]
[c] Values extrapolated to zero-time hydrolysis.
[d] Number of residues per 100,000 g.
[e] Determined as hexosamine.

$\pm$ 4700, as compared to a value of about 140,000 for both enzymes with Sephadex G-200 filtration. In order to avoid intermolecular S-S bridge formation between subunits during disk electrophoresis using various concentrations of polyacrylamide containing SDS, the exposed sulfhydryl groups were S-carboxymethylated by iodoacetate. Hex A dissociated into one major subunit (MW $\sim$18,000) and two other protein bands corresponding to molecular weights of about 35,000 and 55,000; whereas Hex B

CRUDE EXTRACT

Tissue homogenized in H_2O and citrate–PO_4 buffer pH 4.5

|

$(NH_4)_2$ SO_4 FRACTIONATION (5×)

Precipitate formed between 25 and 65% saturation

|

LYOPHYLIZATION (7.5×)

Precipitate dissolved and dialyzed in H_2O and lyophilized

|

SEPHADEX G-200 GEL FILTRATION (51×)

Equilibrated and eluted with 10 mM Na/KPO_4 buffer pH 5.0 containing 100 mM $(NH_4)_2SO_4$

|

DEAE-CELLULOSE COLUMN CHROMATOGRAPHY

Active fraction dialyzed against 10 mM Na/K PO_4 buffer pH 7.0 and eluted from column with 10 mM Na/KPO_4 buffer pH 6.0 and with 0–200 mM NaCl gradient in PO_4 buffer pH 6.0

HEX-A FRACTION (154×)

Fractions from 120 to 150 mM NaCl–PO_4 buffer pooled and dialyzed against 10 mM PO_4 buffer pH 6.0

|

DEAE-CELLULOSE COLUMN CHROMATOGRAPHY (268×)

Eluted with 0–200 mM NaCl gradient in 10 mM PO_4 buffer pH 6.0 and dialyzed against 10 mM PO_4 buffer pH 7.5

|

ECTEOLA-CELLULOSE COLUMN (1547×)

Eluted with 0 to 200 mM NaCl gradient in 10 mM PO_4 buffer pH 7.5, adjusted to pH 6.0 and concentrated to 5 ml by ultrafiltration

|

SEPHADEX G-200 GEL FILTRATION (2613×)

Column equilibrated and eluted with 10 mM PO_4 buffer pH 5.0 containing 100 mM $(NH_4)_2SO_4$ and active fractions dialyzed against 10 mM PO_4 buffer pH 5.0

|

ELECTROFOCUSING

Used Ampholine pH 4–6, IEP = 5.4 and pooled active fractions

|

SEPHADEX G-200 GEL FILTRATION

Column equilibrated and eluted with 10 mM PO_4 buffer pH 5.0 containing 100 mM $(NH_4)_2SO_4$

|

ULTRAFILTRATION (3963×)

Active fractions concentrated to 5 ml with Amicon apparatus

HEX-B FRACTION (84×)

Fractions not absorbed on column plus those eluted at 20 mM NaCl in PO_4 buffer pH 6.0 were pooled and dialyzed against 10 mM PO_4 buffer pH 5.0

|

CM-52 COLUMN CHROMATOGRAPHY (252×)

Eluted with 0–900 mM NaCl gradient in 10 mM PO_4 buffer pH 5.0

|

ULTRAFILTRATION

Concentrated active fraction

|

ELECTROFOCUSING

Used Ampholine pH 7–9, IEP = 7.9 and pooled active fractions

|

SEPHADEX G-200 GEL FILTRATION (2032×)

Column equilibrated and eluted with 10 mM PO_4 buffer pH 5.0 containing 100 mM $(NH_4)_2SO_4$

dissociated into one major subunit of about 18,000. Similar subunit formation was obtained with polyacrylamide gel electrophoresis when Hex A and Hex B were treated with guanidine hydrochloride or with maleic anhydride in the presence of SDS. With urea–starch gel electrophoresis, Hex A dissociated into three major bands and Hex B into two bands, with one of them having an identical electrophoretic mobility to one of the Hex A bands. Both Hex A and Hex B were found to have blocked amino-terminal groups. The carboxyl-terminal amino acid in Hex A was found to be serine and of Hex B to be aspartic acid or asparagine. These differences, together with significant variations in their amino acid composition (Table 3), led the authors to conclude that Hex B does not have the same protein structure as Hex A and that the two isoenzymes do not differ solely in their number of sialic acid residues, as has been suggested by some investigators.[44,65] Their conclusions are also in agreement with the studies of van Someren and van Henegouwen,[68] who used man–Chinese hamster hybrid cells to rule out the possibility that Hex B was an intermediate in the formation of Hex A. However, their amino acid data do not agree with the results obtained by Wetmore and Verpoorte[58] for porcine kidney Hex A and Hex B and by Verpoorte[59] for beef spleen Hex A and Hex B, which showed no significant differences in the amino acid composition of the isoenzymes from each tissue.

Dawson, Propper, and Dorfman[69] published a preliminary report on the use of an affinity column chromatographic method for the partial purification of Hex A from human liver or skin fibroblasts. By sequential treatment of bovine nasal septum proteoglycan with trypsin, chymotrypsin, 0.05 N HCl in dry methanol (desulfation), testicular hyaluronidase, and β-glucuronidase, a glycopeptide was derived which was coupled to Sephadex-4B in the presence of cyanogen bromide. Human liver was sonified in four volumes of 0.1 M citrate–phosphate buffer, pH 4.4, and the extract centrifuged. The extract was applied to the column and the column washed with the same buffer until no enzymic activity was detected in concentrated samples of the eluant. The column was then eluted with 0.1% Triton X-100 in the same buffer and the active fractions were pooled. Based upon heat-denaturation studies (50°C for 2 h), 95% of the activity was shown to be Hex A. Starch gel electrophoresis demonstrated a single band for the fraction eluted with Triton-X-100, while 80% of the hexosaminidase activity of the nonbound material was present in an electrophoretic band corresponding in mobility to Hex B. No additional data are given on degree of purifi-

---

FIGURE 7. Scheme for the purification of Hex A and Hex B from human placental tissues. Numbers in parenthesis indicate degree of purification at each stage of the procedure. For more explicit experimental details, see Scrivastava et al.[64]

cation of Hex A or Hex B obtained with this technique or of the kinetic or structural properties of the purified enzymes.

The preparation of another affinity adsorbent for Hex A has been described by Grebner and Parikh.[70] The p-aminophenyl-N-acetyl-β-D-thio-glucosamine was synthesized and coupled to succinylated diaminodipro-pylaminoagarose to produce the affinity adsorbent. These investigators first utilized their previously described method[71] for the separation and partial purification of Hex A and Hex B from human urine. The isoenzymes were then concentrated by $(NH_4)_2SO_4$ precipitation, dialyzed against 0.06 M phosphate buffer, and an aliquot applied to the affinity column. All of the Hex A activity was adsorbed by the column, while most of the nonenzyme protein material passed through with the void volume. Hex A was then sub-sequently eluted by the addition of 0.2 M borate buffer, pH 8.0, but only about 50% of the enzyme activity was recovered from the column. Recombining the enzyme with the nonenzymatic protein portion, or the ad-dition of 0.1% bovine serum albumin, stimulated enzyme activity by about 50%. Polyacrylamide gel electrophoresis of the urinary Hex A fraction, after affinity chromatography, showed it still to be heterogeneous, with between three to six minor protein bands. When the Hex B fraction was ap-plied to the affinity column under identical conditions as for Hex A, its movement was only slightly retarded. The authors state that while their adsorbent can be used for significant purification of Hex A, it must be combined with other procedures if a homogeneous product is desired.

The extraction and purification of Hex A and Hex B from human sources has made possible the preparation of highly specific antisera for these enzymes and their utilization in an immunological approach toward solving some of the problems of ganglioside disorders. Toward this end, Sri-vastava and Beutler[72] purified Hex B from placental tissue utilizing a procedure similar to that described previously,[64] cf. Figure 7, and prepared an antiserum in rabbits against the purified preparation. They found the antiserum to react equally well with Hex B and with Hex A as was shown be agar gel immunodiffusion and antigen–antibody precipitation of enzyme activity from solution. These studies indicated that the two isoenzymes are closely related structurally and were consistent with the concept that Hex B may be a precursor of Hex A, differing perhaps only by virtue of the attach-ment of additional carbohydrate molecules.

Carroll and Robinson[62,73] also considered the possibility that Hex A and Hex B might be differentiated by their immunological properties. They raised antisera in rabbits to the highly purified isoenzymes from human liver as well as to a partially purified preparation of human liver hexosaminidase. All three antisera precipitated the enzyme in an active form which could be located on immunodiffusion and immunoelectrophoretic gels by staining with naphthol AS-BI N-acetyl-β-D-glucosaminide. The antisera to the purified isoenzymes, anti-(human Hex A) and anti-(human Hex B), were shown to react with hexosaminidases from human liver, kidney, brain, and spleen, but did not cross-react with human liver β-glucosidase, β-galactosidase, α-mannosidase, β-xylosidase, arylsulfatase, or acid phosphatase. Hex A and B were found to be immunologically identical, in agreement with the findings of Srivastava and Beutler,[72] again demonstrating their close structural, functional, and genetic relationships. This reaction of complete immunological identity also extended to the minor intermediate component (Hex I) of the tissue hexosaminidases.[74]

In a subsequent publication, Srivastava and Beutler[75] prepared antisera in rabbits against both purified human placental Hex A and Hex B[64] and found each antiserum to be equally reactive against both isoenzymes with agar gel immunodiffusion. Both Carroll and Robinson[62,73] and Srivastava and Beutler[72,75] have proposed a model to explain their immunological findings in which both Hex A and Hex B share a common subunit, the minimum size of which is about 17,600,[67] and that such a model is consistent with either the two-locus model[76] or a three-locus model,[75] although the latter is in better agreement with the experimental data of van Someren and van Henegouwen.[68]

Once an enzyme, or isoenzyme, is available in highly purified form, measurement of its kinetic properties becomes feasible. For this purpose, continuously monitored spectrophotometric assays are preferable to static, fixed-time assays for several reasons: (1) The change in reaction rate caused by decreasing substrate and increasing product concentrations, if it inhibits the reaction, is not readily determined in fixed-time assays and the measured rate may be less than the initial rate. (2) Short fixed-times are difficult to measure, while simple examination of the recorder trace can often detect erroneous experimental runs. (3) In addition, in continuous assays the entire kinetic course of the reaction can be obtained with one small sample. Sandhoff and Wässle[60] studied the kinetic properties of purified human liver Hex A and Hex B using p-nitrophenyl-N-acetyl-β-D-glucosaminide and -galactosaminide as substrates in which they utilized continuous spectrophotometric analysis of the alkalized incubation solution. A general method for a continuously monitored spectrophotmetric assay of glycosidases, including hexosaminidases, at all pH values, using p-nitrophenyl glycosides has been presented by Ford et al.[77] Rosenthal and Saifer[78] published a method for the continuous UV monitoring of fluorogenic 4-methylumbelliferyl-N-acetyl-β-D-glycosides based upon differences in the absorption spectra between substrate and product, i.e., 4-methylumbelliferone, at 350 nm. With the use of this automated technique, the K_i, K_m, and V_{max} of purified liver Hex A and Hex B and crystalline Jack Bean meal hexosamini-

TABLE 4. Kinetic Parameters of Human N-Acetyl-β-D-hexosaminidases at pH 4.5 and 37.5°C[a]

Enzyme	Source	Substrate	$K_m(\mu M)$	$\dfrac{V(\text{Glc-substrate})}{V(\text{Gal-substrate})}$
Hex A	Liver	4-MUF-GlcNAc[b]	1000	6.1
		4-MUF-GalNAc[b]	160	
		p-NP-GlcNAc[c]	700	
		p-NP-GalNAc[c]	160	12.0
		4-MUF-GlcNAc[d]	830	
		Asialo-G_{M2}[d]	1110	
		Globoside[d]	400	
Hex A	Spleen	4-MUF-Glc-NAc[e]	670	
Hex A	Brain	p-NP-Glc-NAc[f]	590	
		p-NP-Gal-NAc[f]	170	
		4-MUF-GlcNAc[g]	560	
		4-MUF-GalNAc[g]	80	
Hex A	Placenta	4-MUF-GlcNAc[h]	500	
		4-MUF-GlcNAc[i]	1100	
		4-MUF-GalNAc[i]	400	9.1
Hex A	Plasma	4-MUF-GlcNAc[j]	580	
		4-MUF-GalNAc[j]	108	13.0
		p-NP-GlcNAc[j]	830	
		pNP-GalNAc[j]	170	6.3
		4-MUF-GlcNAc[k]	650	
Hex A	Cultured fibroblasts	4-MUF-GlcNAc[l]	833	8.3
		4-MUF-GalNAc[l]	116	
		p-NP-GlcNAc[l]	829	
		p-NP-GalNAc[l]	208	7.3
Hex B	Liver	4-MUF-GlcNAc[b]	830	
		4-MUF-GalNAc[b]	180	8.3
		p-NP-GlcNAc[c]	700	
		p-NP-GalNAc[c]	160	15.0
		4-MUF-GlcNAc[d]	830	
		p-NP-GalNAc[d]	400	
		Asialo-G_{M2}[d]	1110	
		Globoside[d]	120	
Hex B	TSD liver	4-MUF-GlcNAc[d]	1250	
		pNP-GalNAc[d]	2500	
		Asialo-G_{M2}[d]	2000	
Hex B	Spleen	4-MUF-GlcNAc[e]	670	
Hex B	Brain	p-NP-GlcNAc[f]	690	
		p-NP-GalNAc[f]	100	
		4-MUF-GlcNAc[g]	770	
		4-MUF-GalNAc[g]	50	
Hex B	Placenta	4-MUF-GlcNAc[h]	500	
		4-MUF-GlcNAc[i]	1000	
		4-MUF-GalNAc[i]	450	9.3

TABLE 4. (Continued)

Enzyme	Source	Substrate	$K_m(\mu M)$	$\dfrac{V(\text{Glc-substrate})}{V(\text{Gal-substrate})}$
Hex I₂ (or P)	Serum	4-MUF-GlcNAc[k]	550	
Hex B	Cultured fibroblasts	4-MUF-GlcNAc[l]	830	
		4-MUF-GalNAc[l]	110	8.6
		p-NP-GlcNAc[l]	833	
		p-NP-GalNAc[l]	312	6.4

[a] 4-MUF-GlcNAc = 4-methylumbelliferyl-N-acetyl-β-D-glucosaminide; 4-MUF-GalNAc = 4-methylumbelliferyl-N-acetyl-β-D-galactosaminide; p-NP-GlcNAc = p-nitrophenyl-N-acetyl-β-D-glucosaminide; p-NP-GalNAc = p-nitrophenyl-N-acetyl-β-D-galactosaminide; Asialo-G$_{M2}$ = asialo derivative of G$_{M2}$-ganglioside.
[b] Data from Rosenthal and Saifer.[78]
[c] Data from Sandhoff and Wässle.[60] (This paper also contains data on the apparent inhibition constants K_i of a large number of substances.)
[d] Data from Wenger et al.[113]
[e] Data from Robinson and Stirling.[44]
[f] Data from Sandhoff et al.[111]
[g] Data from Robinson et al.[85]
[h] Data from Srivastava et al.[67]
[i] Data from Tallman et al.[166]
[j] Data from Verpoorte.[63]
[k] Data from Stirling.[96]
[l] Data from Kanfer and Spielvogel.[90]

dase were determined. The method was also used to determine the apparent inhibition constants of a number of structurally related compounds. Kanfer and Spielvogel[79] studied the inhibition of β-N-acetylhexosaminidase by lactones. Nearly all available experimental evidence with inhibitors indicates an identity of N-acetylglucosaminidase and N-acetylgalactosaminidase activity. However, they observed a difference in the nature of the inhibition with D-gluconolactone and L-ascorbic acid for these substrates with a purified enzyme preparation, suggesting that there is a dissimilarity. Some of the data presented in these and previously mentioned publications are summarized in Table 4.

Isoenzymes of N-Acetyl-β-D-hexosaminidase in Biological Fluids and Tissues

With the discovery of the presence of two isoenzymes of N-acetyl-β-D-hexosaminidase, i.e., Hex A and Hex B, in human spleen with both N-acetyl-β-glucosaminidase and N-acetyl-β-galactosaminidase activity,[44] interest in these enzymes was stimulated by the demonstration of a specific deficiency of Hex A in biological fluids and tissues of patients with Tay–Sachs disease[43,45,46] and a deficiency of both Hex A and Hex B in a variant form of the disease.[45] Okada and O'Brien[43] confirmed the previously reported finding of Sandhoff *et al.*[12] that *total* hexosaminidase (N-acetyl-β-D-glucosaminidase and -galactosaminidase) activity was markedly elevated in cerebral tissues of patients with TSD when the assays were performed with synthetic substrates. Starch gel electrophoresis at pH 6.0 of brain homogenates from control subjects showed that one component (Hex A) had migrated rapidly toward the anode while another component (Hex B) had moved slightly toward the cathode when visualized with 4-methylum-belliferyl-β-D-N-acetylglucosaminide as the substrate and UV light. Similar results were obtained with homogenates of liver, kidney, and skin. They reported that plasma from normal individuals contained mostly Hex A with only traces of Hex B, while their leukocytes contained both Hex A and Hex B in a ratio of 73%:27%.

Quantitative data were obtained by incubating the gels at 37°C with the naphthol AS-BI derivative of β-D-N-acetylglucosaminide or its cor-responding-galactosaminide derivative and densitometric measurement of the colored spots produced when the substrate was coupled with fast garnet GBC salt. The glucosaminide derivative gave from 3 to 8 times greater readings than did the galactosaminide compound for both Hex A and Hex B. When the same tissues and biological fluids obtained from patients with TSD were analyzed by starch gel electrophophoresis, no Hex A component was detected. Hex A was readily detectable in homogenates of the cerebral cortex from three closely related neuronal lipid storage disorders, i.e., generalized gangliosidosis, Hurler's syndrome, and late infantile amaurotic idiocy. When tissue homogenates from controls and TSD patients were mixed in equal proportions, the activity of the Hex A was the average of their separate activities, indicating that soluble endogenous inhibitors were not responsible for Hex A inactivity in TSD. These investigators also made the important observations that plasma and leukocyte Hex A levels in het-erozygous carriers of the Tay–Sachs gene were intermediate between those of homozygous TSD patients and control subjects and that both Hex A and Hex B were present in readily detectable amounts in normal amniotic fluid cells obtained by amniocentesis early in pregnancy.

Sandhoff *et al.*[80] found that total hexosaminidase activity is not decreased in patients with classical TSD, except for one unusual case, i.e., Sandhoff's disease. These findings led them to suggest that some structural alteration of hexosaminidase might be the cause of TSD. In a subsequent publication, Sandhoff[45] separated the N-acetyl-β-D-hexosaminidases, isolated from normal brain tissue according to the method of Frohwein and Gatt,[81] into two components by isoelectric point focusing. The major fraction (Hex A) had an isoelectric point of about pH 5.0, while a minor fraction (Hex B) was present at an isoelectric point of pH 7.3. When the same procedure was applied to brain tissue from a typical Tay–Sachs case, Hex A was missing and Hex B was markedly increased. He also applied the method to brain tissue from two other non-Jewish children with clinical symptoms similar to TSD and with G_{M2}-ganglioside storage in nervous tissue. In one case both Hex A and Hex B were absent,[80] while in the other both Hex A and Hex B were present in greater than normal amounts. Thus, the introduction of a new analytical technique, i.e., isoelectric focusing applied to hexosaminidase isoenzyme analysis, helped to uncover two new variants of TSD.

Almost simultaneously with the reports of Okada and O'Brien[43] and of Sandhoff[45] that Hex A was the inactive enzyme which might be responsible for the accumulation of the G_{M2}-ganglioside, Hultberg[46] also utilized isoelectric focusing to show that one of the two hexosaminidase bands found in human control tissue, e.g., liver and cerebral cortex, was missing in TSD. The isoelectric point was pH 4.95 for Hex A and pH 7.0 for Hex B. Both enzymes had similar pH optima (pH 4.0) with 4-methylumbelliferyl-N-acetyl-β-D-galactosaminide as a substrate and similar molecular size as determined by gel filtration on Sephadex G-150. Hex B was stable on incubation for 30 min at 50°C in 1 M acetate buffer, pH 5.0, whereas Hex A lost 60% of its activity under these same conditions. Treatment of Hex A with neuraminidase resulted in the appearance of a new component with identical electrophoretic mobility to Hex B. The kinetic parameters of Hex B obtained by isoelectric focusing from the liver homogenate of a patient with TSD were identical to those of the controls.

The presence of two isoenzymes of N-acetyl-β-D-glucosaminidase in another human tissue, i.e., the kidney, was demonstrated by Dance et al.[82] employing 4-methylumbelliferyl-β-D-glucosaminide as the substrate. The two forms, Hex A and Hex B, were readily separated from kidney homogenates or in a more highly purified form, after fractional precipitation with ammonium sulfate, by chromatography on DEAE-cellulose as previously described for human spleen.[44] Hex A constituted 74% of the total hexosaminidase activity of the kidney tissue homogenate. Two bands of N-acetyl-β-D-glucosaminidase activity also were obtained when whole kidney homogenates, or its subcellular fractions,[57] were subjected to starch gel electrophoresis.[83] The anionic and cationic components obtained corresponded to the Hex A and Hex B forms described in human spleen[44] and were present in all the subcellular fractions. The separated kidney Hex A and Hex B forms were treated with neuraminidase R.D.E. in 0.1 M phosphate–citrate buffer, pH 5.6, containing 20 mM calcium chloride, at 37°C for several hours. With starch gel electrophoresis, the mobility of Hex B remained unchanged while Hex A split into two forms, one of which had an identical mobility to that of Hex B. When normal human urine samples were concentrated by vacuum dialysis (50 ml to 1.0 ml) and subjected to starch gel electrophoresis in phosphate buffer, pH 7.0, the major band which appeared corresponded to that of kidney Hex A, while only in a few cases was there a second faint zone of activity evident in the same position as Hex B. The authors concluded from their data that an increase of total N-acetyl-β-D-glucosaminidase activity accompanied by the appearance of increased amounts of Hex B in the urine is a good indication that the enzyme originates from a damaged kidney. The quantitative distribution of Hex A and Hex B in various human organs and body fluids is shown in Figure 8.

The fact that human biological fluids and tissues may contain small amounts of hexosaminidase isoenzymes other than Hex A and Hex B was first reported by Young and her co-workers.[84] Starch gel electrophoresis[83] separated the hexosaminidase components of normal brain homogenates into two broad bands, Hex A and Hex B. However, the presence of *three* minor peaks of activity in brain tissue was demonstrated after fractionation by NaCl-gradient elution from DEAE-cellulose columns[83] and was also indicated by isoelectric focusing.[45] These investigators utilized DEAE-cellulose chromatography for the fractionation of the N-acetyl-β-D-hexosaminidases from brains of five children with G_{M2}-gangliosidosis. Three of the patterns obtained were similar and consisted of an absent Hex A peak, a greatly elevated Hex B peak, a shoulder on the Hex B peak, and an increased peak eluted prior to where Hex A would appear. The authors considered this pattern to be typical of the classical infantile type of TSD and suggested the nomenclature: G_{M2}-gangliosidosis type A_OB_H, where H stands for high. The fourth case showed no hexosaminidase activity and was labeled G_{M2}-gangliosidosis type A_OB_O, or Sandhoff's disease.[80] The fifth case was of late infantile onset[11] and showed an essentially normal chromatographic pattern except for a Hex A peak with about one third the normal activity; they categorized this case as G_{M2}-gangliosidosis type A_LB_N where L stands for low.

The presence of at least four isoenzymes of N-acetyl-β-D-hexosaminidase in calf and human brains was also reported by Robinson and colleagues.[85] Normal human brain homogenates gave two bands with starch-gel electrophoresis at pH 5.8, corresponding to the Hex A and Hex B components, although in some experiments the diffuse anodic Hex A band was resolved into two closely migrating species. Brain samples from TSD patients lacked the Hex A band, but there were indications of an inter-

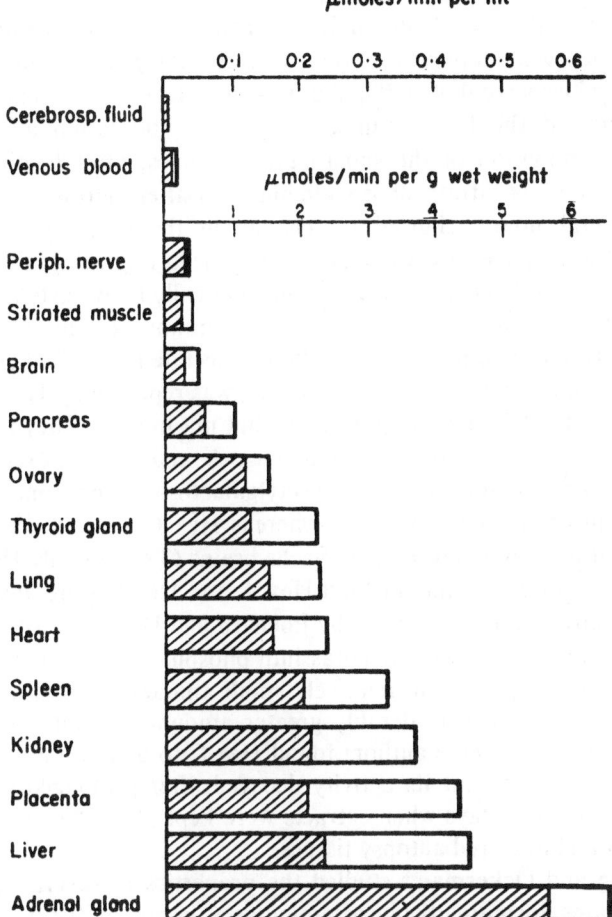

FIGURE 8. Quantitative distribution of Hex A and Hex B in various human organs and body fluids. The cross-hatched area = Hex A; the clear area = Hex B. From Sandhoff and Jatzkewitz.[112]

mediate band between Hex B and the origin. Analysis of the N-acetyl-β-D-hexosaminidases of normal and Tay–Sachs infant brains by isoelectric focusing and DEAE-cellulose ion-exchange chromatography in pH 5.8, 10 mM phosphate buffer showed about 5–10% of a third component which had an isoelectric point of about pH 6.0 and was eluted from the DEAE-cellulose column at 0.02 M NaCl. All three of the hexosaminidases obtained from normal and Tay–Sachs brains had similar pH activity profiles in 0.2 M citrate–phosphate buffer. The pH optimum was 4.6, and the K_m values in the same buffer using 4-methylumbelliferyl-β-D-glucosaminide as the substrate was: Hex B (TSD) = 0.77 mM, Hex B (normal) = 0.32 mM, and Hex A (normal) = 0.56 mM. When 4-methylumbelliferyl-β-D-galactosaminide was employed as the substrate, the pH optimum was 4.4 and the K_m values were 0.05, 0.05, and 0.08 mM, respectively indicating the higher affinity of the hexosaminidases for the glucosaminide substrate. Starch–gel examination of the supernatant enzymes, after heating for 30 min at 50°C in 0.1 M citrate–phosphate buffer or after dialysis or storage at 4°C for several hours, showed no change in the mobility of Hex B. However, Hex A gave rise to a new component migrating between the origin and Hex B and which may be an enzymatically active artefact.

Another isoenzyme of N-acetyl-β-D-hexosaminidase (Hex C) with less cathodic electrophoretic mobility on cellulose acetate strips than either Hex A or Hex B in 0.08 M acetate buffer, pH 5.0, was reported by Hooghwinkel et al.[86] to be present in human brain tissue but not in liver. They found that in normal human brain and liver both Hex A and Hex B exert activity against the 4-methylumbelliferyl-N-acetylgalactosaminide and the cor-responding-glucosaminide substrates, whereas Hex C showed activity only against the latter compound. In Tay–Sachs brains (3 cases) only Hex B was present in above-normal amounts and Hex A and Hex C were absent. This finding was subsequently confirmed by Poenaru and Dreyfus[87] with cellulose acetate electrophoresis in 0.04 M potassium phosphate buffer, pH 6.5. They found Hex C to be present in relatively small amounts in both adult liver and brain tissue but in considerably greater amounts in embryonic brain, liver, and lung tissue. These authors found Hex C to be more unstable than either Hex A or B in that its activity decayed after prolonged storage at −70°C or after a few days when extracts were kept at −20°C, so that it is not usually found in stored autopsy tissues.

Hultberg and Öckerman[88] studied the properties of several lysosomal acid glycosidases, including the hexosaminidases, in human tissues with arti-ficial substrates. On Sephadex G-150 filtration, N-acetyl-β-D-glucosamini-dase and N-acetyl-β-D-galactosaminidase activities were identical and homogeneous for all tissues studied except that enzyme activity was much greater with the glucosaminide substrate. Varying buffer, pH, and ionic strength did not influence the activity level or the gel-filtration pattern. With isoelectric focusing two bands formed, Hex A (isoelectric point, pH 5.0) and Hex B (isoelectric point, pH 7.0), which were present in liver, brain, kidney, spleen, leukocytes, urine, and plasma. In a subsequent publication from this research group,[89] the distribution of four acid hydrolases, including the hexosaminidases, was studied in human kidney tissue and urine by isoelectric focusing and with the use of artificial substrates for the assays. Kidney tissue homogenates and concentrated normal urines were found to contain both Hex A and Hex B, with the latter comprising 40% of the tissue and 10–20% of urinary total activity. Urine from a patient with TSD exhibited high Hex B but no Hex A activity.

Kanfer and Spielvogel[90] investigated the hexosaminidase activity of cultured human skin fibroblasts. They determined the K_m and V values for the four substrates most commonly employed for assaying hexosaminidase activity, i.e., 4-methylumbelliferyl or p-nitrophenyl derivatives of β-D-N-acetylglucosamine or β-D-N-acetylgalactosamine, with partially purified Hex A and Hex B and crude extracts of normal human fibroblasts grown in tissue culture. Hex A and Hex B were separated by DEAE-cellulose column chromatography of the sonicated water extract of the cultured cell pellet. The pH optimum for skin fibroblast hexosaminidase activity in citrate–phosphate buffer was 4.0. As previously reported,[91] the presence of serum albumin enhanced hexosaminidase activity while acetate ions inhibited it. The K_m values ($\sim 8.3 \times 10^{-4}$ M) were identical with all three enzyme sources for 4-methylumbelliferyl- (and p-nitrophenyl-) N-acetylglucosaminides as was the K_m value ($\sim 1.16 \times 10^{-4}$ M) for the 4-methylumbelliferyl-N-acetylgalactosaminide substrate. However, when p-nitrophenyl-N-acetylgalactosaminide was employed as a substrate, the K_m values of Hex A and Hex B were higher than that of the original extract, suggesting "that a cooperativity may exist between Hex A and B, resulting in an altered affinity for the different substrates." Hex A, in contrast to Hex B, was found to hydrolyze the 4-methylumbelliferyl derivatives nearly twice as effectively as the p-nitrophenyl derivatives. The N-acetylglucosaminides were cleaved to a greater extent than the N-acetylgalactosaminides with all three enzyme sources. In view of the low state of purity of the Hex A and Hex B preparations obtained from the cultured skin fibroblasts, the kinetic data in this publication are of questionable validity.

Two additional N-acetyl-β-D-hexosaminidase isoenzymes, other than Hex A and Hex B, were found by Price and Dance[74] in normal human serum by means of DEAE-cellulose chromatography and fluorometric substrate analysis.[92] With this separation technique, the major fraction of the serum hexosaminidase activity ($\sim 60\%$) had similar properties to that of Hex A of human tissues. About 10% of the activity was equivalent to Hex B, and there were two new peaks named Hex I_1 ($\sim 10\%$) and Hex I_2 ($\sim 20\%$) which also had intermediate electrophoretic mobilities between Hex A and Hex B on starch gel electrophoresis.[83] As compared to serum, only trace amounts of Hex B were found in freshly drawn plasma by either DEAE-cellulose chromatography or by starch gel electrophoresis. The Hex I_2 could not be separated chromatographically from the Hex P form present in the sera of pregnant women,[93] and its concentration showed a marked increase on prolonged storage or when a diabetic serum was analyzed. Heat treatment of diluted serum, such as that commonly employed in TSD heterozygote detection (50°C for 4 h [94]), showed that Hex B, Hex I_1, and Hex I_2 had similar heat stability and that the heat-labile Hex A fraction could be converted to both the Hex B and Hex $(I_1 + I_2)$ forms with this procedure. With starch gel electrophoresis of a TSD serum, only one visible hexosaminidase band appeared which corresponded in mobility to that of the Hex I_2 form. It is difficult to reconcile the experimental results of these authors with those of other investigators[43-46,94,95], especially those obtained with starch gel electrophoresis, with respect to the low ratio of Hex B in normal serum and its absence in TSD sera.

The fact that there is a marked increase in total N-acetyl-β-D-hexosaminidase activity in serum during pregnancy[49,51,95] was known for almost a decade before the discovery of multiple forms of this enzyme. Stirling[93,96] found that this increase could be largely explained by the appearance in serum of an isoenzyme which he called N-acetyl-β-D-hexosaminidase P (Hex P). After four weeks of pregnancy, Hex P contributes about 60% of the total activity, and it shows a continuous increase up to the time of delivery.[97] Hex P was separated from Hex A in maternal serum by its slower anodic mobility in starch gel electrophoresis at pH 7.0.[83] Hex A and Hex P were also readily separable by DEAE-cellulose chromatography but not by filtration on Sephadex G-200, indicating their similar molecular weights, i.e., about 140,000. Both Hex A and Hex P have pH optima of 4.5 in 0.05 M citrate buffer and the latter shows greater stability against denaturation by heat or low pH ($\sim pH$ 3.0), behaving in these respects in a manner similar to Hex B. Inhibition studies did not differentiate Hex A from Hex P, but there were differences in their K_m values. Hex A had a K_m value of 0.65 mM, while that of Hex P was 0.55 mM. Attempts to produce Hex P by the addition of purified liver Hex A or Hex B to serum did not result in new electrophoretic forms. Neither was it possible to detect Hex P in fetal or maternal tissues, so that the origin of the enzyme is in doubt. It is quite possible that Hex P does not represent a new hexosaminidase isoenzyme but is an elaboration of Hex I_2, which is found in small amounts in normal serum.[74] In a similar study, Huddleston et al.,[98] utilizing discontinuous-buffer starch gel electrophoresis, found the Hex B of normal serum to be increased in gestational serum but that placental tissue was not the source of this increase.

In an attempt to clarify some of the confusion concerning the number of serum hexosaminidase isoenzymes, Hayase and Kritchevsky[99] utilized polyacrylamide gel electrophoresis and electrofocusing to resolve the three main forms of hexosaminidase (Hex A, Hex B, and Hex I_2 or P) into a number of subbands. These investigators found that by gel electrophoresis, an extract of human aortic tissue could be separated into two major bands, Hex A and Hex B, and a minor band, Hex P (or I_2) closely associated with the Hex B component.[100] By means of gel electrofocusing, Hex A was further subdivided into 5 or 6 bands and Hex I_2 and Hex B into 4 bands each. All the bands were found to possess both N-acetyl-β-D-galactosaminide as well as N-acetyl-β-D-glucosaminide activity, with the latter being predominant. The increase in total hexosaminidase during pregnancy was found to be progressive and related to the number and intensity of bands formed especially in the Hex I_2 (or P) region. Since similar changes are found in hyperlipidemic and cancer sera, such changes are not specific for pregnancy. Heat treatment (50°C for 3 h at pH 4.4) of sera resulted in the disappearance of the Hex A bands and of 1 to 2 bands located between the Hex A and Hex I_2 (or P) forms, some of them being converted into bands of Hex I_2 or Hex B mobility. Analysis of a single Tay–Sachs serum by gel electrofocusing showed it to contain two major bands in the Hex B region and 3 minor ones in the Hex I_2 region. Upon heat treatment, one major Hex B band was converted into the another with the lowest mobility while there was a partial disappearance of the minor bands but with no change in the total hexosaminidase activity.

In my opinion, the work of these authors[99] has increased, rather than clarified, the confusion concerning the number of isoenzyme forms of hexosaminidase which exist in biological fluids and tissues. They offer no satisfactory explanation for the fact that no staining was obtained with α-naphthol-AS-BI-N-acetyl-β-D-glucosaminide for normal serum Hex A although it constitutes about 70% of the total serum hexosaminidase activity, and they continue to use the term Hex P, as proposed by Stirling,[96] although it is apparent that the same isoenzymes are increased in many debilitating disorders. Experimental results from our Institute are in agreement with their conclusion that Tay–Sachs serum does not contain solely Hex I_2, as was stated by Price and Dance,[74] but that it contains both Hex B and a number of other heat-stable forms. It is also possible that some of the serum hexosaminidase subfractions obtained with the acrylamide gel electrofocusing technique are due to artefacts resulting from the procedure.[101]

The existence of two Hex A components in human serum, one major and one minor, with the latter having properties resembling that found in human liver and other tissues, was reported by Ikonne and Ellis.[102] By means of a multiple-pass technique through a Sephadex G-150 column, the major serum Hex A component and liver Hex A obtained in purified form by DEAE-cellulose chromatography could be separately eluted. Liver and serum Hex A were also differentiated by their differences in susceptibility to the action of neuraminidase from *Cl. perfringens*. Liver Hex A and the minor serum Hex A component were not changed by such treatment, whereas, the major serum Hex A component was modified to a form less tightly bound by DEAE-cellulose. The Hex A from tears was found to be similar to that of serum while Hex A from human brain, spleen, kidney, adrenal, pancreas, lymph nodes, lymph, leukocytes, and urine were similar to the liver form. Saliva gave a hexosaminidase DEAE-cellulose chromatographic pattern corresponding to both serum and liver forms. A study of the sera of patients with TSD demonstrated the absence of both liver and serum Hex A, whereas hexosaminidase components B, I_1, and I_2 were all present. The authors suggest that serum Hex A may be derived from liver Hex A by glycosylation prior to excretion.

The presence of more than one type of Hex A in human male, but not in female, urine was reported by Grebner and Tucker,[71] who analyzed the hexosaminidases present by means of DEAE-cellulose chromatography. All the urine samples contained large amounts of Hex A, while Hex B generally comprised 15–25% of the total enzyme activity, although in two out of twelve samples the B form was barely detectable. A third minor acidic peak was eluted after the Hex A at a higher concentration of the salt gradient. It was found in appreciable amounts in four out of five male urines tested and was designated by them as Hex M. Hex M could also be separated from Hex A and Hex B by means of acrylamide gel electrophoresis, where it is the most acidic component. Examination of the pH optimum, heat stability, and substrate specificity of Hex M showed it to be closely related to the properties of Hex A rather than Hex B. In urine samples from a single Tay–Sachs patient, Hex A and Hex M were always absent while either a single Hex B peak or a double peak (Hex B plus Hex I_1 or I_2) was always found by DEAE-cellulose chromatography. Urines from five known carriers of TSD showed no variation from a normal pattern except that Hex B increased to 30–40% of the total enzyme activity. The authors[71] believe that Hex M from urine is not the same acidic isoenzyme as the Hex C from brain extracts described by Hooghwinkel et al.[86] since the latter was unreactive with 4-methumbelliferyl-β-D-galactosaminide. Nor did Hex M appear to be the same as the Hex C from fetal tissues reported by Poenaru and Dreyfus[87] since they found Hex C to be absent from urine. We have not been able to confirm the presence of Hex M in normal male urine with an automated DEAE-cellulose chromatographic system (G. W. Parkhurst and A. Saifer, unpublished data).

Following the important observations by Okada and O'Brien[3] that Hex A was present in normal amniotic cells and by Schneck et al.[103] that this isoenzyme was inactive in the amniotic fluid and cells of a fetus with confirmed TSD, Murphy[104] compared the properties of Hex A from cellfree amniotic fluid with those of serum Hex A. He stated that "If these enzymes are the same, then the determination of Hex A of amniotic fluid could be a valuable tool in the prenatal diagnosis of TSD." He found the total hexosaminidase of amniotic fluid to have similar heat-denaturation patterns, the same pH optima (pH 4.4 in 0.04 M citrate–phosphate buffer), similar K_m values at pH 4.4 (1.0 $\times$ 10^{-3} M), and identical acrylamide gel electrophoretic patterns (separation into Hex A and Hex B) as does serum or leukocytes.

Interconversion of Acidic to Basic Hexosaminidases

From the very first publication by Robinson and co-workers[44,82] concerning the existence in human tissues of two forms of N-acetyl-β-D-hexosaminidase, i.e., Hex A and Hex B, it was postulated that Hex B is convertible into Hex A by neuraminyltransferase. This interpretation was based on the experimental fact that by neuraminidase treatment they were able to convert purified Hex A into a number of degradation products increasingly resembling Hex B in mobility on starch gel electrophoresis. This suggested that Hex A could be a glycoprotein consisting of Hex B with up to 12 short carbohydrate side chains with terminal sialic acid residues. Since this initial publication, the effect of neuraminidase action on Hex A has been a controversial matter among investigators in that some subsequent publications have confirmed their findings while others have not.

Hultberg[46] also reported that Hex A isolated from human liver could also be converted to a form resembling Hex B by treatment with neuraminidase, a finding that was later confirmed with a more highly purified liver Hex A preparation by Sandhoff and Wässle.[60] Goldstone *et al.*[65] studied the N-acetylhexosaminidase activity of rat kidney lysosomes and found the soluble fraction to contain Hex A as the major and Hex B as the minor components, but that only the latter occurred in the bound fraction. Neuraminidase treatment converted most of Hex A to Hex B, while incubation without added neuraminidase resulted in a similar conversion but to a much lesser extent. Murphy and Craig[66] separated small amounts of Hex A and Hex B from human leukocytes by acrylamide gel electrophoresis. Leukocyte Hex A was treated with neuraminidase from *Cl. perfringens* in 0.1 mM citrate–phosphate buffer (pH 5.6) containing 20 mM CaCl$_2$ and the product formed studied by heat denaturation and electrophoresis. These investigators found that after 6 hours of incubation neuraminidase-treated Hex A behaved like Hex B both with respect to its decreased mobility with acrylamide gel electrophoresis[105] and its increased resistance to heat denaturation.[43] Shorter periods of incubation, i.e., 2, 4, and 5 h, showed gradually increasing amounts of a presumed "Hex B" band, as well as Hex A, but no bands of intermediate electrophoretic mobility, as had been reported by Robinson and Stirling.[44] Incubation of Hex B with neuraminidase produced no changes in its physical properties. In a subsequent publication,[106] the same authors studied the effect of human cerebral neuraminidase on Hex A obtained from human liver or placental tissue. They found that most of the Hex A could be converted from a heat-labile to a heat-stable enzyme which behaved like Hex B with acrylamide gel electrophoresis.[105] This change in physical properties occurred concurrently with the release of increasing amounts of N-acetylneuraminic acid. Neuraminidase treatment of Hex B produced little change in its physical properties and released an insignificant amount of N-acetylneuraminic acid. Murphy and Craig[106] concluded from their experimental data that neuraminidase acts directly on Hex A to convert it into an enzyme behaving like Hex B and that changes in the heat-lability and electrophoretic-migration properties of the two isoenzymes result from differences in their N-acetylneuraminic acid content.

Contrary to the findings of the investigators quoted above, Ikonne and Ellis[102] found that human liver Hex A was not effected by the action of neuraminidase (*Cl. perfringens*) but that human serum Hex A was changed into a form resembling Hex B in being less tightly held by DEAE-cellulose. Srivastava *et al.*[64] were not able to convert placental Hex A to Hex B by treatment with neuraminidase from *Cl. perfringens*. Less than 5% of the enzyme was converted to a heat-stable form by incubation for 18 h at 37°C but a similar change took place without the addition of neuraminidase. They state that differences in the amino acid composition of placental Hex A and Hex B "clearly indicate the Hex B cannot be the aneuraminyl derivative of Hex A." This conclusion is questioned by Murphy and Craig,[106] who point out that not all commercially available bacterial neuraminidase samples are effective and that Wetmore and Verpoorte[58] and Verpoorte[59] obtained no significant differences in the amino acid composition of Hex A as compared to Hex B when the isoenzymes were purified from porcine kidney[58] or from beef spleen.[59]

In my opinion, the weight of experimental evidence favors the viewpoint that Hex A is convertible by neuraminidase to an enzyme with physical properties similar to that of Hex B but that it would be best to use a neuraminidase prepared from human brain tissue.[107]

Hydrolysis of the Tay–Sachs (G_{M2}-) Ganglioside by N-Acetyl-β-D-hexosaminidase A

The discovery that Hex A is deficient in the biological fluids and tissues of children with the classical form of TSD was based upon measurements of its enzyme activity with synthetic substrates such as p-nitrophenyl-(or 4-methylumbelliferyl-) N-acetyl-β-D-glucosaminide.[44-46] It is only in recent years, with the availability of highly purified hexosaminidases from human tissues, that the substrate specificities of Hex A and Hex B toward various naturally occurring sphingoglycolipids, e.g., G_{M2}-ganglioside, have been studied.

The earliest attempt in this direction was that of Frohwein and Gatt,[81] who prepared a partially purified enzyme from calf brain which was capable of removing the N-acetylgalactosyl residue from the G_{M2}-ganglioside. Kolodny et al.[42] then demonstrated that when rat brain G_{M2}-ganglioside, tritium-labeled in the N-acetylneuraminic acid moiety, was used as a substrate, the enzyme which catalyzes the hydrolysis of this molecular entity was equally active in control and TSD human muscle preparations. However, with a G_{M2}-ganglioside preparation, tritium-labeled in both the N-acetylneuraminyl and N-acetylgalactosaminyl residues, the hexosaminidase which catalyzes the hydrolysis of this amino sugar was present in the control tissue but absent in TSD human muscle preparations. Although the data of these authors[42] clearly established an abnormality of ganglioside catabolism localized at the N-acetylgalactosaminyl residue of the G_{M2}-ganglioside in TSD, their experimental design did not enable them to determine whether the N-acetylneuraminyl moiety of the G_{M2}-ganglioside must be cleaved *prior* to the hydrolysis of the N-acetylgalactosamine. In addition, their labeled G_{M2}-ganglioside was from rat and not human brain and their enzyme preparations were nonpurified tissue extracts.

In two more detailed and extensive publications, Tallman et al.[108,109] presented data on catabolic studies with lysosomal enzymes from rat brain and from normal human and Tay–Sachs children's brain tissue which extended and confirmed the results of their investigation with skeletal muscle biopsies[42] that the enzymatic defect in TSD is a deficiency of the N-acetylhexosamine-cleaving enzyme which is normally available for brain ganglioside catabolism. In their studies they used G_{M2}-ganglioside specifically labeled with tritium in the N-acetylneuraminic acid moiety and with ^{14}C in the N-acetyl-β-D-galactosaminyl residue. Their findings indicate the presence of two alternate pathways, one initiated via G_{M2}-sialidase and the other via G_{M2}-hexosaminidase, in mammalian brain for the catabolism of the Tay–Sachs ganglioside. Since in Tay–Sachs brain the activity of neuraminidase on the G_{M2}-ganglioside is normal while that of hexosaminidase is negligible,[109] this implies that the first step in the degradation of the Tay–Sachs ganglioside is hydrolysis by hexosaminidase.[64] These investigators also found hexosaminidase activity with artificial substrates to be 600 times greater than with the G_{M2}-ganglioside in the absence of detergents.

Sandhoff[110] purified Hex A and Hex B, 3000-fold and 1000-fold, respectively, from human liver and found that Hex A could catabolize the Tay–Sachs ganglioside, which was tritium-labeled in the sphingosine moiety, to the G_{M3}-ganglioside (*cf.* Figure 1), while Hex B showed no significant degradation. As compared to artificial substrates, the reaction rate with the natural substrate, i.e., Tay–Sachs ganglioside, is extremely slow (10^6 to 1). In two subsequent publications,[111,112] Sandhoff and his colleagues extended their investigations on the ability of hexosaminidases from normal tissues to degrade the glycolipids which accumulate in tissues of cases with TSD. Although the rate was slow, they were able to demonstrate the degradation of the Tay–Sachs ganglioside by highly concentrated preparations containing both Hex A and Hex B obtained from normal human liver. No comparable breakdown of the G_{M2}-ganglioside occurred when it was treated with corresponding enzyme preparations from livers of patients with Tay–Sachs disease or its variants.

The basic conclusions of these investigators[42,108,110,111,112] that hydrolysis of the N-acetylgalactosaminyl residue of the Tay–Sachs ganglioside by Hex A was the primary mechanism of its catabolism was challenged by Wenger et al.[113] They isolated partially purified Hex A and Hex B from normal human liver using DEAE-cellulose column chromatography and biosynthetically prepared asialo-G_{M2}-ganglioside radioactively labeled in the N-acetylgalactosaminyl moiety with ^{14}C. Liver Hex A and Hex B equally well catalyzed the synthetic N-acetylglycosaminides, while Hex B from a Tay–Sachs liver had a slightly higher Michaelis constant toward these substrates. Similar results were obtained for the isoenzymes when either tagged asialo-G_{M2}-ganglioside or globoside was used as the substrate, confirming the results of Sandhoff et al.[60,111] Under their incubation conditions, neither Hex A or Hex B catalyzed the hydrolysis of the N-acetylgalactosaminyl residue from G_{M2}-ganglioside. However, in the presence of neuraminidase (Cl. perfringens) plus Hex A or Hex B at pH 3.8 there was significant enzymatic hydrolysis of G_{M2}-ganglioside to ceramide lactose. These experimental results led the authors to postulate that $G_{\overline{M2}}$-ganglioside could be metabolized in vivo only "by a complex between brain neuraminidase and hexosaminidase."

In order to elucidate the relationship between the excessive storage of G_{M2}-ganglioside in neural tissue and the absence of Hex A in TSD, Li and co-workers,[61] carried out an extensive examination of the actions of N-acetyl-β-D-hexosaminidases isolated from human liver and urine upon the Tay–Sachs ganglioside. They found that a crude hexosaminidase fraction prepared by $(NH_4)_2SO_4$ precipitation of normal human liver extract or urine was able to convert the Tay–Sachs ganglioside to the G_{M3}-ganglioside. After separation of these crude fractions into Hex A and Hex B by DEAE-cellulose chromatography, only freshly prepared Hex A hydrolyzed the G_{M2}-ganglioside, although both Hex A and Hex B were active toward artificial substrates. A heat-stable, nondialyzable preparation, obtained from the crude liver hexosaminidase fraction, stimulated the hydrolysis of the G_{M2}-ganglioside by purified Hex A, but not by Hex B, obtained from both liver and urine. Extensive purification or aging of Hex A preparations tended to reduce the capacity to hydrolyze the G_{M2}-ganglioside, even in the presence of the heat-stable preparation. Their results serve to explain why highly purified Hex A has been reported by previous investigators to hydrolyze G_{M2}-ganglioside only with great difficulty and helps to establish the inactivity of Hex A as the major cause of the G_{M2}-ganglioside accumulation in the tissues of patients with classical TSD.

Sandhoff's Disease [G_{M2} (0)]

By analogy with the demonstration of deficiencies of catabolic enzymes in such sphingolipid disorders as Gaucher's disease (glucocerebrosidase), Niemann–Pick disease (sphingomyelinase), and Fabry's disease (ceramide trihexosidase), it was assumed that a similar metabolic defect was present in TSD and that the most likely possibility was a defective hexosaminidase.[114] However, *total* hexosaminidase activity was found to be severalfold greater than normal in brain tissue of children with the classical type of TSD.[12] It was not until 1968 that Sandhoff et al.[12,80] and Pilz et al.[16] described a disease with essentially no total hexosaminidase activity and which was characterized by neural and visceral accumulation of the G_{M2}-ganglioside, its asialo derivative, and of globoside (NAcgal-Gal-Gal-Glc-Cer)* in the non-Jewish affected children, cf. Figure 1. The clinical features and course of this disorder are almost identical to that of TSD. Since all the accumulated sphingolipids contained a terminal β-linked N-acetylgalactosamine, the absence of both Hex A and Hex B[80] provided a logical explanation for the storage of these substances in body tissues. Recent reviews on the biochemistry and chemical pathology of Sandhoff's disease (variant 0) have been published by Sandhoff and Jatzkewitz,[112] Kolodny,[115] and by Desnick and co-workers.[116] The relationship between the stored glycosphingolipids in this disease resulting from deficient Hex A and Hex B activities[116] is shown in Figure 9.

The same publications which reported the variant 0 of TSD (Sandhoff's disease) also reported a single case of another variant, AB (or type $A_H B_H$) [45,111,112] in which there was an even greater accumulation of the G_{M2}-ganglioside and of the asialo-ganglioside than is generally found in classical TSD (variant B or type $A_0 B_H$). The correlation between the alterations of the hexosaminidase pattern in these three variants of TSD and the glycosphingolipid accumulation is illustrated in Figure 10. The acid

---

* NAcgal–N-acetylgalactosamine, Gal–galactose, Glc–glucose, and Cer–ceramide.

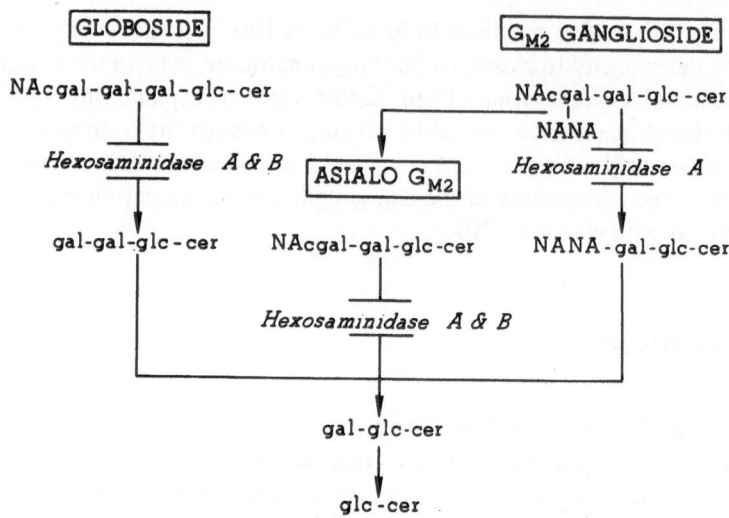

FIGURE 9. The glycosphingolipids with *N*-acetylgalactosamine terminal residues which accumulate in Sandhoff's disease due to deficiencies of both Hex A and Hex B. Here cer = ceramide, gal = galactose, glc = glucose, NAcgal = *N*-acetylgalactosamine, NANA = *N*-acetylneuraminic acid. From Desnick *et al.*[116]

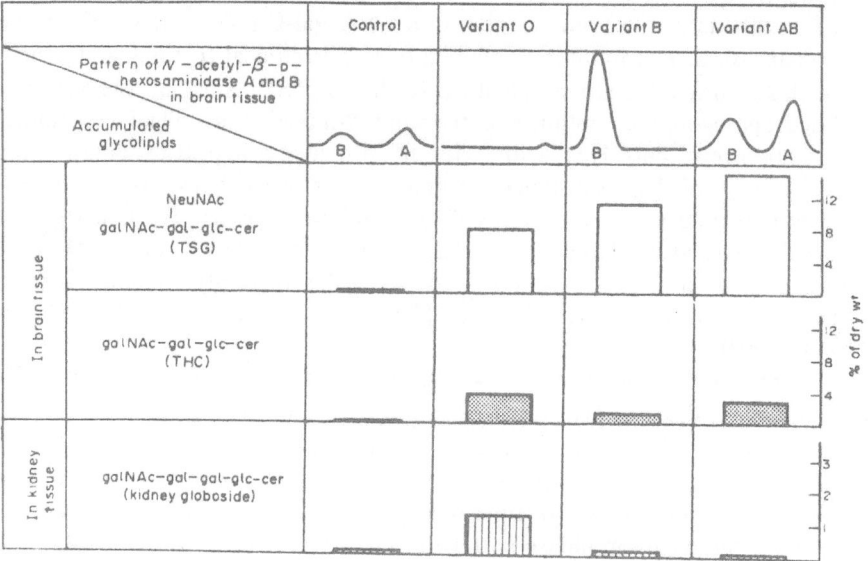

FIGURE 10. Correlation between the changes of the *N*-acetyl-β-D-hexosaminidase patterns and glycosphingolipid accumulation in the three variants of Tay–Sachs disease. From Sandhoff *et al.*[111]

TABLE 5. Acid Hydrolase Activities in Brain Tissue of Three Variants of Tay–Sachs Disease in Comparison to Other Neurological Disorders and Normal Controls[a]

Subjects	Acid phosphatase	β-Galactosidase	β-Glucosidase	β-N-Acetylglucosaminidase	
				A	B
Tay–Sachs tissue					
Normal controls	0.75	0.08	0.025	0.32	0.21
Variant 0	1.38	0.18	0.37	0.04	0.004
Variant B	1.16	0.12	0.23	<0.02	1.71
Variant AB	1.30	0.13	0.18	0.88	0.86
Other pathological tissues					
G_{M1}-gangliosidosis	0.89	0.012	0.09	1.46	0.54
Gaucher (infantile)	0.92	0.06	0.007	0.38	0.34
Gargoylism	1.18	0.04	0.05	1.12	0.48
Juvenile amaurotic idiocy	0.71	0.07	0.05	0.30	0.18
Niemann–Pick	0.84	0.09	0.08	0.76	0.79

[a] Data from Sandhoff *et al.*[111]

hydrolase activities in the brain tissue of the three variants of TSD, in comparison to other neurological disorders and to normal controls, are presented in Table 5.

The Relationship between Glycosphingolipid Accumulation in Tay–Sachs Disease Variants and Their Hexosaminidase Activity Patterns

Any comprehensive examination of the pathogenesis of classical TSD should present a reasonable explanation for the accumulation of the G_{M2}-ganglioside in the brain tissue of the afflicted children and the lack of such storage, and that of the asialo derivative, in peripheral tissues. The nature of the genetic defect in Sandhoff's and Tay–Sachs disease has been the subject of many recent publications.[73,75,76,111,112,115-120] One explanation which has been proposed to account for the existence of these two genetic diseases is based upon the possibility that Hex B is the precursor of Hex A through the action of one or more sialyltransferases.[119] As pointed out by Kolodny,[115] the manner in which the gene for Sandhoff's disease is expressed in the carrier state does not support this hypothesis. There is a greater reduction in the amount of Hex B than of Hex A in heterozygotes with the disease. If Hex B is the precursor of Hex A, then one would expect the reverse to be true. This model also does not conform with the reported differences in the amino acid composition of Hex A and Hex B by Srivastava et al.[75] or their finding of Hex A antigen in the absence of Hex B antigen in one case of Sandhoff's disease.

The model which seeks to explain the obvious close genetic relationship between Hex A and Hex B which is favored by a number of investigators[73,75,76,116] is that both isoenzymes share a common subunit. Sandhoff's disease would result from a mutation of the active site of the common subunit while TSD would be due to a mutation affecting formation of a subunit present only in Hex A. A possible model for the genetic relationship between Hex A and Hex B based on three genetic loci has been proposed by Srivastava et al.[75] and is illustrated in Figure 11. An autosomal structural mutation in the $(\alpha\beta)_3$ subunit would render Hex A catabolically inactive on natural and artificial substrates. Sandhoff et al.[111] have shown that both Hex A and Hex B degrade asialo-G_{M2}-ganglioside and globoside but that only Hex A hydrolyzes the terminal N-acetylgalactosamine from G_{M2}-ganglioside. The inactivity of Hex A and increased activity of Hex B plus the presence of normal amounts of neuraminidase would account for the marked accumulation of G_{M2}-ganglioside and the lesser accretion of its asialo derivative. Brady et al.[118] have pointed out that the concentration of gangliosides in most visceral organs is about 1% of that in brain. They suggest that the presumed lesser quantity of G_{M2}-ganglioside turned over in

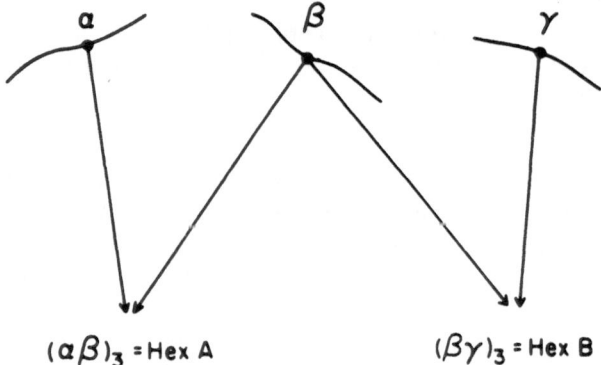

FIGURE 11. A possible model for the genetic relationship between Hex A and Hex B. Here α, β, and γ represent the three genetic loci which may code for the three types of subunits comprising the two types of hexosaminidase. From Srivastava et al.[76]

these organs can be catabolized via sialidase and Hex B to a sufficient extent to prevent any appreciable storage of the Tay–Sachs ganglioside in the extraneural tissues.

In Sandhoff's disease[116] a single, autosomal, structural mutation in the common $(\beta)_3$ unit (Figure 11) alters the active sites of both Hex A and Hex B and renders them catabolically inactive with both natural and synthetic substrates. These enzymatic deficiencies are consistent with the deposition of G_{M2}-ganglioside, its asialo derivative, and globoside which accumulate in both the brain tissue and visceral organs of patients with Sandhoff's disease (Figure 9).

It is somewhat more difficult to explain the accumulation of G_{M2}-ganglioside, its asialo derivative, and globoside in variant AB of TSD. Sandhoff and co-workers[45,111,112] found both Hex A and Hex B activities to be markedly increased above normal when artificial substrates were utilized, but that both isoenzymes were only partially active against natural substrates (Figure 10 and Table 5). Desnick et al.[116] have suggested that the structural defect in this new variant results from an amino acid substitution in the common $(\beta)_3$ unit. They have assumed that this mutation is located at a site which alters the catabolic activity of both enzymes toward natural substrates so as to decrease their reaction velocities. The cells respond to the resulting increase in the amounts of unreacted sphingolipid substrates by increasing the number and area of lysosomal membranes, with a con-comitant increase in the activity of lysosomal enzymes, including hexosaminidases, per gram of tissue. If the normal catalytic activity of the hexosaminidases toward synthetic substrates remained unaltered then an ap-parent increase in Hex A and Hex B activity would result.

This reviewer is in agreement with the statement of Brady et al.[118] that "we still have much to unravel before the pathogenesis of TSD (and its variants) is completely understood."

Detection of Tay–Sachs and Sandhoff's Disease Homozygotes and Heterozygotes

Sandhoff's disease[111,112,115,116,120] is characterized enzymatically by a de-ficiency of Hex A and Hex B, or total hexosaminidase, in the body fluids and tissues of the affected children. Sandhoff and Jatzkewitz[112] reported total hexosaminidase values for tissue extracts from brain, liver, kidney, and spleen, utilizing p-nitrophenyl-β-D-N-acetylglucosaminide as a substrate, which were about 10% of those obtained for control tissues. Tateson and Bain[117] found a reduction of total hexosaminidase activity per gram wet weight of liver, spleen, and brain in Sandhoff's disease to 0.25% of the normal levels. Total hexosaminidase values of essentially zero were reported by Suzuki et al.[120] for brain gray matter, liver, spleen, and leukocytes in a single patient with Sandhoff's disease. For two cases of Sandhoff's disease Kolodny[115] obtained values of liver hexosaminidase which were about 1.5% of the values of the controls with 4-methylumbelliferyl glycosides as substrates, and zero values were obtained when asialo-G_{M2}-ganglioside, or globoside, was used as the substrate. Desnick et al.[116] found the following total hexosaminidase levels (nmol/ml/h) utilizing 4-methylumbelliferyl-N-acetyl-β-D-glucosaminide as the substrate: in liver, <1%; cultured skin fibroblasts, 5%, cerebrospinal fluid, 8%; and plasma, 2% of the matched control values for a homozygote with Sandhoff's disease. He found total hexosaminidase values in liver or plasma for an infant heterozygote to be about 50% of that of a normal-infant control.

The initial diagnosis of the Sandhoff variant of G_{M2}-gangliosidosis is generally made after low levels of total hexosaminidase are found in the child's serum. For this purpose, as well as for heterozygote detection, most investigators[115,116,120,121] have utilized the fluorometric procedure of Leaback and Walker[50] as modified by O'Brien et al.[94] which employs 4-methylumbelliferyl-β-D-N-acetylglucosaminide as the substrate (see Appendix B). The total serum hexosaminidase values for seven patients with Sandhoff's disease and for nine heterozygotes are given in Table 6 together with control data. In three of the cases, the percentage of Hex A of the total hexosaminidase activity is also given, and those values are above normal or in the upper end of the normal range. While the heterozygotes tend to have values which are considerably below the average of the controls, there is a good deal of overlap between the normal and the carrier ranges. Kolodny[115] has provided evidence that the criteria of low total hexosaminidase and a high percentage of Hex A in serum is a useful one for detecting the heterozygotes among the close relatives of a patient with Sandhoff's disease. At present, the lack of a well-defined ethnic group with a high carrier rate does not warrant the effort required to screen the general population for the genetic carriers of Sandhoff's disease, although the automated systems required to conduct such surveys are commercially available as an integral part of the equipment needed for TSD-carrier detection.

TSD is characterized enzymatically by the inactivity of Hex A in the biological fluids and tissues of children (homozygotes) who have inherited it as an autosomal recessive trait from their carrier parents, i.e., obligatory heterozygotes.[43,122] While both of the major forms of the enzymes, Hex A and Hex B, are present in readily detectable quantities in fluids from normal individuals,[94,105] heterozygotes show Hex A activities intermediate between those of normal controls and TSD patients.[94,105,123,-125] As compared

TABLE 6. Serum Total Hexosaminidase and Hexosaminidase A Values in Normal Controls, Heterozygotes, and Homozygotes with Sandhoff's and Tay-Sachs Disease

Subject	Total hexosaminidase, nmol/ml/h	Hexosaminidase A, % of total
Controls[a] (33)	333–775 (Av = 575)	49–68 (Av = 57.3)
Controls[b] (436)	330–2144 (Av = 536)	53–86 (Av = 66.2)
Controls[c] (170)	347–983 (Av = 665)	58–79 (Av = 67.3)
Sandhoff (No. 1)[d]	11.3	58.3
Sandhoff (No. 2)[d]	33.9	60.1
Sandhoff (No. 3)[d]	32.0	——
Sandhoff (No. 4)[d]	9.5	78.0
Sandhoff (No. 5)[d]	22.0	35.0
Sandhoff (No. 6)[d]	10.0	48.0
Sandhoff Heterozygotes	333–545	68.5–81.3
Tay–Sachs disease[a] (9)	284–1232 (Av = 539)	0–4 (Av = 1.7)
Tay–Sachs disease[c] (9)	242–1242 (Av = 742)	0–16 (Av = 7.8)
TSD heterozygotes[a] (26)	288–644 (Av = 450)	26–45 (Av = 37.5)
TSD heterozygotes[b] (15)	337–1336 (Av = 659)	37–46 (Av = 44.1)
TSD heterozygotes[c] (27)	257–945 (Av = 601)	35–60 (Av = 47.5)

[a] Heat denaturation at 50°C (manual). O'Brien et al.[94]
[b] Heat denaturation at 60°C (automated). Lowden et al.[133]
[c] pH inactivation at 37°C (automated). Saifer and Perle.[135]
[d] Data compiled from articles by Kolodny,[115] Desnick et al.,[116] Yabuuchi et al.,[121] and O'Brien et al.[122]

to the extremely low (or zero) levels of Hex A obtained for the TSD children, the ability to detect TSD carriers by mass screening of the high-risk Ashkenazic Jewish segment of a community is based on the quantitative measurement of the Hex A activity of a particular biological fluid. Fluids which have been used for this purpose include serum,[94,124] leukocytes,[105,123,124] urine,[126] and tears.[127] The quantitative determination of Hex A in a biological fluid usually involves the difference obtained between the total hexosaminidase activity and that of Hex B or the "heat- or pH-stable" fraction. The fluorogenic substrate, 4-methylumbelliferyl-N-acetyl-β-D-glucosaminide, is reacted upon with equal velocity by both the Hex A and Hex B components of a biological fluid or tissue extract at pH 4.5 to release the highly fluorescent 4-methylumbelliferone which serves as a measure of the total hexosaminidase activity.[94]

For assay of Hex A activity of a biological fluid by manual or semiautomated procedures, three general principles have been used: (1) Denaturation of Hex A: Hex A is relatively labile to heat, i.e., 3–4 h at 50°C at pH

4.4, as compared to Hex B, or the heat-stable, fraction.[94,128] Hex A activity can also be destroyed by means of pH inactivation. Incubation of a fluid for 5 min in pH 2.80 glycine hydrochloride buffer at 37°C denatures Hex A without appreciably affecting the activity of Hex B.[129] After destruction of the Hex A activity of the biological sample, the fluorescent assay is performed in the same manner as for the total hexosaminidase procedure. The remaining enzyme activity of the "heat-or pH-stable" fraction has been designated as "Hex B," although recent publications have reported the presence of a number of additional isoenzymes in serum, urine, and other biological fluids, $cf.$ pages 73–83. Although hexosaminidase values can be calculated as nmol/ml/h, it is often more convenient to express the results as the percentage of Hex A of the total activity. Detailed descriptions of the manual heat-denaturation method of O'Brien et $al.$[94] and the manual pH-inactivation procedure of Saifer and Rosenthal[129] are provided in Appendix B of this volume. (2) Separation of Hex A from Hex B as a result of differences in their electrophoretic mobility at pH 8.1 in such media as acrylamide gel[105] or cellulose acetate.[124,130] The acrylamide gel electrophoretic procedure of Friedland et $al.$[105] is also described in detail in Appendix B of this volume. (3) Separation of Hex A from the other hexosaminidases present in biological fluids by means of DEAE-cellulose chromatography. Although Young et $al.$[84] reported the presence of three additional minor peaks with hexosaminidase activity in normal brain tissue extracts and Price and Dance[74] demonstrated that serum hexosaminidase activity could be resolved into four components, A, I_1, I_2, and B by DEAE-cellulose chromatography, it was not until recently that Yabuuchi and co-workers[121] employed micro-DEAE-cellulose columns and buffer–salt gradients to separate and quantitate these four isoenzymes from 20 μl of serum. Their Hex A values for normal adults, heterozygotes of TSD and Sandhoff's disease, and for pregnant women were in good agreement with the results obtained with the heat-denaturation method.[94] They found the intermediate components (Hex I_1 and Hex I_2) to have thermostability similar to that of Hex B and that, contrary to the reports of other investigators,[74,99], heat denaturation under the conditions prescribed by O'Brien et $al.$[94] destroys only Hex A and that during this process there is no interconversion of Hex A to other heat-stable isoenzyme forms. The main drawback to the use of this procedure for the routine investigation of heterozygotes and homozygotes with G_{M2}-gangliosidosis is the tediousness involved in the collection and analysis of some 100 samples for each run. Saifer and Parkhurst[131] have incorporated similar micro-DEAE-columns into a Technicon automated system for performing total hexosaminidase assays, the manifold for which is illustrated in Figure 12. This equipment enables a single operator to perform eight or more column analyses per working day on a continuous

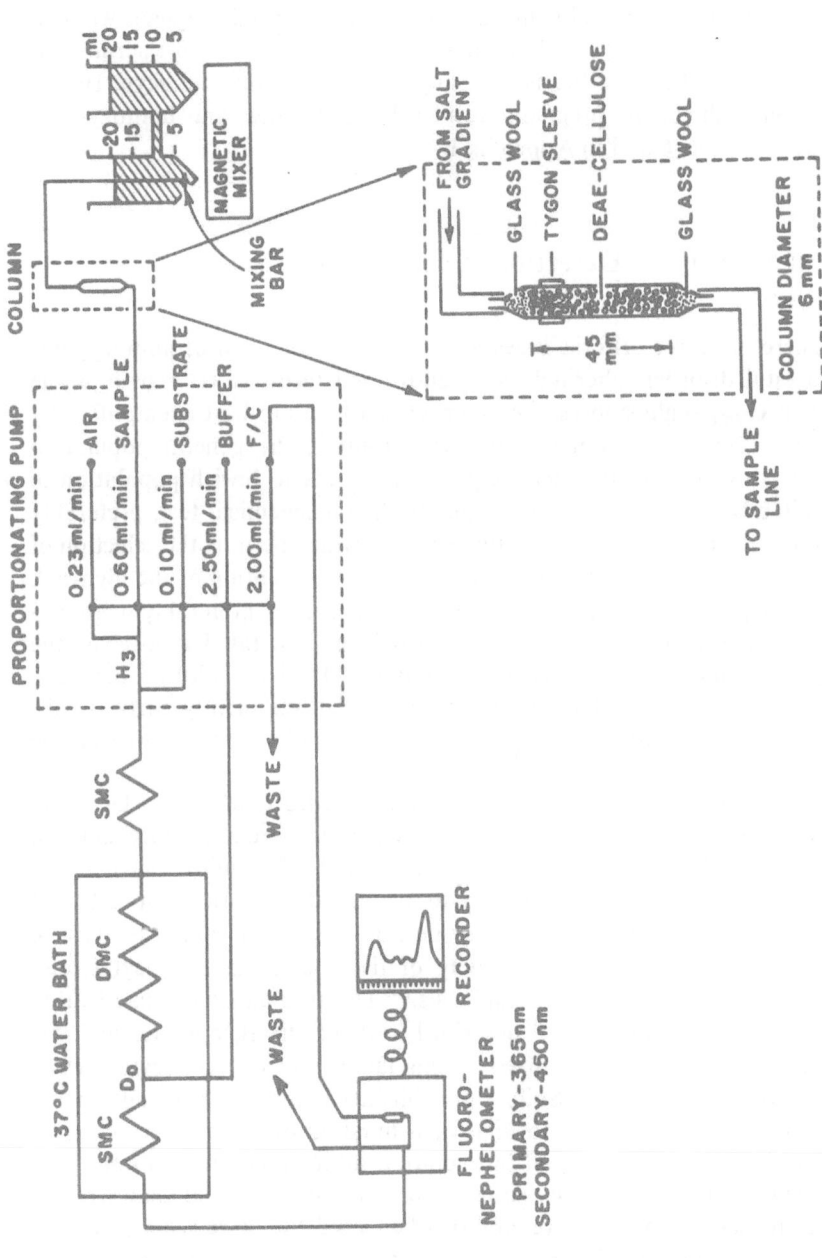

FIGURE 12. Flow diagram for automated measurement of effluent from DEAE-cellulose microcolumn for *N*-acetyl-*β*-D-hexosaminidase activity with 4-methylumbelliferylacetamido-2-deoxy-D-glucopyranoside as the substrate. From Saifer and Parkhurst.[131]

basis with little attention required once a run has been started. Hexosamini-dase isoenzyme patterns obtained with this procedure for serum and leukocytes from normal individuals, TSD carriers, normal pregnant women, pregnant carriers, and TSD children are shown in Figure 13 for serum and Figure 14 for leukocytes. Statistical ranges for serum and leukocyte Hex A for normal individuals, pregnant women, heterozygotes, and homozygotes are listed in Table 6 and in Appendix B.

Pre- and Postnatal Detection of Tay–Sachs Disease

There are three criteria necessary to prevent the birth of homozygotes with a fatal disorder inherited as an autosomal recessive trait such as the G_{M1}- and G_{M2}-gangliosidoses. These criteria, which are best exemplified by TSD, are: (1) a well-defined, high-risk group in the general population which carries the defective gene, e.g., the Ashkenazic Jewish population in the United States.[132] (2) A simple, quantitative biochemical test, preferably based on the analysis of the defective enzyme, which permits the selection of heterozygotes from the general population and the isolation of the high-risk carrier couples, e.g., the assay of Hex A in serum preferably with au-tomated fluorometric procedures.[133-135] (3) The prenatal diagnosis of the diseae by enzymatic analysis of the amniotic fluid or cultured amniotic cells obtained from the fetuses of carrier couples sufficiently early (weeks 14–16 of gestation) to give the parents the choice of safely terminating the pregnancy.[103]

In the automated Hex A procedures of Lowden et al.[133] and Delvin et al.[134] the isoenzyme is rendered inactive by heating serum at more elevated temperatures (55–60°C) for shorter time periods (5–6 min). Such higher temperatures have a greater tendency to increase the denaturation of Hex B and the other stable isoenzymes of serum, but also, they cannot be used to determine the hexosaminidase activity of tissue extracts, leukocytes, cul-tured fibroblasts, and amniotic fluid cells.[133] The automated pH-inactivation method of Saifer and Perle,[135] described in Appendix B, operates at 37°C and has been successfully utilized in this laboratory for leukocyte Hex A analysis (G. Perle and A. Saifer, unpublished data). Such an automated system enables a technician to analyze a hundred or more serum samples per working day and has been in operation in our laboratory for the past year. Automated assays have distinct advantages over manual analyses with respect to speed, cost, and reliability when used for large-scale screening programs. Automated hexosaminidase procedures have thus solved the

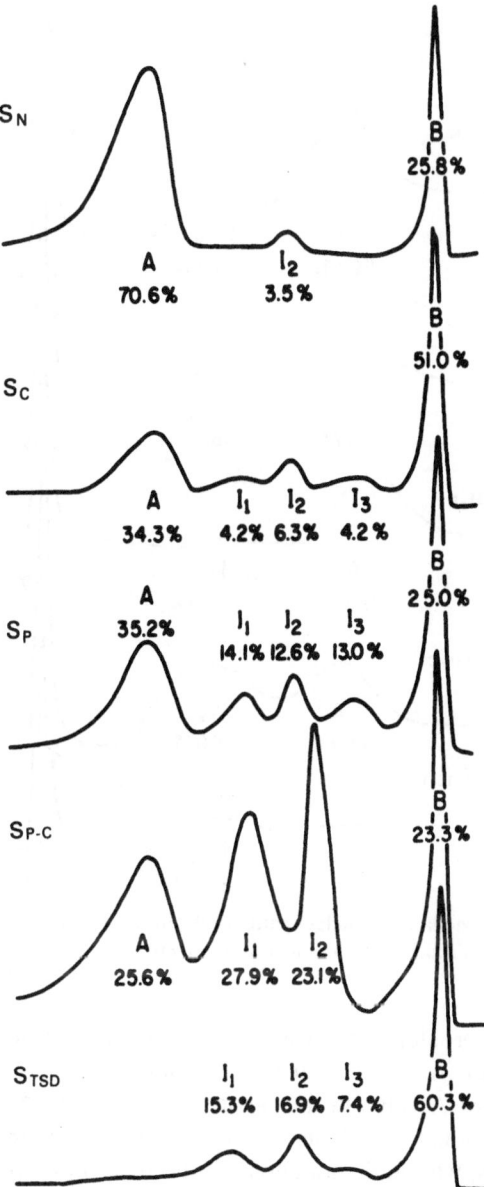

FIGURE 13. Serum hexosaminidase patterns obtained with a DEAE-cellulose microcolumn automated system. S_N = normal serum, S_C = serum from a TSD carrier, S_P = pregnancy serum, S_{P-C} = serum from a pregnant carrier, and S_{TSD} = serum from a patient with TSD. From Saifer and Parkhurst.[181]

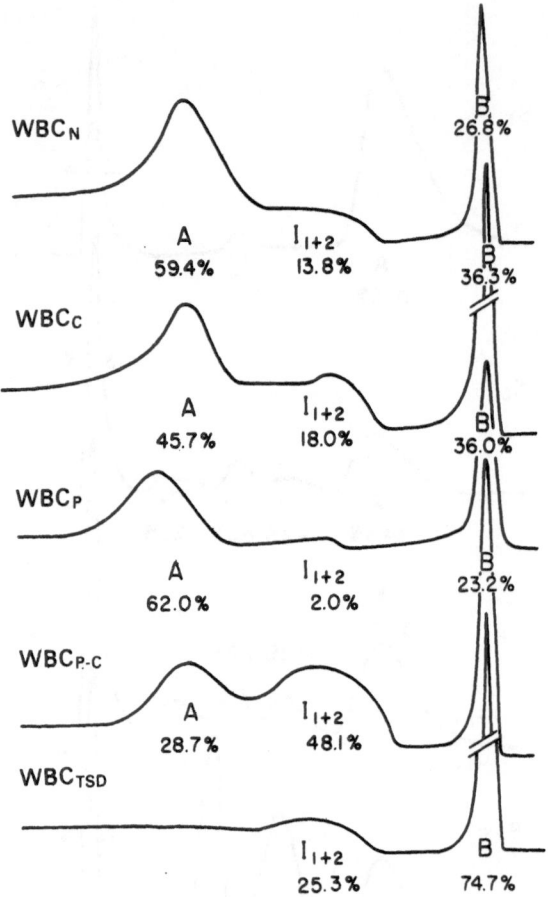

FIGURE 14. Leukocyte hexosaminidase patterns obtained with DEAE-cellulose microcolumn automated system. Nomenclature is the same as in Figure 13. From Saifer and Parkhurst.[131]

major logistical problem concerned with the identification of heterozygotes of TSD among the Ashkenazic Jewish population.

A serum Hex A value in the carrier range, i.e., 39–59%, serves only to identify an individual as a "suspected or potential carrier" of TSD. That these individuals, who make up about 5% of the test group, are actually carriers is best confirmed by Hex A analysis of their leukocytes. This is due to the fact that there are a number of clinical conditions such as pregnancy, diabetes, and other debilitating diseases in which the serum Hex A values fall within the carrier range.[97,125,135,136] The heat-denaturation method of O'Brien and associates[94] has been applied to the determination of the Hex A content of leukocytes and amniotic fluid cells by Padeh and Navon.[123] In our experience, assays of such fluids based on heat denaturation yield positive values for Hex A (Figure 15) even when other techniques, such as gel electrophoresis (Figure 16) or DEAE-cellulose column chromatography (Figure 14), show it to be absent. For the determination of the Hex A content of leukocytes, amniotic fluids, and cultured amniotic cell extracts, it is preferable to utilize a procedure which separates the two isoenzymes such as acrylamide gel[105] or cellulose acetate[124,130] electrophoresis or DEAE-cellulose chromatography.[121,131] While such techniques are useful for confirmatory analysis of suspected heterozygotes and homozygotes, they are not suited for mass-screening procedures.

Interference with the serum Hex A carrier-detection test due to pregnancy constitutes a serious problem since many couples do not become concerned about the prospect of a genetically defective child until after the wife is pregnant. If the serum value of the father falls into the "suspected-carrier" range, then the leukocytes of both parents should be analyzed for their Hex A content with the acrylamide gel (Figure 16) or micro-DEAE-cellulose column (Figure 14) procedures. The use of leukocytes with these methods gives almost complete differentiation between the pregnant and carrier groups and therefore it constitutes the most suitable biological ma-

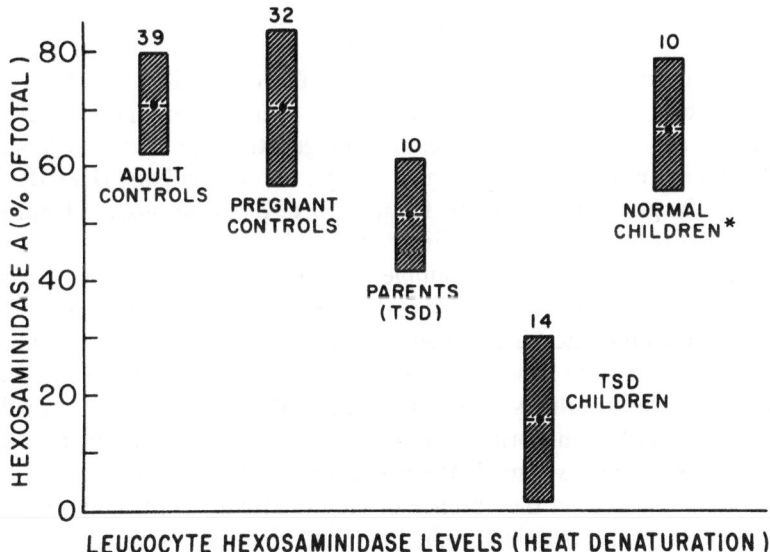

LEUCOCYTE HEXOSAMINIDASE LEVELS (HEAT DENATURATION)

FIGURE 15. Statistical data [mean (—●—) ± 2 SD] of leukocyte Hex A levels obtained by heat denaturation for: 39 adult (normal) controls, 32 pregnant controls, 10 Tay–Sachs disease carrier parents, 14 Tay–Sachs children, and 10 control (nonneurological) children. From Saifer *et al.*[136]

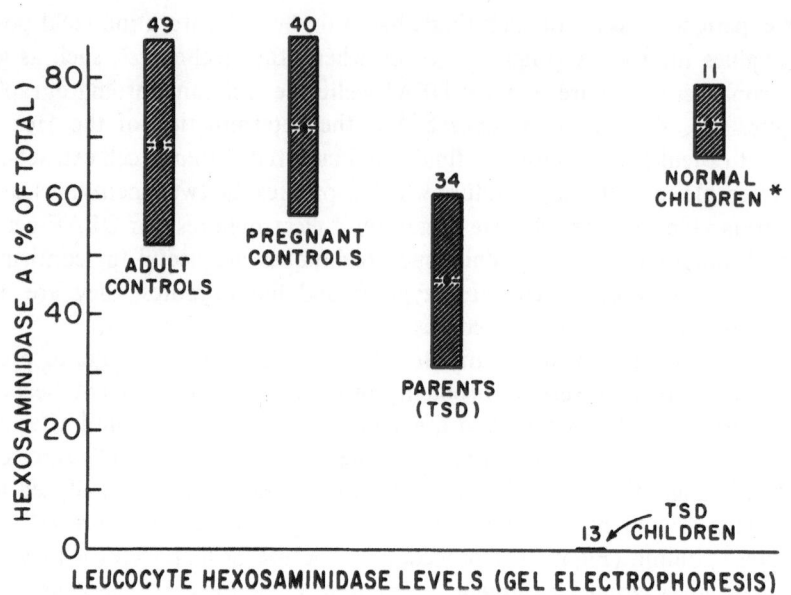

FIGURE 16. Statistical data [mean (—•—) ± 2 SD] of leukocyte Hex A levels obtained by acrylamide gel electrophoresis for: 49 adult (normal) controls, 40 pregnant controls, 34 Tay–Sachs disease carrier parents, 13 Tay–Sachs children, and 11 control (nonneurological) children. From Saifer et al.[186]

terial for determining whether a pregnant woman is a carrier. Gel electrophoresis and micro-DEAE-cellulose column chromatography of leukocytes are also the most reliable diagnostic tests for determining whether an infant has TSD since only a single fluorescent band (Hex B) will appear in the gel pattern (Figure 17) and Hex A will be missing from the DEAE-cellulose column pattern (Figure 14).

TSD constitutes an ideal example of a genetic disorder which fits the criterion discussed above for prenatal detection by means of enzymatic analysis of the amniotic fluid or cultured amniotic cells obtained by amniocentesis. Okada and O'Brien[43] had shown that Hex A was absent in all the tissues and biological fluids of patients with TSD but was present in readily detectable quantities in normal amniotic cells. Following up on this lead, Schneck and colleagues[103] made the first prenatal diagnosis of TSD in a 20-week-old fetus based on the absence of Hex A activity in its amniotic fluid and amniotic cells. Since this original case, 40 high-risk pregnancies of carrier couples have been monitored at this Institute, mostly from women who had one or more affected children. There is a 25% chance of a child being born with TSD from such a mating with each pregnancy. Based on Hex A analysis of the amniotic fluid, TSD was diagnosed in 12 out of 40 pregnancies (Figure 18). Recently micro-DEAE-cellulose column chromatography[131] has been employed to study the hexosaminidase isoenzyme patterns of amniotic fluids (Figure 19) and extracts of cultured amniotic cells (Figure 20) obtained from normal, presumed carrier, and TSD fetuses. Every child predicted to be normal prenatally proved to be free of TSD upon subsequent clinical and laboratory examination. In every instance, where fetal tissue was available for analysis, the prenatal diagnosis of TSD was confirmed by the absence of Hex A in the biological fluids and tissues of the fetus, the presence of "membranous cytoplasmic bodies" in

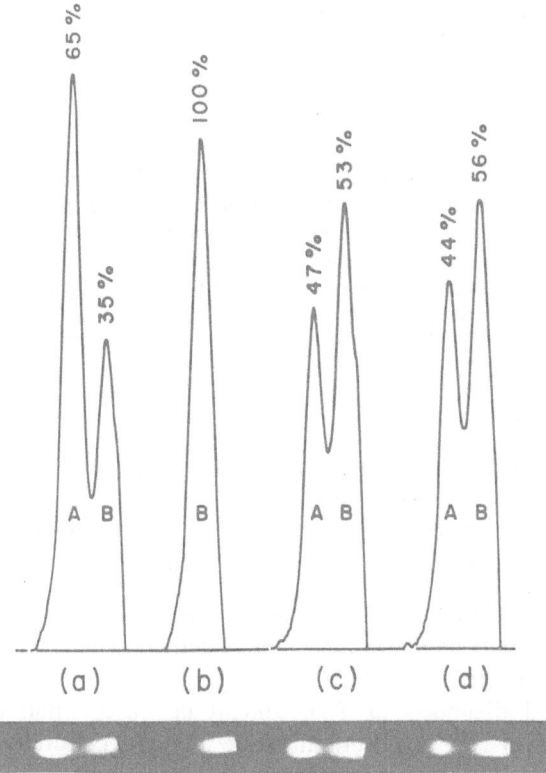

FIGURE 17. Automated fluorometric scan of acrylamide gels obtained by electrophoresis of leukocyte preparations and incubation with 4-methylumbelliferyl-β-D-glucosaminide substrate. (a) Normal adult pattern, (b) a Tay–Sachs child's (homozygote) pattern, (c) a male parent's (heterozygote) pattern, and a female parent's (heterozygote) pattern. From Friedland et al.[105]

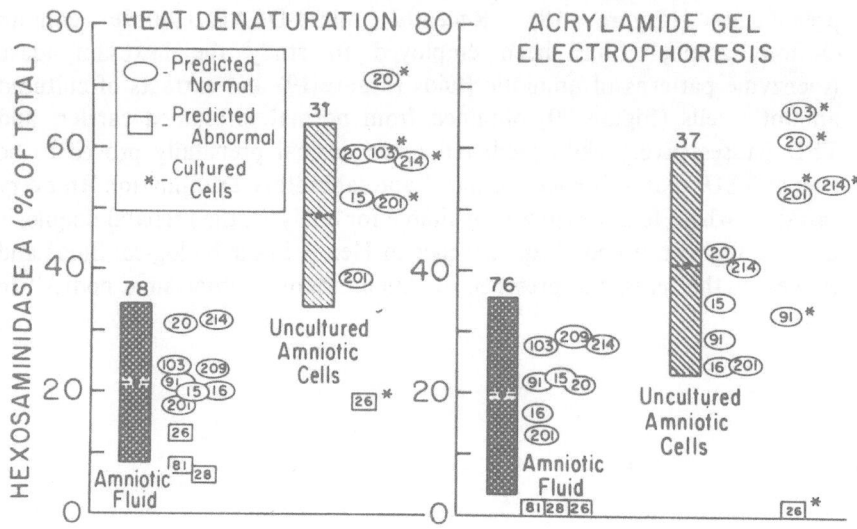

FIGURE 18. Statistical data [mean (—•—) ± 2 SD] of normal amniotic-fluid and uncultured-cell Hex A levels obtained with the heat denaturation and acrylamide gel electrophoretic techniques (see Appendix B). Hex A values are also given for all amniotic fluids and cells (uncultured and cultured) obtained from the fetuses of carrier couples, of which 9 (AF No. 15, 16, 20, 91, 103, 201, 204, 209, 214) were predicted normal and 3 (AF No. 26, 28, 81) were predicted as Tay–Sachs disease. From Saifer et al.[186]

the brain tissue as visualized by electron microscopy, and an increase in the percentage of cerebral G_{M2}-ganglioside.[103,137]

As a result of our extensive experience in the prenatal diagnosis of TSD, we can make the following recommendations:[138]

1. Uncultured amniotic cells should not be used for the antenatal diagnosis of TSD based on their Hex A activity, since in many instances these cells are nonviable.[130]

2. Prenatal diagnosis of TSD should be based upon the complete absence of Hex A in both amniotic fluid and cultured amniotic cells as determined by a procedure which separates Hex A from its other isoenzymes, e.g., acrylamide gel electrophoresis or DEAE-cellulose column chromatography.

3. As much reliance can be placed on the Hex A values obtained with two or more amniotic-fluid samples, in making an antenatal diagnosis of TSD, as on the analysis of cultured cell extracts provided

that the analysis is performed by acrylamide gel electrophoresis or automated micro-DEAE-column chromatography. Such results can be obtained in less than 24 hours for the amniotic fluid but may require 3–4 weeks for amniotic cell growth.[139]

4. When the heat-denaturation procedure is used for Hex A analysis of amniotic fluid samples, it is best to use only cultured cells since this material provides the best differentiation between a normal and Tay–Sachs fetus.

5. A portion of each sample tested should be sent to another genetic laboratory for confirmatory analysis before reaching a final decision.

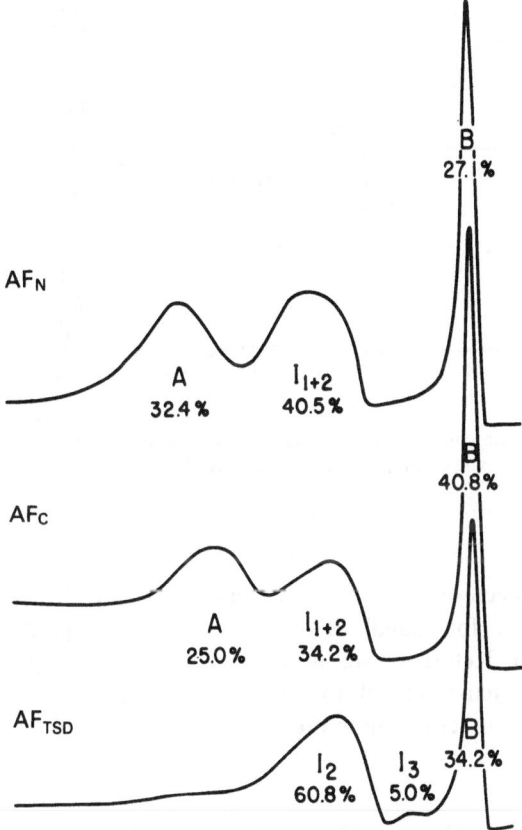

FIGURE 19. Amniotic-fluid hexosaminidase patterns obtained with DEAE-cellulose microcolumn automated system. AF_N = normal amniotic fluid, AF_C = presumed-carrier amniotic fluid, and AF_{TSD} = amniotic fluid from a predicted Tay–Sachs disease fetus. From Saifer and Parkhurst.[131]

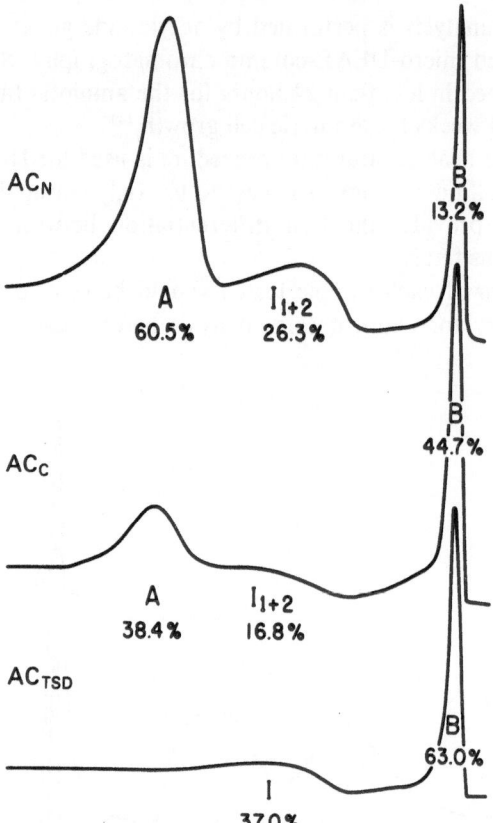

FIGURE 20. Amniotic cultured-cell patterns obtained with a DEAE-cellulose microcolumn automated system. Nomenclature is the same as Figure 19. From Saifer and Parkhurst.[181]

There has been only one reported instance in which the prenatal diagnosis of a fetus for Sandhoff's disease was attempted. Kolodny and associates (their Reference 42 in Reference 115 here) have successfully monitored a pregnancy of risk for this disease which resulted in the birth of a nonaffected infant, confirming the prenatal assessment.[125]

Bernheimer–Seitelberger Disease [G_{M2} (A,B)]

Patients with late infantile (or juvenile) G_{M2}-gangliosidosis are readily distinguished from those with TSD or Sandoff's disease since the onset of the disease occurs between 2 and 6 years of age and all the patients have been of non-Jewish origin. The clinical features of the disease are similar to Batten–Spielmeyer–Vogt disease and have been described in five patients from three families.[10,11,140] Cerebral levels of G_{M2}-ganglioside are considerably smaller (40–90 times normal) than in TSD and Sandhoff's disease and there is a small increase (5–10 times normal) of the asialo-G_{M2}-ganglioside.[13] A partial deficiency of Hex A in this disorder was reported by Suzuki and Suzuki,[141] Schneck et al.,[142] and Okada et al.[140] The partial enzyme defect was found to be present in brain, liver,[125,141] spleen,[141] serum,[140] and in cultured skin fibroblasts.[91] Diagnosis is best made by a serum Hex A assay wherein the values obtained fall within the range of TSD heterozygotes (Table 6). If the deficiency of Hex A is measured using natural, i.e., G_{M2}-ganglioside, substrates rather than synthetic ones, the deficiency might be more pronounced since the observed decrease in Hex A activity in this disorder is insufficient to account for the G_{M2}-ganglioside storage. O'Brien et al.[122] have presented the concept that the mutation in late infantile G_{M2}-gangliosidosis may involve a different region of the polypeptide chain of the same protein that is altered in TSD, so as to produce a similar but less marked decrease in Hex A activity against artificial substrates. The testing of this hypothesis awaits further enzyme studies of the disease.

O'Brien[125] performed amniocentesis on the pregnant mother of his patient with Bernheimer–Seitelberger disease. Assay of cultured amniotic cells for Hex A yielded normal values, indicating the fetus to be free of the disease, and a normal infant was born.

G_{M1}-Gangliosidoses

Norman–Landing Disease [G_{M1} (0)]

Although patients resembling those with generalized gangliosidosis had been described in the literature by Norman et al.[143] and other clinicians, it was not until 1964 that Landing and colleagues[13] established this genetic disorder as a clinicopathological entity. The disease is much rarer than TSD since information on only about 25 cases has been compiled in the review articles by O'Brien.[14,122,125] These patients exhibit psychomotor retardation from birth. Other clinical manifestations, which occur during the first year of life, include liver enlargement, foam cells in the bone marrow, thinning of the bones, and skeletal deformities. Their facial features resemble the appearance of infants with mucopolysaccharide storage diseases, such as

Hurler's syndrome. Death occurs at about 2 years of age. There is a high degree of consanguinity in reported sibships, no sexual preference in the frequency of the disease, a pattern of familial occurrence, and an absence of disease symptomology in the parents. All these factors indicate that the disease is probably inherited as an autosomal recessive trait.

The principal substances that accumulate in the brain tissue and viscera of children with Norman–Landing disease [G_{M1} (0)] include the G_{M1}-ganglioside [Cer-Glc-Gal-(NeuNAc)-GalNAc-Gal],* its asialo derivative, and a mucopolysaccharide structurally similar to keratan sulfate.[41] The accumulation of the G_{M1}-ganglioside is about 10 times normal in brain gray matter and 20–50 times normal in liver. Asialo-G_{M1}-ganglioside is also increased to levels 10 times that of normal in the brain. In liver there is storage of the keratan-type mucopolysaccharide to an extent 50 times greater and of a sialomucopolysaccharide 10 times larger than the amount of G_{M1}-ganglioside found.

Derry's Disease (G_{M1} (A))

O'Brien[14,122,125] has collated the clinical and biochemical findings concerning 11 patients with Derry's disease, which was first delineated into an entity distinct from Norman–Landing disease by Derry et al.[15] The clinical, electroencephalographical, pathological, and biochemical features of an additional case of Derry's disease and another of Norman–Landing disease occurring in Hindu and Muslim patients has recently been described by Taori et al.[144]

Derry's disease is differentiated from the similar disorder, Norman–Landing, by its later onset (after one year of age), its more slowly progressive course without visceromegaly or bony deformities and with death occuring between 4 and 10 years of age. The familial occurrence has been reported at least twice and the consanguinity of parents noted in one of the affected kindred.[15,145]

G_{M1}-ganglioside, and its asialo derivative (Figure 1), accumulate in the brain tissue of the affected children only to a slightly lesser degree in Derry's as compared to Norman–Landing disease. There is considerably less storage of G_{M1}-ganglioside in the livers of patients with Derry's disease than those afflicted with Norman–Landing disease. Suzuki et al.[146] have shown that the accumulation of both G_{M1}-ganglioside and mucopolysaccharide in the livers and spleens of Norman–Landing patients exceeded that of the

---

* See legend of Fig. 9 on p. 88.

patients with Derry's disease. Recent biochemical studies support the concept that both types of G_{M1}-gangliosidosis are genotypically distinct entities.

Enzymatic Defect in G_{M1}-Gangliosidosis

Based on the premise that all of the structures which accumulate in G_{M1}-gangliosidosis probably contain a terminal galactose, it was postulated that the deficient degradative enzyme was probably a β-galactosidase. Using both radioactively tagged G_{M1}-ganglioside and synthetic galactosides as substances, Okada and O'Brien[147] found a deficiency of a G_{M1}-ganglioside-β-galactosidase which was 3% of normal in brain and about 5% of normal in liver of patients with Norman–Landing disease. In the brain tissue of such infants a three times greater enzyme deficiency was found when G_{M1}-ganglioside was employed as a substrate as compared to the use of a p-nitrophenylgalactoside.[147] The β-galactosidase deficiency in G_{M1}-gangliosidosis has been confirmed by other investigators using labeled G_{M1}-ganglioside[148] and artificial β-galactosides[146,149,150] as substrates. It was demonstrated by Okada and O'Brien[147] that the lack of activity of β-galactosidase was not due to inhibition by G_{M1}-ganglioside or to soluble endogeneous inhibitors. Other lysosomal enzymes, including N-acetyl-β-D-hexosaminidase, β-glucosidase, and acid phosphatase, are present in either normal or increased amounts in the body fluids and tissues of patients with Norman–Landing disease.[125, 146] If one assumes the presence of normal amounts of neuraminidase in brain and visceral organs in this disorder, as occurs in TSD,[42] then the accumulation of the G_{M1}-ganglioside and its asialo derivative is due to the inactivity of a β-galactosidase that normally catabolizes this glycosphingolipid (Figure 1).

MacBrinn and colleagues[151] isolated the stored mucopolysaccharide from the liver of a patient with G_{M1}-gangliosidosis. Suzuki et al. (41) had found the keratan-type mucopolysaccharide in this disease to contain almost equimolar quantities of galactose and glucosamine, which, if present in a 1,4-β-linkage, should be degraded by a β-galactosidase. MacBrinn et al.[151] determined the rate of cleavage of galactose from the mucopolysaccharide with purified liver homogenates and found it to be 10% of normal in Norman–Landing-type gangliosidosis. These investigators[151] also prepared sialic acid-free fetuin by mild acid hydrolysis so as to yield a glycoprotein with a terminal galactose residue. When this modified glycoprotein was incubated with purified preparations of β-galactosidase from the liver of a patient with the Norman–Landing variant and from a normal control for 18 h at 37°C, only the latter produced detectable amounts of galactose. Therefore, both mucopolysaccharide and glycoprotein storage in the visceral tissues of Norman–Landing-type G_{M1}-gangliosidosis can also be explained on the basis of a specific β-galactosidase deficiency. The high order of specificity of this enzyme for the G_{M1}-ganglioside is demonstrated by work of Brady et al.,[152] who found normal or increased β-galactosidase activity for brain tissue acetone powder extracts from a patient with generalized gangliosidosis for such galactose-containing substrates as cerebroside (ceramide galactose), ceramide lactoside (ceramide glucose galactose), and ceramide trihexoside (ceramide glucose galactose galactose). In a recent publication, Suzuki and Suzuki,[153] using crude liver extracts, confirmed the increased galactosylceramide-β-galactosidase activity reported by Brady et al.[152] but found low activity of lactosylceramide-β-galactosidase in their five patients. Electrofocusing patterns of their hepatic β-galactosidases gave no detectable residual activities of G_{M1}-ganglioside- and asialo-G_{M1}-ganglioside-β-galactosidases.

The clinical diagnosis of Norman–Landing disease is best confirmed by β-galactosidase analysis of leukocytes,[154] urine,[155] and of extracts from cultured skin fibroblasts.[148] Since the use of artificial substrates is more convenient and practical than the use of natural ones for the quantitative determination of β-galactosidase levels, both p-nitro-β-D-galactopyranoside[147,154,155] and 4-methylumbelliferyl-β-D-galactopyranoside[153,156,157] have been used for this purpose. We have utilized the latter substrate and a procedure similar to that published by Hultberg and Öckerman[56] in our laboratory for the fluorometric analysis of β-galactosidase except that 0.1 M NaCl is incorporated into the assay medium[158] in order to achieve full stimulation and stabilization of the enzymatic procedure.[157] When Singer and Schafer[154] found leukocyte β-hexosaminidase levels of obligatory carriers to fall in a range intermediate between homozygote and normal control values, heterozygote detection in the families and close relatives of patients with this disease became feasible. They reported values of β-hexosaminidase activity (nmol p-nitrophenol/min/mg protein) of 0.6 for Norman–Landing disease, 0.8 for Derry's disease, 2.4–4.5 for heterozygotes, and 5.4–11.8 for controls. In addition, they made the important observation that the reported deficiency of a specific β-galactosidase in Hurler's syndrome (types 1 and 3)[59] was not the same as that found in Norman–Landing disease since essentially normal values are found in patients with mucopolysaccharidoses.[150,154]

β-Galactosidase activity was found to be present in the cultured amniotic cells obtained by amniocentesis in the second trimester of pregnancy. The enzyme assay can therefore be utilized to diagnose homozygotes prenatally. One pregnancy was monitored in a women who had previously given birth to a child with generalized gangliosidosis. β-Galactosidase assay indicated that the fetus was not homozygous and the child exhibited no disease symptoms at 8 months of age.[122]

Isoenzymes of β-Galactosidases in Norman–Landing Disease and Derry's Disease

Using 4-methylumbelliferyl-β-D-galactopyranoside as the substrate, O'Brien[125] determined the pH activity curves of liver β-galactosidases in two control subjects, three patients with Norman–Landing, and one patient with Derry's disease. The curves showed two pH optima, a major one at pH 4–5 and a minor one at pH 6.6. Both of the peaks were decreased in the former but only the major one was missing in the single case of the latter studied. Enzymatic differences between the two types of G_{M1}-gangliosidoses have also been demonstrated in cultured skin fibroblasts by Pinsky et al.[160] They found the residual β-galactosidase activity in cells of the two clinical subtypes had different pH optima and reacted differently after heat treatment at 42°C for 20 min. Except for the large difference in total activity, the results obtained with β-galactosidase from cells of patients with Derry's disease closely resembled those obtained with normal, control, enzyme preparations.

Ho and O'Brien[161] separated the β-galactosidases from liver into three components by means of starch gel electrophoresis. This technique resolved the isoenzymes into a fast-moving component (A) and two slower moving components (B and C). In three patients with Norman–Landing disease, β-galactosidases A, B, and C were markedly deficient, but in a single patient with Derry's disease, β-galactosidase A was present in nearly normal amounts. In this publication,[161] the authors described a procedure for the separate assay of "acid" and "neutral" β-galactosidase activity based on the experimental fact that at pH 4.35, 0.02 M citrate–phosphate buffer, 0.2 M NaCl almost completely inhibits the activity of only the "neutral" β-galactosidase. Using this method they found a marked deficiency of all the β-galactosidase isoenzymes in Norman–Landing disease, but only the "acid" β-galactosidase component was found to be absent in a case of Derry's disease.[162]

As mentioned previously, activities of other lysosomal enzymes such as β-glucosidase and N-acetyl-β-D-glucosaminidase are either normal or increased in urine[155] skin biopsies, and cultured skin fibroblasts from both types of G_{M1}-gangliosidosis.[122] Thomas[155] utilized a urinary assay, employing p-nitrophenyl-β-D-galactopyranoside as the substrate, for the quantitative determination of β-galactosidase. He found the ratio of the N-acetyl-β-D-glucosaminidase to that of the β-galactosidase to be over 100 in the urine of a single patient with Norman–Landing disease and less than 20 in the control group which included patients with Hurler's syndrome. O'Brien et al.[122] have presented similar data for skin biopsies and cultured skin fibroblasts from three patients with Derry's disease in which they also reported values over 100 for the homozygotes and of less than 20 for both heterozygotes and controls. Again, values for the obligatory heterozygotes, i.e., parents, are above the upper limit of the control range, indicating the possibility of utilizing the ratio of N-acetyl-β-D-glucosaminidase to β-galactosidase values for the purpose of carrier detection among the sibships and close relatives of patients with G_{M1}-gangliosidosis of either type.

Suzuki and co-workers[146] attempted to correlate biochemical findings with the clinical grouping of eight patients with G_{M1}-gangliosidosis. Starch gel electrophoresis of liver β-galactosidase was performed in four of these cases, three of which were classified as Norman–Landing disease on both biochemical and clinical grounds. In all four cases, the slow-moving components B and C were deficient whereas in only one case, classified as Norman–Landing disease, was there a significant amount of the fact-moving component A. In view of the absence of the A isoenzyme in both types of G_{M1}-gangliosidosis, these authors concluded that "no conclusion can be drawn as to the significance of the preserved component A in relation to clinical features." These authors also point out that there is an absence of β-galactosidase components B and C, with preservation of component A, in Hurler's and Hunters's syndromes,[159] which is the same abnormal pattern seen in some cases of G_{M1}-gangliosidosis. However, as was discussed above, these two conditions can be readily distinguished enzymatically by means of the value of the ratio of N-acetyl-β-D-glucosaminidase to β-galactosidase, it being less than 100, as was discussed above.

In two recent, subsequent publications, Suzuki and Suzuki[153,157] delineated procedures for the standard assay of glycosphingolipid-β-galactosidase and their characterization by electrofocusing and gel filtration in normal human liver[157] and in livers from five patients with G_{M1}-gangliosidosis.[153] In the first phase of their study,[157] these investigators determined that optimal conditions of assay for the glycosphingolipid-β-galactosidases required the presence of 10 mM NaCl as an activator and stabilizer of enzyme activity and that sodium taurocholate was the most effective stimulator of such activity of any of the detergents utilized in the assay system. In the second phase of their investigation, they separated the total β-galactosidase activity of low-speed supernatants of human liver by means of gel-filtration and electrofocusing techniques and studied the hydrolytic activities of the separated components on radioactively labeled galactosylceramide, lactosylceramide, G_{M1}-ganglioside, and its asialo derivatives, as substrates.

Their finding that Sephadex G-200 gel filtration separated the total β-galactosidase into three peaks of well-defined activity was similar to the results of other previous investigators.[161,163]

They employed an electrofocusing procedure to separate the liver 4-methylumbelliferyl-β-galactosidase activities into three fractions, which they designated as α (pH 4.1–4.2), β (pH 4.5–4.6), and γ (pH 4.8–4.9), in order of increasing isoelectric points. Electrofocusing of gel filtration Peaks II and III showed them to be equivalent to the β and γ peaks, respectively, while the results obtained with peak I were inconclusive. The hydrolytic activity of each fraction, obtained with both separation procedures, was determined against the tagged natural glycosphingolipid substrates, and the results are summarized in Table 7. Their results are in general agreement with those of Hultberg et al.[163] except that their peak II did not hydrolyze galactosylceramide. While no simple relationship exists between the β-galactosidase activities of the fractions separated by electrofocusing and those obtained by gel filtration, the data should be useful for the investigation of genetic disorders, e.g., G_{M1}-gangliosidosis, characterized by deficiencies of specific β-galactosidases.

Suzuki and Suzuki[153] studied the hepatic β-galactosidases of four patients with Norman–Landing disease and one patient with Derry's disease by means of the electrofocusing method they had utilized in their prior publication to investigate these isoenzymes in low-speed supernatants of sonicated liver homogenates.[157] In these studies, the residual activities

TABLE 7. β-Galactosidases from Normal Human Liver Low-Speed Supernatant Fractionated by Electrofocusing and Sephadex G-200 Gel Filtration[a]

	Substrates				
Components	4-Methylumbelliferyl-β-galactoside	Galactosylceramide	Lactosylceramide	G_{M1}-Ganglioside	G_{M1}-Ganglioside
Electrofocusing peaks					
α (pH 4.1–4.2)	+	−	+	+	−
β (pH 4.5–4.6)	+	+	+	+	+
γ (pH 4.8–4.9)	+	+	+	+	+
Gel filtration peaks					
I	+	+	+	+	ND[b]
II	+	−	+	+	ND
III	+	−	−	−	ND

[a] Data from Suzuki and Suzuki.[157]
[b] ND = not determined.

of G_{M1}-ganglioside- and asialo-G_{M1}-ganglioside-β-galactosidases, after electrofocusing, were too low to be detectable. However, the electrofocusing patterns of galactosylceramide- and lactosylceramide-β-galactosidases were unexpectedly abnormal. The activities of galactosylceramide-β-galactosidase of the patient with Derry's disease were generally higher than normal but the electrofocusing pattern was similar to that of the controls with β and γ activity peaks, cf Table 8. In two patients with Norman-Landing diseaes, there were no galactosylceramide- or lactosylceramide-β-galactosidase activities at the isoelectric point of the γ peak. In addition to high activities at the β peak, these specimens showed another peak at more acidic isoelectric points, i.e., the α region at lower pH values where there is little activity of 4-methylumbelliferyl-β-galactosidase (Table 8). As a result of these experiments the authors[153] concluded "that the genetic mutation in G_{M1}-gangliosidosis results not only in loss of activities of some β-galactosidases but also in abnormal changes in the nature of other β-galactosidases which do not show deficient total activities." Although it can reasonably be assumed that there should be enzymatic differences between the two

TABLE 8. Electrofocusing Patterns of Hepatic β-Galactosidases in G_{M1}-Gangliosidosis[a]

		Electrofocusing peaks[c]		
Sample	Substrate[b]	α	β	γ
Controls	4-MU	+	+	+
	C-gal	0	+	+
	C-lact	+	+	+
	Asialo-G_{M1}	+	+	+
Patient 1 (Norman–	4-MU	0	+ ($\downarrow\downarrow$)	0
Landing disease)	C-gal	+ ($\uparrow\uparrow$)	+ ($\uparrow\uparrow$)	0
	C-lact	+ ($\downarrow\downarrow$)	+ ($\downarrow\downarrow$)	0
	Asialo-G_{M1}	0	0	0
Patient 3 (Norman–	4-MU	0	+ ($\downarrow$)	0
Landing disease)	C-gal	+ ($\uparrow\uparrow\uparrow$)	+ ($\uparrow\uparrow\uparrow$)	0
	C-lact	+ ($\downarrow$)	+ ($\downarrow\downarrow$)	0
	Asialo-G_{M1}	0	0	0
Patient 5 (Derry's disease)	4-MU	0	0	0
	C-gal	0	+ ($\uparrow$)	+ ($\uparrow$)
	C-lact	0	$\pm$	+ ($\downarrow\downarrow$)
	Asialo-G_{M1}	0	0	0

[a] Data from Suzuki and Suzuki.[153]

[b] 4-MU = 4-methylumbelliferyl β-galactoside; C-gal = galactosylceramide; C-lact = lactosylceramide; Asialo-G_{M1} = asialo-G_{M1}-ganglioside.

[c] + = present; 0 = absent; $\pm$ = questionably present. Arrows indicate the degree of increase or decrease compared to normal controls.

phenotypes, the fact that each of the previous studies[160-162,164] included only one case of Derry's disease makes it difficult to define the enzymatic criteria necessary for distinguishing the two types of G_{M1}-gangliosidosis.

Summary and Conclusions

1. Earlier studies of cytoplasmic glycolytic and transaminating enzymes permitted definitive diagnosis of TSD prior to the development of well-defined clinical symptoms. Elevated levels of these enzymes in serum and cerebrospinal fluid are associated with a parallel depression of tissue enzyme values, suggesting that the rise in their enzymatic activity reflects a nonspecific neurocytolysis.

2. Serum isoenzyme LDH patterns obtained with agar gel electrophoresis showed that the ratio of LDH-3: LDH-5 provided a useful statistical indicator for differentiating brain ganglioside storage disorders from other sphingolipidoses.

3. Elucidation of normal and Tay–Sachs ganglioside structures resulted in a rational evaluation of those metabolic pathways in which a deficient enzyme would result in storage of the particular glycosphingolipids found in the brain or visceral organs of patients with each type of gangliosidosis.

4. While in most lipidoses, including the gangliosidoses, the enzyme found to be deficient was that which had been predicted, e.g., lack of total hexosaminidase activity in Sandhoff's disease, in the case of TSD the activity of total N-acetyl-β-D-hexosaminidase against artificial substrates was increased above normal.

5. The important finding that normal human spleen contains two major hexosaminidase isoenzymes, Hex A and Hex B, led several experimenters to reinvestigate the problem of the deficient enzyme in TSD and to conclude that it was Hex A.

6. The introduction of the fluorogenic substrate, 4-methylumbelliferyl-N-acetyl-β-D-glucosaminide, provided a sensitive and convenient method for the assay of hexosaminidase activity of biological fluids and tissues. Many of the conditions which give rise to elevated serum total hexosaminidase levels, e.g., pregnancy and debilitating diseases, will generally yield Hex A values in the TSD-carrier range.

7. Highly purified plasma and tissue preparations, i.e., from one-hundredfold to several thousandfold, of Hex A and Hex B permitted measurements of their MWs, amino acid composition, and their kinetic properties, including inhibition studies. Antisera prepared against either isoenzyme was

found to react equally well with the other as was shown by agar gel immunodiffusion and antigen–antibody precipitation of enzyme activity from solution.

8. The application of newer analytical techniques such as gel electrophoresis, isoelectric focusing, DEAE-cellulose column chromatography, etc., to hexosaminidase isoenzyme analysis helped to uncover two new variants of TSD. One of these variants, i.e., Sandhoff's disease, in which there is a deficiency of total hexosaminidase activity, has been the subject of much recent investigation.

9. While there are many isoenzymic forms of hexosaminidase in human biological fluids and tissues, the number obtained depends on the separation techniques employed as well as on the material being analyzed. Present evidence indicates that the serum isoenzyme which increases markedly during pregnancy (Hex P) is the same as that which increases in diabetes and other debilitating disorders (Hex I_2) although much more investigative work is needed in this area.

10. The weight of experimental evidence favors the viewpoint that Hex A is convertible by neuraminidase to an enzyme with physical properties similar to that of Hex B although several recent studies with purified liver and placental Hex A have reported negative findings.

11. Highly purified Hex A has been shown to hydrolyze G_{M2}-ganglioside with great difficulty as compared to its action on artificial substrates (1 to 10^6). Recent work has indicated that extensive purification and aging of Hex A, or removal of nondialyzable cofactors, may markedly diminish its ability to catabolize the Tay–Sachs ganglioside.

12. Diagnosis of Sandhoff's disease is confirmed by the low levels of total hexosaminidase found in the suspected infant's serum; heterozygotes are detected by the criteria of low total hexosaminidase and a high percentage of Hex A in their serum.

13. Diagnosis of TSD is best made by essentially zero leukocyte Hex A levels obtained by acrylamide gel electrophoresis or DEAE-cellulose chromatography. Detection of heterozygotes in the Ashkenazic Jewish population should be performed with automated systems for serum Hex A analysis based on heat- or pH-inactivation of Hex A and the use of sensitive fluorogenic substrates. Carrier detection in pregnant women is best performed by Hex A analysis of their leukocyte extracts by either automated micro-DEAE-cellulose column chromatographic analysis or acrylamide gel electrophoresis.

14. Prenatal diagnosis of TSD should be based upon the complete absence of Hex A in both amniotic fluid and cultured amniotic cells as determined with a procedure which separates Hex A from its other isoenzymes.

15. Bernheimer–Seitelberger disease is characterized enzymatically by a partial deficiency of Hex A against synthetic substrates. Since the observed decrease in Hex A in this disorder is insufficient to account for the G_{M2}-ganglioside storage, it has been suggested that the defect would be more pronounced if the enzyme activity was measured against a natural substrate.

16. Both types of G_{M1}-gangliosidosis (Norman–Landing and Derry's diseases) are characterized by a deficiency of specific β-galactosidases when measured against both artificial and natural substrates. This enzymatic defect results in the accumulation of the G_{M1}-ganglioside and its asialo derivative in brain and visceral organs, and of a keratan-type mucopolysaccharide and of a sialomucopolysaccharide in liver and spleen.

17. Liver β-galactosidases have been separated into three isoenzymes by starch gel electrophoresis, Sephadex G-200 gel filtration, and isoelectric focusing.

18. Because each previous study included only one case of Derry's disease, it is difficult at present to define the exact enzymatic criteria necessary for distinguishing the two types of G_{M1}-gangliosidosis. However, there is substantial experimental evidence, in a number of studies, for different β-galactosidase isoenzyme patterns for each type of G_{M1}-gangliosidosis.

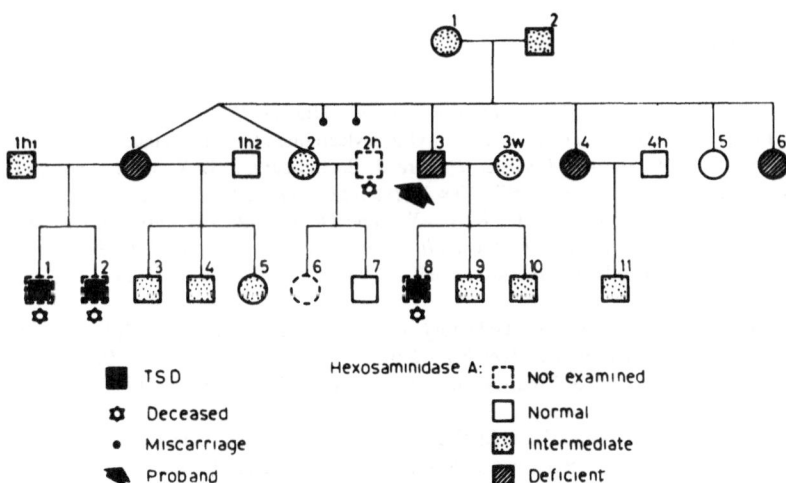

FIGURE 21. Pedigree of an Ashkenazic Jewish family some of whose adult members show an absence of Hex A activity with 4-methylumbelliferyl-β-D-glucosaminide as a substrate and no clinical symptoms. Mating of these individuals with carriers of the Tay–Sachs gene has resulted in the birth of children with the classical form of Tay–Sachs disease (variant B). The levels of Hex A shown in this figure are those determined on samples of peripheral leukocytes. From Navon *et al.*[165]

After this review was completed two papers appeared in the literature which are of the utmost importance to the subject under discussion. First, was a report by Navon *et al.*[165] of an apparent deficiency of Hex A in healthy members of a family with TSD. The pedigree of this family, including some biochemical data, is shown in Figure 21. Of four siblings, with essentially zero Hex A levels as determined with a synthetic fluorogenic substrate, two have had TSD offspring. The authors suggest that the exceptional phenotype may be due to compound heterozygosity for the common mutant TSD gene and a rare allele which causes an apparent enzymatic deficiency but does not lead to TSD. Since in such families the possibility exists of a false-positive prenatal diagnosis of TSD it is important that once a diagnosis of TSD is made, the leukocyte Hex A levels of the infant's parents and other close relatives be determined.

Second, was the publication by Tallman *et al.*[166] on the isolation and properties of highly purified placental Hex A and Hex B in which they propose a working model for the interrelationship of the hexosaminidases.

At this point one can only paraphrase the previously quoted statement of Brady *et al.*[118] that much experimental biochemical work remains to be done in this area if the pathogenesis of TSD and its variants are to be fully comprehended.

References

1. Stoffel, W., *Sphingolipids, Annu. Rev. Biochem.* **40**:57 (1971).
2. Fredrickson, D. S. and Sloan, H. R., Glucosylceramide lipidoses. Gaucher's disease, in: *The Metabolic Basis of Inherited Disease,* J. B. Stanbury, J. B. Wyngaarden, and D. S. Fredrickson, eds., McGraw-Hill, New York, 3rd ed., pp. 730–759 (1972).
3. Sweeley, C. C., Klionsky, B., Krivit, W., and Desnick, R. J., Fabry's disease. Glycosphingolipid lipidosis, in: *The Metabolic Basis of Inherited Disease*, J. B. Stanbury, J. B. Wyngaarden, and D. S. Fredrickson, eds., McGraw-Hill, New York, 3rd ed., pp. 663–687 (1972).
4. Suzuki, K. and Suzuki, Y., Galactosyl ceramide lipidosis: Globoid cell leucodystrophy (Krabbe's disease), in: *The Metabolic Basis of Inherited Disease,* J. B. Stanbury, J. B. Wyngaarden, and D. S. Fredrickson, eds., McGraw-Hill, New York, 3rd ed., pp. 760–782 (1972).
5. Dawson, G., Matalon, R., and Stein, A. O., Lactosylceramidosis: Lactosylceramide galactosyl hydrolase deficiency and accumulation of lactosylceramide in cultured skin fibroblasts, *J. Pediatr.* **79**:423 (1971).
6. Moser, H. W., Sulfatide lipidoses: Metachromatic leukodystrophy, in: *The Metabolic Basis of Inherited Disease*, J. B. Stanbury, J. B. Wyngaarden, and D. S. Fredrickson, eds., McGraw-Hill, New York, 3rd ed., pp. 688–729 (1972).
7. Fredrickson, D. S. and Sloan, H. R., Sphingomyelin lipidoses: Niemann–Pick disease, in: *The Metabolic Basis of Inherited Disease,* J. B. Stanbury, J. B. Wyngaarden, and D. S. Fredrickson, eds., McGraw-Hill, New York, 3rd ed., pp. 783–807 (1972).

8. Durand, P., Barrone, C., Della Cella, G., and Philippart, M., Fucosidosis, *Lancet* **1**:1198 (1968).
9. Volk, B. W., Schneck, L., and Adachi, M., Clinic pathology and biochemistry of Tay–Sachs disease, in: *Handbook of Clinical Neurology*, P. J. Vinken, and G. W. Bruyn, eds., North-Holland, Amsterdam, Vol. 10, pp. 385–426 (1970).
10. Bernheimer, H. and Seitelberger, F.: Über das Verhalten der Ganglioside im Gehirn bei 2 Fällen von spatinfantiler amaurotischer Idiotie. *Wien Klin. Wochenschr.* **80**:163 (1968).
11. Volk, B. W., Adachi, M., Schneck, L., Saifer, A., and Kleinberg, W., G-5 variant of systemic late infantile lipidosis, *Arch. Pathol.* **87**:393 (1969).
12. Sandhoff, K., Andreae, U., and Jatzkewitz, H., Deficient hexosaminidase activity in an exceptional case of Tay–Sachs disease with additional storage of kidney globoside in visceral organs, *Life Sci.* **7**:283 (1968).
13. Landing, B. H., Silverman, F. N., Craig, M. M., Jacoby, M. D., Lahey, M. E., and Chadwick, D. L., Familial neurovisceral lipidosis, *Am. J. Dis. Child.* **108**:503 (1964).
14. O'Brien, J. S., G$_{M1}$-gangliosidoses, in: *The Metabolic Basis of Inherited Disease*, J. B. Stanbury, J. B. Wyngaarden, and D. S. Fredrickson, eds., McGraw-Hill, New York, 3rd ed., pp. 639–662 (1972).
15. Derry, D. M., Fawcett, J. S., Andermann, F., and Wolfe, L. S., Late infantile systemic lipidosis. Major monosialogangliosidosis, delineation of two types, *Neurology* **18**:340 (1968).
16. Pilz, H., Müller, D., Sandhoff, K., and ter Meulen, V., Tay–Sachssche Krankheit mit Hexosaminidase-Defekt. Klinische, morphologische und biochemische Befunde bei einem Fall mit viszeraler Speicherung von Nierenglobosid, *Dtsch. Med. Wochenschr.* **39**:1833 (1968).
17. Klenk, E., The pathological chemistry of the developing brain, in: *Biochemistry of the Developing Nervous System*, E. Waelsch, ed., Academic Press, New York, pp. 397–409 (1955).
18. Svennerholm, L., The nature of the gangliosides in Tay–Sachs disease, in: *Cerebral Lipidosis*, L. van Bogaert, J. N. Cumings, and A. Lowenthal, eds., Blackwell, Oxford, pp. 139–145 (1957).
19. Saifer, A. and Wishnow, D. E., Disturbances of lipid metabolism and their relationship to the lipidoses, in: *Handbook of Clinical Neurology*, P. J. Vinken, and G. W. Bruyn, eds., North-Holland, Amsterdam, Vol. 10, pp. 265–324 (1970).
20. King, J., *Practical Clinical Enzymology*, Van Nostrand, Princeton, N. J. (1965).
21. Svennerholm, L., The chemical structure of normal human brain and Tay–Sachs gangliosides, *Biochem. Biophys. Res. Commun.* **9**:436 (1962).
22. Svennerholm, L., Chromatographic separation of human brain gangliosides, *J. Neurochem.* **10**:613 (1963).
23. Saifer, A., The biochemistry of Tay–Sachs disease, in: *Tay–Sachs Disease*, B. W. Volk, ed., Grune & Stratton, New York, pp. 97–103 (1964).
24. Aronson, S. M., Saifer, A., Perle, G., and Volk, B. W., Studies on enzyme alterations in the infantile sphingolipidoses. Correlation with pathologic changes, *Am. J. Clin. Nutr.* **9**:103 (1961).
25. Aronson, S. M., Saifer, A., Kanof, A., and Volk, B. W., Progression of amaurotic family idiocy as reflected by serum and cerebrospinal fluid changes, *Am. J. Med.* **24**:390 (1958).
26. Siegel, A. and Bing, R. J., Plasma enzyme activity in myocardial infarction in dog and man, *Proc. Soc. Exp. Biol. Med.* **91**:604 (1956).
27. Saifer, A., Schneck, L., Perle, G., and Volk, B. W., Lactate dehydrogenase isoenzyme distribution in the cerebral sphingolipidoses and other neurological disorders, *Neurology* **19**:147 (1969).

28. Aronson, S. M., Perle, G., Saifer, A., and Volk, B. W., Biochemical identification of the carrier state in Tay–Sachs disease, *Proc. Soc. Exp. Biol. Med.* **111**:664 (1962).
29. Schneck, L., Perle, G., and Volk, B. W., Fructose tolerance in Tay–Sachs' disease, *Pediatrics* **36**:272 (1965).
30. Klenk, E., Beiträge zur Chemie der Lipoidosen, Niemann–Pick'sche Krankheit und amaurotische Idiotie, *Hoppe-Seyler's Z. Physiol. Chem.* **262**:128 (1939–1940).
31. Klenk, E., Über die Ganglioside des Gehirns bei der infantilen am-aurotischen Idiotie von Typus Tay–Sachs, *Ber. Dtsch. Chem. Ges.* **75**:1632 (1942).
32. Svennerholm, L., The gangliosides, *J. Lipid Res.* **5**:145 (1964).
33. Gatt, S. and Berman, E. R., Studies on brain lipids in Tay–Sachs disease. I. Isolation of two sialic acid-free glycolipids, *J. Neurochem.* **10**:43 (1963).
34. Suzuki, K., Ganglioside patterns of normal and pathological brain, in: *Inborn Disorders of Sphingolipid Metabolism,* S. M. Aronson, and B. W. Volk, eds., Pergamon Press, New York, pp. 215–230 (1967).
35. Klenk, E., Liedtke, U., and Gielen, W., Das Gangliosid des Gehirns bei der infantilen amaurotischen Idiotie vom Typ Tay–Sachs, *Hoppe-Seyler's Z. Physiol. Chem.* **334**:186 (1963).
36. Makita, A. and Yamakawa, T., The glycolipids of the brain of Tay–Sachs disease. The chemical structures of a globoside and main ganglioside, *Jpn. J. Exp. Med.* **33**:361 (1963).
37. Ledeen, R., The chemistry of gangliosides: A review, *J. Am. Oil Chem. Soc.* **43**:57 (1966).
38. Wiegandt, H., Glycoside, *Ergeb. Physiol. Biol. Chem. Exp. Pharmakol.* **57**:190 (1966).
39. Volk, B. W., ed., *Tay–Sachs' Disease,* Grune & Stratton, New York, (1964).
40. Stanbury, J. B., Wyngaarden, J. B., and Fredrickson, D. S., eds., *The Metabolic Basis of Inherited Disease,* McGraw-Hill, New York, Chaps. 1 and 2 (1972).
41. Suzuki, K., Suzuki, K., and Kamoshita, S., Chemical pathology of G_{M1}-gangliosidosis (generalzied gangliosidosis), *J. Neuropathol. Exp. Neurol.* **28**:25 (1969).
42. Kolodny, E. H., Brady, R. O., and Volk, B. W., Demonstration of an alteration of ganglioside metabolism in Tay–Sachs disease, *Biochem. Biophys. Res. Commun.* **37**:526 (1969).
43. Okada, S. and O'Brien, J., Tay–Sachs disease: Generalized absence of a β-D-N-acetylhexosaminidase component, *Science* **165**:698 (1969).
44. Robinson, D. and Stirling, J. L., N-Acetyl-β-glucosaminidases in human spleen, *Biochem. J.* **107**:321 (1968).
45. Sandhoff, K., Variation of β-N-acetylhexosaminidase-pattern in Tay–Sachs disease, *FEBS Lett.* **4**:351 (1969).
46. Hultberg, B., N-acetylhexosaminidase activities in Tay–Sachs disease, *Lancet* **2**:1195 (1969).
47. Helferich, B. and Iloff, A., Über Emulsion. XIII. Darstellung und fermentative Spaltung von Glykosiden des N-Acetyl-glucosamins und der 2-Desoxyglucose, *Hoppe-Seyler's Z. Physiol. Chem.* **221**:252 (1933).
48. Caygill, J. C. and Jevons, F. R., β-Glucosaminidase activity in human synovial fluid, blood, plasma and leucocytes, *Clin. Chim. Acta* **13**:61 (1966).
49. Furiya, S. and Fukuda, A., Estimation of serum β-acetylaminodeoxyglucosidase, *J. Biochem.* **54**:398 (1963).
50. Leaback, D. H. and Walker, P. G., Studies on glucosaminidase. 4. The fluorimetric assay of N-acetyl-β-glucosaminidase, *Biochem. J.* **78**:151 (1961).
51. Woollen, J. W. and Turner, P., Plasma N-acetyl-β-glucosaminidase and β-glucuronidase in health and disease, *Clin. Chim. Acta* **12**:671 (1965).

52. Price, R. G., Dance, N., Richards, B., and Cattell, W. R., The excretion of N-acetyl-β-glucosaminidase and β-galactosidase following surgery to the kidney, *Clin. Chim. Acta* **27**:65 (1970).

53. Sandman, R., Margules, R. M. and Kountz, S. L., Urinary lysosomal glycosidases after renal allotransplantation: Correlation of enzyme excretion with allograft rejection and ischemia, *Clin. Chim. Acta* **45**:349 (1973).

54. Walker, P. G., Woollen, J. W., and Heyworth, R., Studies on glucosaminidase. 5. Kidney N-acetyl-β-glucosaminidase and N-acetyl-β-galactosaminidase, *Biochem. J.* **79**:288 (1961).

55. Li, S.-C. and Li, Y.-T., Studies on the glycosidases of Jack Bean meal. 3. Crystallization and properties of β-N-acetylhexosaminidase, *J. Biol. Chem.* **245**:5153 (1970).

56. Mega, T., Ikenaka, T., and Matsushima, Y., Studies on N-acetyl-β-D-glucosaminidase of *Aspergillus oryzae*, *J. Biochem.* **68**:109 (1970).

57. Frohwein, Y. Z. and Gatt, S., Isolation of β-N-acetylhexosaminidase, β-N-acetylglucosaminidase, and β-N-acetylgalactosaminidase from calf brain, *Biochemistry* **6**:2775 (1967).

58. Wetmore, S. J. and Verpoorte, J. A., The partial purification of two β-N-acetyl-D-hexosaminidases from porcine kidney, *Can. J. Biochem.* **50**:563 (1972).

59. Verpoorte, J. A., Purification of two β-N-acetyl-D-glucosaminidases from beef spleen, *J. Biol. Chem.* **247**:4787 (1972).

60. Sandhoff, K. and Wässle, W., Anreicherung und Charakterisierung zweier Formen der menschlichen N-acetyl-β-D-hexosaminidase, *Hoppe-Seyler's Z. Physiol. Chem.* **352**:1119 (1971).

61. Li, Y.-T., Mazzotta, M. Y., Wan, C.-C., Orth, R., and Li, S.-C., Hydrolysis of Tay–Sachs ganglioside by β-hexosaminidase A of human liver and urine, *J. Biol. Chem.* **248**:7512 (1973).

62. Carroll, M. and Robinson, D., Immunological properties of N-acetyl-β-D-glucosaminidase of normal human liver and of G_{M2}-gangliosidosis liver, *Biochem. J.* **131**:91 (1973).

63. Verpoorte, J. A., Isolation and characterization of the major β-N-acetyl-D-glucosaminidase from human plasma, *Biochemistry* **13**:793 (1974).

64. Srivastava, S. K., Awasthi, Y. C., Yoshida, A., and Beutler, E., Studies on human β-D-N-acetylhexosaminidases. I. Purification and properties, *J. Biol. Chem.* **249**:2043 (1974).

65. Goldstone, A., Konecny, P., and Koenig, H., Lysosomal hydrolases: Conversion of acidic to basic forms by neuraminidase, *FEBS Lett.* **13**:68 (1971).

66. Murphy, J. V. and Craig, L., Neuraminidase-induced changes in white blood cell hexosaminidase A, *Clin. Chim. Acta* **42**:267 (1972).

67. Srivastava, S. K., Yoshida, A., Awasthi, Y. C., and Beutler, E., Studies on human β-D-N-acetylhexosaminidases. II. Kinetic and structural properties, *J. Biol. Chem.* **249**:2049 (1974).

68. van Someren, H. and van Henegouwen, H. B., Independent loss of human hexosaminidases A and B in man–Chinese hamster somatic cell hybrids, *Humangenetik* **18**:171 (1973).

69. Dawson, G., Propper, R. L., and Dorfman, A., Partial purification of β-N-acetylhexosaminidase A by affinity chromatography, *Biochem. Biophys. Res. Commun.* **54**:1102 (1973).

70. Grebner, E. E. and Parikh, I., An affinity adsorbent for N-acetyl-β-hexosaminidase A, *Biochim. Biophys. Acta* **350**:437 (1974).

71. Grebner, E. E. and Tucker, J., Human urinary N-acetyl-β-hexosaminidases, *Biochim. Biophys. Acta* **321**:228 (1973).

72. Srivastava, S. K. and Beutler, E., Antibody against purified human hexosaminidase B cross-reacting with hexosaminidase A, *Biochem. Biophys. Res. Commun.* **47**:753 (1972).

73. Robinson, D., and Carroll, M., Tay–Sachs disease: Interrelation of hexosaminidases A and B, *Lancet* **1**:322 (1972).

74. Price, R. G. and Dance, N., The demonstration of multiple heat-stable forms of *N*-acetyl-β-glucosaminidase in normal human serum, *Biochim. Biophys. Acta* **271**:145 (1972).

75. Srivastava, S. K. and Beutler, E., Studies on human β-D-*N*-acetylhexosaminidases. III. Biochemical genetics of Tay–Sachs and Sandhoff's diseases, *J. Biol. Chem.* **249**:2054 (1974).

76. Srivastava, S. K., and Beutler, E., Hexosaminidase-A and hexosaminidase-B: Studies in Tay–Sachs and Sandhoff's disease, *Nature (London)* **241**:463 (1973).

77. Ford, J. R., Nunley, J. A., Li, Y.-T., Chambers, R. P., and Cohen, W., A continuously monitored spectrophotometric assay of glycosidases with nitrophenyl glycosides, *Anal. Biochem.* **54**:120 (1973).

78. Rosenthal, A. L. and Saifer, A., Continuous UV monitoring of fluorogenic substrates. I. Kinetic analysis of *N*-acetyl-β-D-hexosaminidases, *Anal. Biochem.* **55**:85 (1973).

79. Kanfer, J. N. and Spielvogel, C. H., The inhibition of β-*N*-acetylhexosaminidases by lactones, *Biochim. Biophys. Acta* **327**:405 (1973).

80. Sandhoff, K., Andreae, U., and Jatzkewitz, H., Deficient hexosaminidase activity in an exceptional case of Tay–Sachs disease with additional storage of kidney globoside in visceral organs, *Pathol. Eur.* **3**:278 (1968).

81. Frohwein, Y. Z. and Gatt, S., Enzymatic hydrolysis of sphingolipids. VI. Hydrolysis of ceramide glycosides by calf brain β-*N*-acetylhexosaminidase, *Biochemistry* **6**:2783 (1967).

82. Dance, N., Price, R. G., Robinson, D., and Stirling, J. L., β-Galactosidase, β-glucosidase and *N*-acetyl-β-glucosaminidase in human kidney, *Clin. Chim. Acta* **24**:189 (1969).

83. Robinson, D., Price, R. G., and Dance, N., Separation and properties of β-galactosidase, β-glucosidase, β-glucuronidase and *N*-acetyl-β-glucosaminidase from rat kidney, *Biochem. J.* **102**:525 (1967).

84. Young, E. P., Ellis, R. B., Lake, B. D., and Patrick, A. D., Tay–Sachs disease and related disorders: Fractionation of brain *N*-acetyl-β-hexosaminidase on DEAE-cellulose, *FEBS Lett.* **9**:1 (1970).

85. Robinson, D., Jordan, T. W., and Horsburgh, T., The *N*-acetyl-β-D-hexosaminidases of calf and human brain, *J. Neurochem.* **19**:1975 (1972).

86. Hooghwinkel, G. J. M., Veltkamp, W. A., Overdijk, B., and Lisman, J. J. W., Electrophoretic separation of β-*N*-acetylhexosaminidases of human and bovine brain and liver and of Tay–Sachs brain tissue, *Hoppe-Seyler's Z. Physiol. Chem.* **353**:839 (1972).

87. Poenaru, L. and Dreyfus, J. C., Electrophoretic study of hexosaminidases. Hexosaminidase C, *Clin. Chim. Acta* **43**:439 (1973).

88. Hultberg, B. and Öckerman, P. A., Artificial substrates in the assay of acid glycosidases, *Clin. Chim. Acta* **39**:49 (1972).

89. Hultberg, B., Öckerman, P. A., and Norden, N. E., Isoenzymes of four acid hydrolases in human kidney and urine, *Clin. Chim. Acta* **52**:239 (1974).

90. Kanfer, J. N. and Spielvogel, C., Hexosaminidase activity of cultured human skin fibroblasts, *Biochim. Biophys. Acta* **293**:203 (1973).

91. Okada, S., Veath, M. L., Leroy, J., and O'Brien, J. S., Ganglioside G_{M2} storage diseases: Hexosaminidase deficiencies in cultured fibroblasts, *Am. J. Hum. Genet.* **23**:55 (1971).

92. Woolen, J. and Walker, P. G., The fluorimetric estimation of *N*-acetyl-β-glucosaminidase and β-galactosidase in blood plasma, *Clin. Chim. Acta* **12**:647 (1965).

93. Stirling, J. L., A new form of *N*-acetyl-β-glucosaminidase present in pregnancy serum, *Biochem. J.* **123**:11P (1971).

94. O'Brien, J. S., Okada, S., Chen, A., and Fillerup, D. L., Tay-Sachs disease: Detection of heterozygotes and homozygotes by serum hexosaminidase assay, *New Engl. J. Med.* **283**:15 (1970).

95. Walker, P. G., Woollen, M. E., and Pugh, D., N-Acetyl-β-glucosaminidase activity in serum during pregnancy, *J. Clin. Pathol.* **13**:353 (1960).

96. Stirling, J. L., Separation and characterisation of N-acetyl-β-glucosaminidases A and P from maternal serum, *Biochim. Biophys. Acta* **271**:154 (1972).

97. Lowden, J. A. and LaRamee, M. A., Problems in prenatal diagnosis using sphingolipid hydrolase assays, in: *Sphingolipids, Sphingolipidoses and Allied Disorders*, B. W. Volk and S. M. Aronson, eds., Plenum Press, New York, pp. 257–267 (1972).

98. Huddleston, J. F., Lee, G., and Robinson, J. C., Electrophoretic characterization of glucose dehydrogenase, β-glucuronidase, and N-acetyl-β-glucosaminidase from placenta and gestational serum, *Am. J. Obstet. Gynecol.* **109**:1017 (1971).

99. Hayase, K. and Kritchevsky, D., Separation and comparison of isoenzymes of N-acetyl-beta-D-hexosaminidase of pregnancy serum by polyacrylamide gel electrofocusing, *Clin. Chim. Acta* **46**:455 (1973).

100. Hayase, K., Reisher, S. R., and Kritchevsky, D., Microheterogeneity of N-acetyl-β-D-hexosaminidase of bull epididymis, *Proc. Soc. Exp. Biol. Med.* **142**:466 (1973).

101. Williamson, A. R., Salaman, M. R., and Kreth, H. W., Microheterogeneity and allomorphism of proteins, *Ann. N. Y. Acad. Sci.* **209**:210 (1973).

102. Ikonne, J. U. and Ellis, R. B., N-Acetyl-β-D-hexosaminidase component A. Different forms in human tissues and fluids, *Biochem. J.* **135**:457 (1973).

103. Schneck, L., Friedland, J., Valenti, C., Adachi, M., Amsterdam, D., and Volk, B. W., Prenatal diagnosis of Tay-Sachs disease, *Lancet* **1**:582 (1970).

104. Murphy, J. V., Hexosaminidases in cell-free amniotic fluid, *Life Sci.* **11**:309 (1972).

105. Friedland, J., Schneck, L., Saifer, A., Pourfar, M., and Volk, B. W., Identification of Tay-Sachs disease carriers by acrylamide gel electrophoresis, *Clin. Chim. Acta* **28**:397 (1970).

106. Murphy, J. V. and Craig, L., Effect of human cerebral neuraminidase on hexosaminidase A, *Clin. Chim. Acta* **51**:67 (1974).

107. Leibovitz, Z. and Gatt, S., Enzymatic hydrolysis of sphingolipids. VII. Hydrolysis of gangliosides by a neuraminidase from calf brain, *Biochim. Biophys. Acta* **152**:136 (1968).

108. Tallman, J. F., Johnson, W. G., and Brady, R. O., The metabolism of Tay-Sachs ganglioside: Catabolic studies with lysosomal enzymes from normal and Tay-Sachs brain tissue, *J. Clin. Invest.* **51**:2339 (1972).

109. Tallman, J. F. and Brady, R. O., The catabolism of Tay-Sachs ganglioside in rat brain lysosomes, *J. Biol. Chem.* **247**:7570 (1972).

110. Sandhoff, K., The hydrolysis of Tay-Sachs ganglioside (TSG) by human N-acetyl-β-D-hexosaminidase A, *FEBS Lett.* **11**:342 (1970).

111. Sandhoff, K., Harzer, K., Wässle, W., and Jatzkewitz, H., Enzyme alterations and lipid storage in three variants of Tay-Sachs disease, *J. Neurochem.* **18**:2469 (1971).

112. Sandhoff, K. and Jatzkewitz, H., The chemical pathology of Tay-Sachs disease, in, *Sphingolipids, Sphingolipidoses and Allied Disorders*, B. W. Volk and S. M. Aronson, eds., Plenum Press, New York, pp. 305–319 (1972).

113. Wenger, D. A., Okada, S., and O'Brien, J. S., Studies on the substrate specificity of hexosaminidase A and B from liver, *Arch. Biochem. Biophys.* **153**:116 (1972).

114. Brady, R. O., The sphingolipidoses, *New Engl. J. Med.* **275**:312 (1966).

115. Kolodny, E. H., Sandhoff's disease: Studies on the enzyme defect in homozygotes and detection of heterozygotes, in: *Sphingolipids, Sphingolipidoses and Allied Disorders*, B. W. Volk and S. M. Aronson, eds., Plenum Press, New York, pp. 321–341 (1972).

116. Desnick, R. J., Snyder, P. D., Desnick, S. J., Krivit, W., and Sharp, H. L., Sandhoff's disease: Ultrastructural and biochemical studies, in: *Sphingolipids, Sphingolipidoses and Allied Disorders,* B. W. Volk and S. M. Aronson, eds., Plenum Press, New York, pp. 351–371 (1972).

117. Tateson, R. and Bain, A. D., G_{M2} gangliosidoses: Consideration of the genetic defects, *Lancet* 2:612 (1971).

118. Brady, R. O., Tallman, J. F., Johnson, W. G., and Quirk, J. M., An investigation of the metabolism of Tay–Sachs ganglioside specifically labeled in critical portions of the molecule, in: *Sphingolipids, Sphingolipidoses and Allied Disorders,* B. W. Volk and S. M. Aronson, eds., Plenum Press, New York, pp. 277–285 (1972).

119. Snyder, P. D., Jr., Krivit, W., and Sweeley, C. C., Generalized accumulation of neutral glycosphingolipids with G_{M2} ganglioside accumulation in the brain, *J. Lipid Res.* 13:128 (1972).

120. Suzuki, Y., Jacob, J. C., Suzuki, K., Kutty, K. M., and Suzuki, K., G_{M2}-gangliosidosis with total hexosaminidase deficiency, *Neurology* 21:313 (1971).

121. Yabuuchi, H., Sumi, K., Okada, S., and Yutaka, T., Chromatograpic study of serum hexosaminidase in normal and G_{M2}-gangliosidosis, *Clin. Chim. Acta* 53:85 (1974).

122. O'Brien, J. S., Okada, S., Ho, M. W., Fillerup, D. L., Veath, M. L., and Adams, K., Ganglioside storage diseases, *Fed. Proc. Fed. Am. Soc. Exp. Biol.* 30:956 (1971).

123. Padeh, B. and Navon, R., Diagnosis of Tay–Sachs disease by hexosaminidase activity in leukocytes and amniotic cells, *Israel J. Med. Sci.* 7:259 (1971).

124. Suzuki, Y., Berman, P. H., and Suzuki, K., Detection of Tay–Sachs disease heterozygotes by assay of hexosaminidase A in serum and leukocytes, *J. Pediatr.* 78:643 (1971).

125. O'Brien, J. S., Ganglioside storage diseases, in: *Advances in Human Genetics,* H. Harris and K. Hirschhorn, eds., Plenum Press, New York, Vol. 3, pp. 39–98 (1972).

126. Navon, R., and Padeh, B., Urinary test for identification of Tay–Sachs genotypes, *J. Pediatr.* 80:1026 (1972).

127. Carmody, P. J., Rattazzi, M. C., and Davidson, R. G., Tay–Sachs disease—The use of tears for the detection of heterozygotes, *New Engl. J. Med.* 289:1072 (1973).

128. Kaback, M. M.: Thermal fractionation of serum hexosaminidases: Applications to heterozygote detection and diagnosis of Tay–Sachs disease, in: *Methods of Enzymology,* V. Ginsburg, ed., Academic Press, New York, Vol. 28, part B, pp. 862–867 (1973).

129. Saifer, A. and Rosenthal, A. L., Rapid test for the detection of Tay–Sachs disease heterozygotes and homozygotes by serum hexosaminidase assay, *Clin. Chim. Acta* 43:417 (1973).

130. Rattazzi, M. C. and Davidson, R. G., Prenatal detection of Tay–Sachs disease, in: *Antenatal Diagnosis,* A. Dorfman, ed., University of Chicago Press, Chicago, Ill., pp. 207–211 (1972).

131. Saifer, A. and Parkhurst, G. W., *N*-Acetyl-β-D-hexosaminidase isoenzyme pattern in Tay–Sachs disease, *Clin. Chem.* 20:881 (1974) (Abstract 139).

132. Kaback, M. M and Zeiger, R. S., Heterozygote detection in Tay–Sachs disease: A prototype community screening program for the prevention of recessive disorders, in: *Sphingolipids, Sphingolipidoses and Allied Disorders,* B. W. Volk and S. M. Aronson, eds., Plenum Press, New York, pp. 613–632 (1972).

133. Lowden, J. A., Skomorowski, M. A., Henderson, F., and Kaback, M., Automated assay of hexosaminidases in serum, *Clin. Chem.* 19:1345 (1973).

134. Delvin, E., Pottier, A., Scriver, C. R., and Gold, R. J. M., The application of an automated hexosaminidase assay to genetic screening. *Clin. Chim. Acta* 53:135 (1974).

135. Saifer, A. and Perle, G., Automated determination of serum hexosaminidase A by *p*H inactivation for detection of Tay–Sachs disease heterozygotes, *Clin. Chem.* 20:538 (1974).

136. Saifer, A., Perle, G., Valenti, C., and Schneck, L., Pre- and postnatal detection of Tay–Sachs disease. A comparative study of biochemical screening methods, in: *Sphingolipids, Sphingolipidoses and Allied Disorders*, B. W. Volk and S. M. Aronson, eds., Plenum Press, New York, pp. 599–611 (1972).

137. Schneck, L., Adachi, M., and Volk, B. W., Chemical pathology of Tay–Sachs disease in the fetus, in: *Sphingolipids, Sphingolipidoses and Allied Disorders*, B. W. Volk and S. M. Aronson, eds., Plenum Press, New York, pp. 385–394 (1972).

138. Saifer, A., Schneck, L., Perle, G., Valenti, C., and Volk, B. W., Caveats of antenatal diagnosis of Tay–Sachs disease, *Am. J. Obstet. Gynecol.* 115:553 (1973).

139. Friedland, J., Perle, G., Saifer, A., Schneck, L., and Volk, B. W., Screening for Tay–Sachs disease *"in utero"* using amniotic fluid, *Proc. Soc. Exp. Biol. Med.* 136:1297 (1971).

140. Okada, S., Veath, M. L., and O'Brien, J. S., Juvenile G_{M2} gangliosidosis: Partial deficiency of hexosaminidase A, *J. Pediatr.* 77:1063 (1970).

141. Suzuki, Y. and Suzuki, K., Partial deficiency of hexosaminidase component A in juvenile G_{M2}-gangliosidosis, *Neurology* 20:848 (1970).

142. Schneck, L., Friedland, J., Pourfar, M., Saifer, A., and Volk, B. W., Hexosaminidase activities in a case of systemic G_{M2} gangliosidosis of the late infantile type, *Proc. Soc. Exp. Biol. Med.* 133:997 (1970).

143. Norman, R. N., Urich, H., Tingey, A. H., and Goodbody, R. A., Tay–Sachs disease with visceral involvement and its relationship to Niemann–Pick's disease, *J. Pathol. Bacteriol.* 72:409 (1959).

144. Taori, G. M., Basu, D. K., Chandi, S., Raman, P. T., Abraham, J., Leelavathy, R., and Job, C. K., G_{M1}-gangliosidosis, *J. Neurol. Sci.* 21:77 (1974).

145. Wolfe, L. S., Callahan, J., Fawcett, J. S., Andermann, F., and Scriver, C., G_{M1} gangliosidosis without chondrodystrophy or visceromegaly: β-Galactosidase deficiency with gangliosidosis and the excessive excretion of a keratan sulfate, *Neurology* 20:23 (1970).

146. Suzuki, Y., Crocker, A. C., and Suzuki, K., G_{M1}-gangliosidosis. Correlation of clinical and biochemical data, *Arch. Neurol. (Chicago)* 24:58 (1971).

147. Okada, S. and O'Brien, J. S., Generalized gangliosidosis: β-Galactosidase deficiency, *Science* 160:1002 (1968).

148. Sloan, H. R., Uhlendorf, B. W., Jacobson, C. B., and Fredrickson, D. S., β-Galactosidase in tissue culture derived from human skin and bone marrow: Enzyme defect in G_{M1}-gangliosidosis, *Pediatr. Res.* 3:532 (1969).

149. Dacremont, G. and Kint, J. A., G_{M1}-ganglioside accumulation and β-galactosidase deficiency in a case of G_{M1}-gangliosidosis (Landing disease), *Clin. Chim. Acta* 21:421 (1968).

150. Van Hoof, F. and Hers, H. G., The abnormalities of lysosomal enzymes in mucopolysaccharidoses, *Eur. J. Biochem.* 7:34 (1968).

151. MacBrinn, M. C., Okada, S., Ho, M. W., Hu, C. C., and O'Brien, J. S., Generalized gangliosidoses. Impaired cleavage of galactose from a mucopolysaccharide and a glycoprotein, *Science* 163:946 (1969).

152. Brady, R. O., O'Brien, J. S., Bradley, R. M., and Gal, A. E., Sphingolipid hydrolases in brain tissue of patients with generalized gangliosidosis, *Biochim. Biophys. Acta* 210:193 (1970).

153. Suzuki, Y. and Suzuki, K., Glycosphingolipid β-galactosidases. IV. Electrofocusing characterization in G_{M1}-gangliosidosis, *J. Biol. Chem.* 249:2113 (1974).

154. Singer, H. S. and Schafer, I. A., White cell β-galactosidase activity, *New Engl. J. Med.* 282:571 (1970).

155. Thomas, G. H., β-D-Galactosidase in human urine: Deficiency in generalized gangliosidosis, *J. Lab. Clin. Med.* 74:725 (1969).

156. Hultberg, B. and Öckerman, P. A., Artificial substrates in the assay of acid glycosidases, *Clin. Chim. Acta* **39**:49 (1972).
157. Suzuki, Y. and Suzuki, K., Glycosphingolipid β-galactosidases. I. Standard assay procedures and characterization by electrofocusing and gel filtration of the enzymes in normal human liver, *J. Biol. Chem.* **249**:2098 (1974).
158. Ho, M. W. and O'Brien, J. S., Stimulation of acid β-galactosidase activity by chloride ions, *Clin. Chim. Acta* **30**:531 (1970).
159. Ho, M. W. and O'Brien, J. S., Hurler's syndrome: Deficiency of a specific beta-galactosidase isoenzyme, *Science* **165**:611 (1969).
160. Pinsky, L., Powell, E., and Callahan, J., G$_{M1}$-gangliosidosis types 1 and 2: Enzymatic differences in cultured fibroblasts, *Nature (London)* **228**:1093 (1970).
161. Ho, M. W. and O'Brien, J. S., Differential effect of chloride ions on β-galactosidase isoenzymes: A method for separate assay, *Clin. Chim. Acta* **32**:443 (1971).
162. O'Brien, J. S., Five gangliosidoses, *Lancet* **2**:805 (1969).
163. Hultberg, B., Öckerman, P.-A., and Dahlqvist, A., Gargoylism: Hydrolysis of β-galactosides and tissue accumulation of galactose- and mannose-containing compounds, *J. Clin. Invest.* **49**:216 (1970).
164. Singer, H. S. and Schafer, I. A., Clinical and enzymatic variations in G$_{M1}$ generalized gangliosidosis, *Am. J. Hum. Genet.* **24**:454 (1972).
165. Navon, R., Padeh, B., and Adam, A., Apparent deficiency of hexosaminidase A in healthy members of a family with Tay–Sachs disease. *Am. J. Hum. Genet.* **25**:287 (1973).
166. Tallman, J. F., Brady, R. O., Quirk, J. M., Villalba, M., and Gal, A. E., Isolation and relationship of human hexosaminidases, *J. Biol. Chem.* **249**:3489 (1974).

PATHOLOGY

MASAZUMI ADACHI AND BRUNO W. VOLK

G_{M2}-Gangliosidoses

Tays–Sachs Disease [G_{M2}(B)]

Gross Pathology

The following observations are based on studies of 30 brain biopsies and 70 postmortem examinations of patients afflicted with Tay–Sachs disease (TSD).

The gross appearance of the brain varies with the duration of the disease. During the first 12–14 months of illness, the leptomeninges over the convexity as well as over the base of the brain are somewhat edematous, opaque, and considerably thickened. The gyri of the frontoparietal lobe show moderate atrophy, with widening of the sulci and gaping of the temporal fissures. The weight of the brain at this time is moderately decreased. On coronal sections, it is rubbery in consistency. The ventricular system, particularly the third ventricle, is moderately distended.

Between months 15 and 24 the brain weight increases slightly. The cerebral hemispheres are somewhat enlarged, especially the parietooccipital lobes, and the gyri are moderately swollen and flattened. The brain cuts with increased consistency. Coronal sections show marked attenuation of

MASAZUMI ADACHI AND BRUNO W. VOLK. Isaac Albert Research Institute of the Kingsbrook Jewish Medical Center and State University of New York, Downstate Medical Center, Brooklyn, New York.

the cortices, especially those of the frontal gyri. This is frequently accompanied by a linear depressed necrotic zone running parallel to the leptomeninges. The white matter of the parietal lobe is usually edematous. In some cases the basal ganglia are pale and ill-defined. The lateral ventricles are compressed because of swelling of the white matter.

After 24 months, the brain weight increases significantly, occasionally up to 2400 g. The cerebral hemispheres are uniformly enlarged, and the gyri, especially those of the temporo-parieto-occipital lobes, are flattened (Figure 1). At the base, the thin-walled third ventricle protrudes ventrally, pushing the optic chiasm downward. The optic nerves are atrophic. The brain is of leathery consistency. On coronal sections, the increased brain weight is due to uniform enlargement of all lobes. The cortices and the deep gray matter are pale. The entire white matter is edematous and shows tannish discoloration (Figure 2). With the progression of the disease, the white matter of the fronto-parietal lobe displays small areas of cystic changes which are well defined and contain a gelatinous gray-white material.

In contrast to the cerebrum, the cerebellar hemispheres are also increased in consistency but are uniformly decreased in volume (Figure 3). These features become progressively pronounced as the disease evolves. Sections show pale, atrophic folia of all lobules and brown discoloration of the white matter (Figure 3). The dentate nuclei are pale.

Histopathology

During the first year, the subarachnoid space is usually distended. Later, the trabeculae of the leptomeninges become thickened and form a meshwork which consists of proliferating fibroblasts filled with macrophages. The leptomeningeal blood vessels frequently show thickening of the adventitia.

The central nervous system exhibits ubiquitous involvement of the neurons without special predilection of any area. However, the degree of neuronal loss and of glial proliferation differs in various anatomical locations and appears closely related to the phylogenetic development. In the

FIGURE 1. Brain of a four-year-old boy afflicted with TSD (weight, 1700 g) showing megalencephaly with flattened gyri of the cerebral temporo-parieto-occipital lobes, while the cerebellum shows considerable atrophy.

FIGURE 2. Coronal sections of the cerebrum shown in Figure 1 exhibiting attenuation of the cortices of the frontal and parietal lobes. All cortices and basal ganglia are pale. The white matter of all lobes is edematous and displays areas of tannish discoloration. The parietal lobe shows more advanced degenerative changes and formation of cavities. The lateral ventricle is slightly dilated.

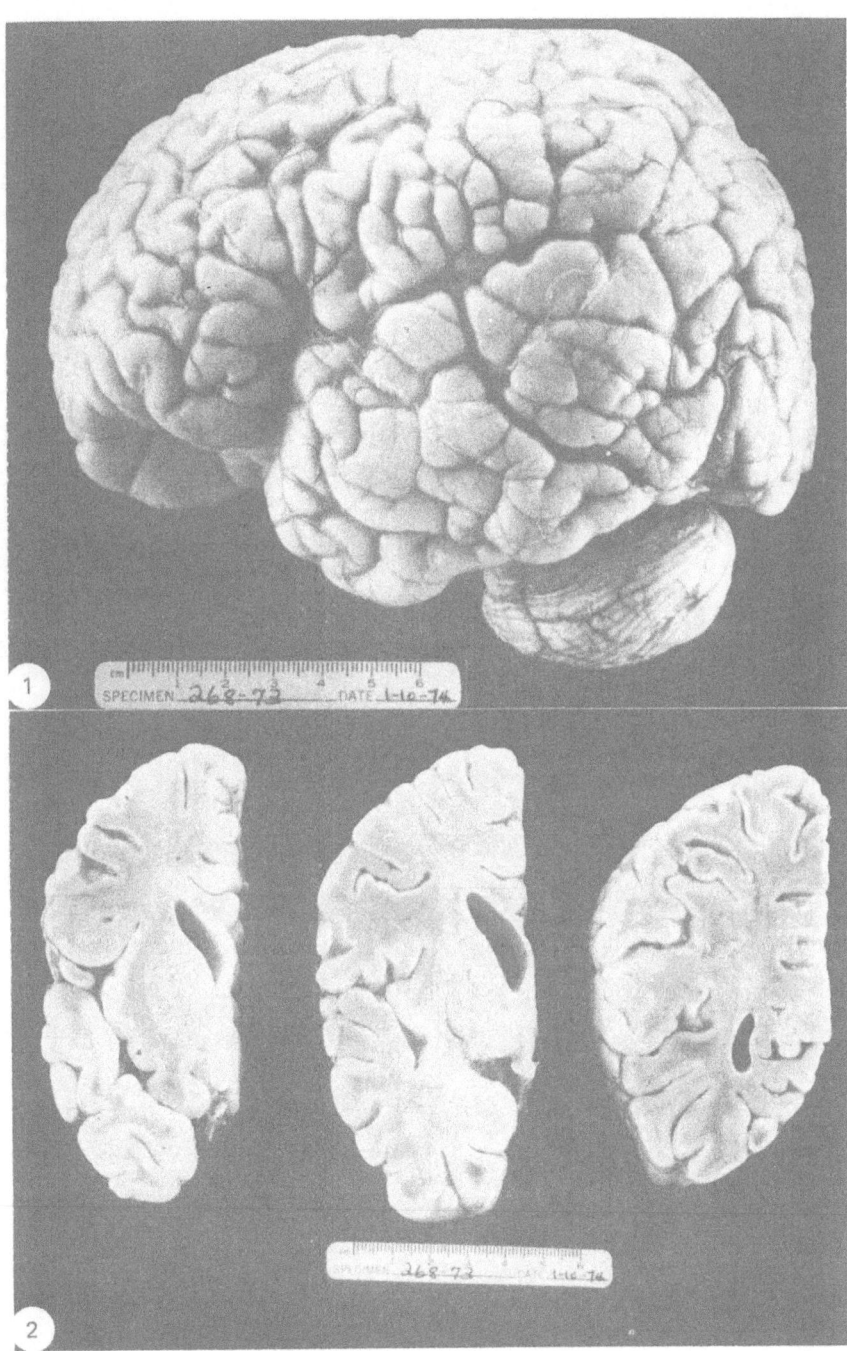

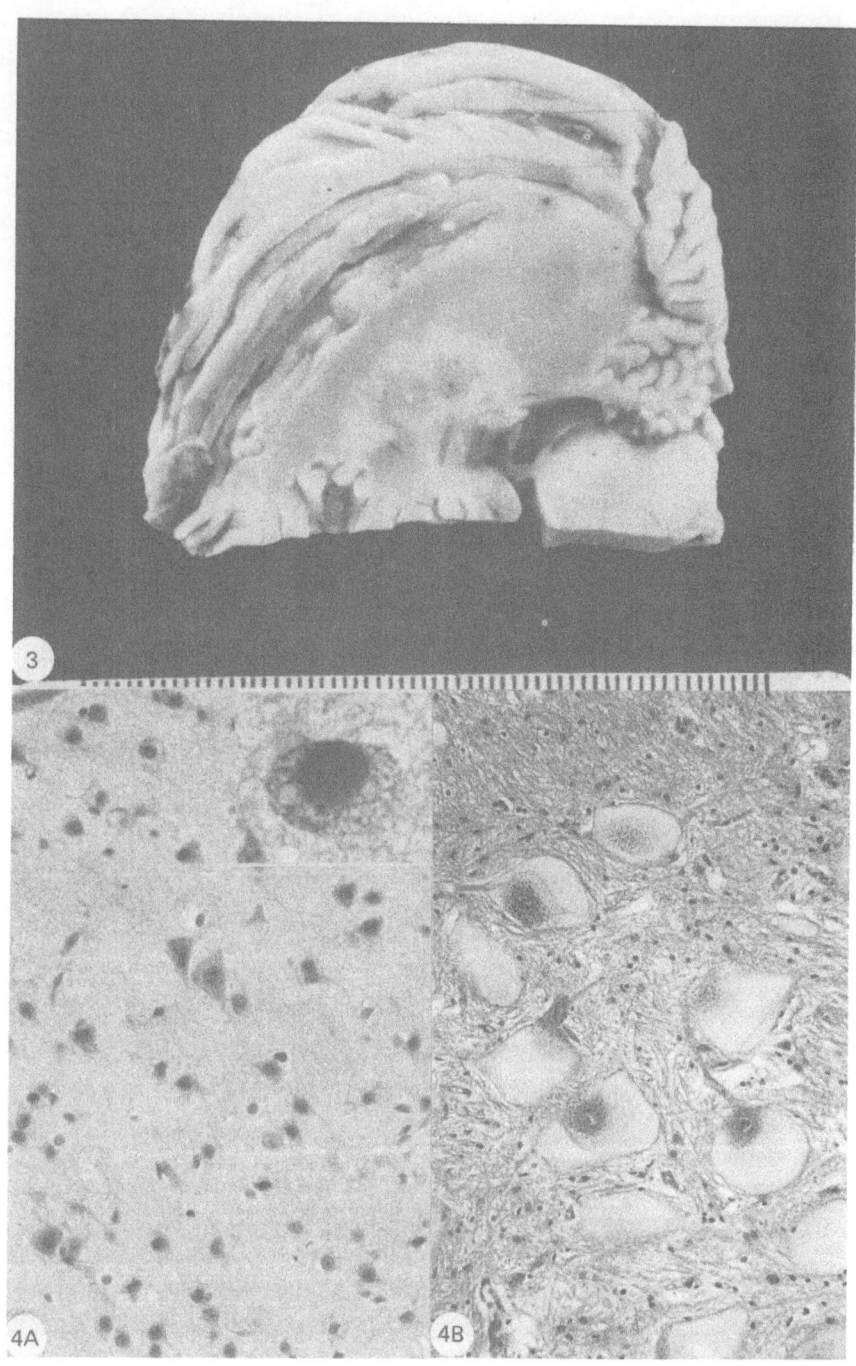

3

4A   4B

cerebral cortex these changes are more severe than those seen in the deep gray matter, brain stem, and spinal cord.

Distinct changes are present as early as 14 weeks. There is moderate reduction in the number of neurons, although they are as yet not distended (Figure 4A). Under higher magnification, the neuronal cytoplasm contains fine vacuoles (Figure 4A, inset). At this stage, the cortex shows only a minimal degree of reactive astrocytosis and microglial proliferation. In the white matter, moderate reduction of axonal fibers can be observed in silver stains, and no visible myelin sheaths are demonstrable in Luxol fast blue PAS and Mahon preparations. Microglial cells and macrophages containing a sudanophilic material are present in small numbers.[1]

At 12-14 months of illness the cerebrum shows marked neuronal distension in the cortex and in the deep gray matter. These neurons have lost their angular or pyramidal shape and have acquired a ballooned out, round, or ovoid outline (Figure 4B). The cytoplasm is filled with a finely granular or vacuolar material, and the Nissl bodies are present only in the perikaryon. The nuclei are eccentrically placed and are often pyknotic. In the white matter there is variable reduction of axonal fibers and myelin sheaths. Reactive astrocytosis and an increase of macrophages are observed in both gray and white matter.

During months 15 to 24 the cytoarchitecture of the cerebral cortex becomes increasingly distorted. It shows augmented cellularity due to marked proliferation of macrophages and reactive astrocytes in the presence of a significant decrease of neurons. The remaining neurons are markedly distended and contain numerous fine granules or vacuoles. The Nissl bodies have disappeared and the nuclei are pyknotic and are often missing (Figure 5). The neuronal processes are focally distended and contain a material which is similar to that seen in the cytoplasm. The neuronal inclusions give moderately positive reactions with PAS (Figure 6A), Sudan black B (Figure 6B), and Luxol fast blue stains (Figure 6C). Macrophages, on the other hand, exhibit intensely positive reactions in the same preparations (Figures 6A-6C). The white matter, especially of the parietal lobes, is edematous and shows extensive loss of axons and severe demyelination accompanied by

FIGURE 3. Section of the cerebellum showing atrophy of the cortical folia and brown discoloration of the white matter. The dentate nucleus is pale, but is well defined.

FIGURE 4. (A) Biopsy from the cerebral frontal cortex of a 14-week-old boy with TSD showing a moderate reduction of the number of neurons. Those remaining are not distended. Under higher magnification, the cytoplasm contains fine vacuoles (inset). Hematoxylin-eosin stain, 280×. Inset: 930×. (B) Portion of frontal cortex of a 16-month-old boy with TSD exhibiting marked distention of the neuronal cytoplasm which contains numerous fine granules or vacuoles. The Nissl bodies are diminished in number and are located around the shrunken nuclei which are displaced to the periphery of the cells. Hematoxylin-eosin stain, 125×.

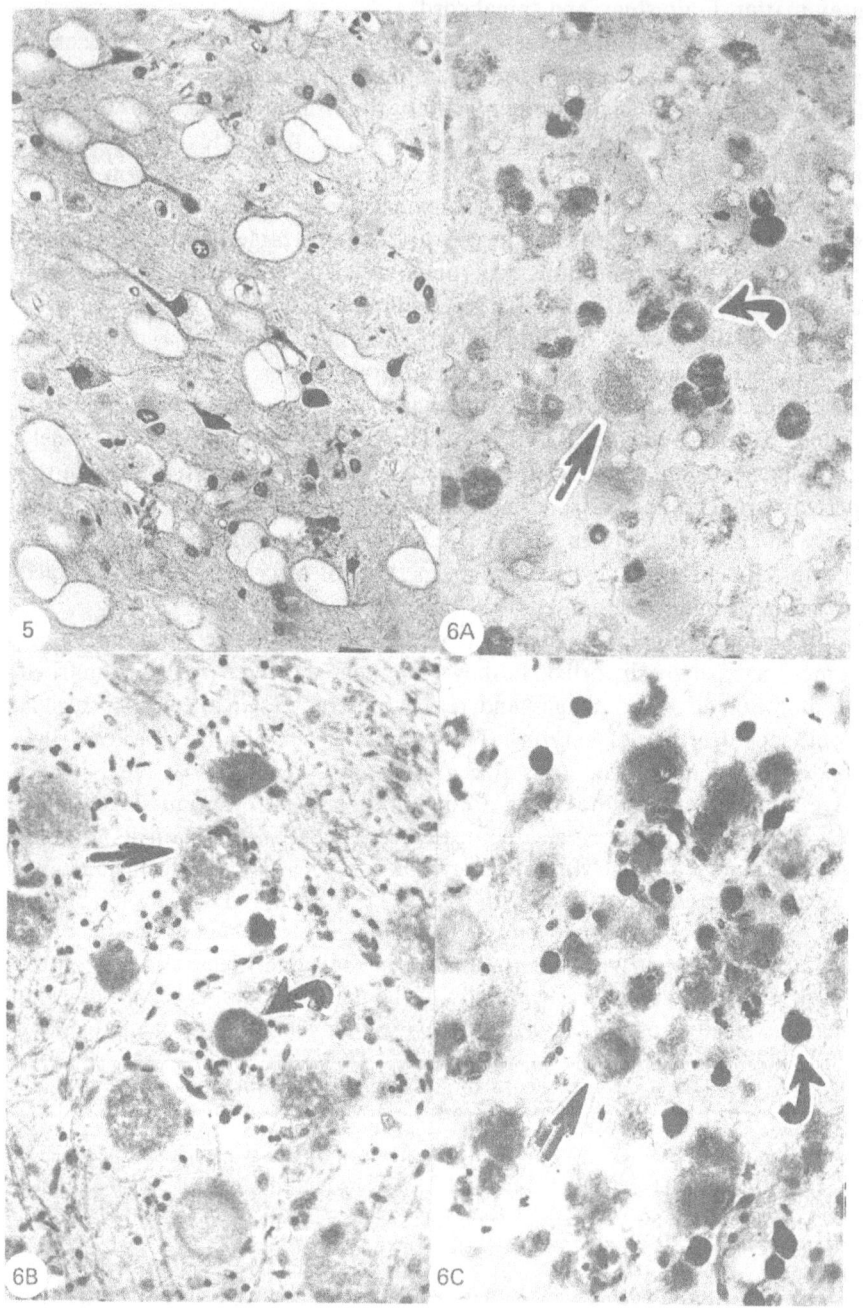

proliferation of protoplasmic astrocytes and macrophages, which are filled with a sudanophilic material. In many areas, clusters of macrophages can be seen in the perivascular areas of the white matter. The capillary endothelial cells are frequently enlarged and contain fine vacuoles.

After 24 months, the cerebral cortex shows more extensive neuronal loss and marked glial proliferation. In contrast, in the deep gray matter and brain stem little loss of neurons can be seen. Moreover, the glial reaction in these areas is less pronounced than in the cortex. The white matter of all lobes is edematous and shows only occasional preservation of axons (Figure 7A). There is diffuse demyelination and reduction of oligodendroglial cells, which are replaced by reactive astrocytes and macrophages (Figure 7B). The blood vessels in both gray and white matter are usually patent but frequently show endothelial proliferation and occasionally contain an intravascular lipid material.

The cerebellum exhibits atrophy of the folia corresponding to reduction of the Purkinje and granular cells. The remaining Purkinje cells are irregularly distributed. Their cytoplasm is distended and contains a lipid material which can be visualized by various fat stains. Their Nissl bodies are absent and the nuclei are pyknotic. The dendrites are distended by abnormal lipids and exhibit an antlerlike pattern (Figure 8). The basket cells, although not decreased in number, are often enlarged and also contain similar lipids. The neurons of the dentate nuclei and other areas of the deep gray matter are markedly reduced in number. Those remaining contain cytoplasmic inclusions. These changes are accompanied by increased glial proliferation. The cerebellar white matter shows moderate reduction of myelin sheaths and axons during the advanced stage of the disease. Microglial and astrocytic reactions in the cerebellum are less conspicuous than those in the cerebrum.

In the spinal cord the characteristic neuronal changes are more pronounced in the anterior horn cells. During the early stage, the degree of neuronal alterations varies from cell to cell. Some appear normal in shape, while others are distended and show reduction of the amount of Nissl

FIGURE 5. Portion of the cerebral medulla of a 24-month-old child with TSD displaying ballooned out neurons with loss of Nissl bodies and pyknotic nuclei. Most cells give a "ghost-like" appearance and are devoid of nuclei. Occasional residual neurons show axonal preservation. Hematoxylin-eosin stain, 285×. From Volk, B. W.: Tay–Sachs Disease. Grune & Stratton, New York, 1964, with permission of the publisher.

FIGURE 6. The cortical neurons (straight arrows) of a child with TSD give moderate reaction of the cytoplasmic material in (A) PAS, (B) Sudan black B, and (C) Luxol fast blue preparations, while the macrophages (curved arrows) stain intensely with these dyes. A, 280×; B, 280×; C, 225×. From Volk, B. W.: Tay–Sachs Disease. Grune & Stratton, New York, 1964, with permission of the publisher.

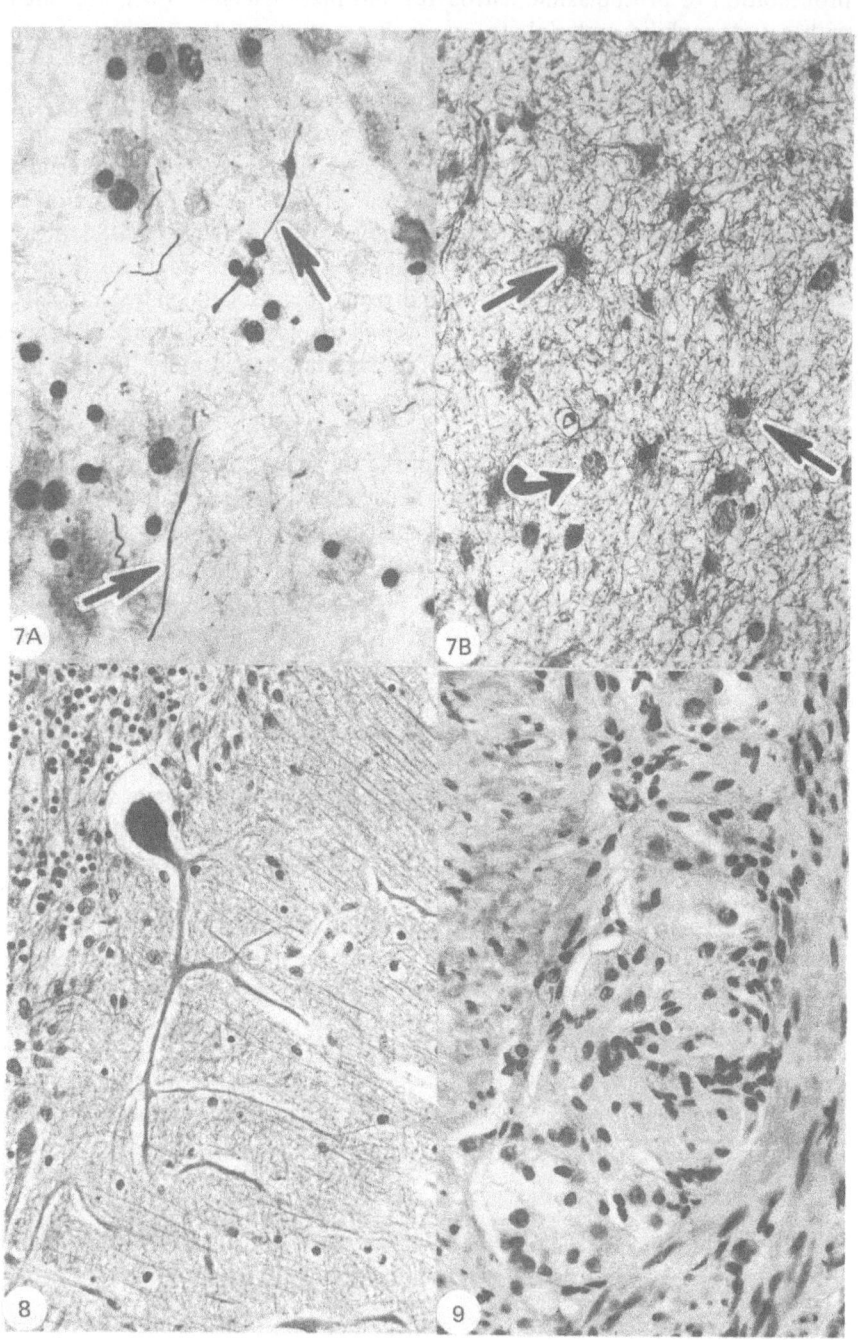

bodies. As the disease progresses, most of the anterior horn cells appear ballooned out and are filled with cytoplasmic inclusions. The changes are similar to those in the cerebrum. However, while there is extensive neuronal loss in the anterior horn, the nerve cells in the posterior and lateral horns are less affected and appear normal in number. In advanced cases, the white matter shows axonal loss and demyelination, especially in both pyramidal tracts. These changes are accompanied by a moderate increase of macrophages and mild astrocytosis.

In the dorsal ganglia, the neurons are distended and filled with vacuoles. There are areas of neuronal loss accompanied by proliferation of the capsular nuclei.

The retina shows varying degrees of loss of ganglion cells. Those still present are swollen and filled by lipids which give similar tinctorial characteristics as those seen in the cerebrum. In many instances, there is loss of the ganglion cells at the margin of the fovea and more so in the macula. The layers of the rods and cones and of both nuclear layers show occasional cellular loss. There are no changes in the choroid or in other parts of the eye. The clinically characteristic cherry-red spot is due to involvement of the ganglion cells and thinning of the nerve-cell layer so that more of the underlying choroidal coat becomes visible on ophthalmologic examination. The opaque whitish macula surrounding this area is thought to be due to edema and swelling of the plexiform layer or due to swelling and necrosis of the ganglion cells. The nerve-fiber layer shows marked loss of fibers when examined in silver stains. The optic nerves in advanced cases show demyelination and axonal loss, especially in the central portion of the fibers. There is also increase of collagen fibers in the peri- and endoneurium.

The neurons of the autonomic nervous system, including those of the sympathetic chain and the visceral plexuses, show similar morphologic and tinctorial alterations as those of the central nervous system (Figure 9).

While Globus described alterations in the posterior lobe of the pituitary gland,[2] in our own material no visible alterations could be observed by optical microscopy in both the anterior and posterior portions. Ul-

---

FIGURE 7. (A) The white matter of the parietal lobe of a patient with TSD exhibits only occasional preservation of axons (arrows) which are focally swollen. (B) There is marked proliferation of reactive astrocytes and their fibers (straight arrows) as well as of macrophages (curved arrow). A, Bodian stain, 500×; PTAH stain, 225×. From Volk, B. W.: Tay–Sachs Disease, Grune & Stratton, New York, 1964, with permission of the publisher.

FIGURE 8. The cerebellar Purkinje cells show antlerlike distention of their dendrites. Romanes stain, 280×.

FIGURE 9. Ganglion cells of the myenteric plexus of a child with Tay–Sachs disease showing ballooned out cytoplasm. Hematoxylin-eosin stain, 280×.

trastructurally, however, cytoplasmic inclusions were noted in both lobes albeit only occasionally.[3]

In light microscopic studies, various authors reported extraneuronal inclusions in lungs, thymus, liver, intestine, spleen, bone marrow, lymph nodes, kidney, and pancreas.[4-10] However, electron microscopic studies have confirmed such material only in the liver.[11,12]

The skeletal muscles show neurogenic atrophy due to gradual degeneration of the anterior horn cells during the progression of TSD. However, since regression of the individual neurons is not uniform, the myofibers show considerable variations in size, although cross striations are maintained. The subsarcolemmal nuclei are frequently increased in number and may show a chainlike pattern. There is an increase of collagen fibers mainly in the perimysium.

In the peripheral blood, small vacuoles have been reported in lymphocytes, the contents of which were sudanophilic and PAS positive.[13,14] These features are present in only 1–4% of lymphocytes, regardless of the duration of the disease.[15,16]

Histochemistry

The cytoplasmic material within the neurons consists of complex proteolipid compounds, the histochemical characteristics of which are summarized in Table 1.[8,17-48] The modified PAS method for cerebroside and protein-bound ganglioside[49] gives a strong reaction in frozen sections, which decreases in intensity in paraffin preparations (Figure 6A). The material stains moderately intense in Sudan black B preparations (Figure 6B) and gives faint or negative reactions with Sudan IV and oil red O stains. It stains positively in Luxol fast blue preparations (Figure 6C). Although neuraminic acid is an important constituent of the gangliosides, the Bial reaction[8] gives uneven results and is frequently negative. This suggests that the gangliosides in TSD are mixed with various amounts of a carbohydrate moiety within the affected cells, resulting in different reactions. The neuronal material also gives positive reactions in modified Smith–Dietrich[50] and Baker preparations[51,52] for phospholipids, and it stains blue in Nile blue sulfate preparations.[53] These results are in keeping with the presence of phospholipids and cerebrosides. The cellular inclusions furthermore give positive stains with the Schultz method[54] for cholesterol and with Feigin's procedure[55] for demonstration of cholesterol esters, indicating that it is a compound lipid. In general, the material is easily soluble in cold alcohol, chloroform, and ether, while in some instances, the deposited substance, or a portion thereof, may resist extraction with lipid solvents. The cytoplasmic inclusions also react strongly with the orcin–sulfuric acid test,[18] indicating

TABLE 1. Histochemistry of Intraneuronal Material in Tay–Sachs Disease

Methods	Reactions	Specificity
Modified periodic acid Schiff[49]	+++	Cerebrosides and, probably, protein-bound gangliosides
Orcin–sulfuric acid[8]	+++	Pentoses and hexoses
Nile blue[53]	++	Phosphoglycerides and sulfatides, blue
Luxol fast blue[48]	++	Nonspecific, perhaps protein-bound lipids
Feigin[55]	++	Cholesterol esters
Schultz[54]	++	Cholesterol and cholesterol esters, pink to red
Perchloric acid–naphthoquinone[56]	++	Cholesterol and cholesterol esters, light blue to dark blue
Smith–Dietrich[50]	+	Phospholipids, black
Baker[51,52]	+	Choline-containing phospholipids, cerebroside (mild reaction)
Phosphomolybdic acid–stannous chloride[56]	+	Lecithin and sphingomyelin
Alcian blue[56]	+	Acid mucopolysaccharide, blue-green
Toluidine blue[56]	Metachromatic	Mainly sulfatides and some acid mucopolysaccharides
Acetic acid–cresyl violet[8]	Metachromatic	Sulfatides, brown
Sudan black B[56]	+	Unsaturated triglyceride esters, unsaturated cholesterol esters, unsaturated free fatty acids, glycolipids, and phospholipids
Oil red O[56]	±	Unsaturated triglyceride esters, unsaturated cholesters, unsaturated free fatty acid, and cerebroside
McManus's periodic acid Schiff[56]	+	Phospho- and glycolipids, steroids, fatty acids, hexose-containing mucopolysaccharides, glycogen
Coupled tetrazonium[56]	±	Aromatic and heterocyclic amino acids: tyrosine, tryptophan, histidine
Benzoylation[56]	±	Histidine-containing proteins
Million[56]	±	Tyrosine-containing proteins
Ninhydrin Schiff[56]	±	Protein-containing reactive NH_2 groups
Bial[8]	−	Neuraminic acid, red
Okamoto[56]	−	Sphingomyelin and lecithin
Performic acid Schiff[56]	−	Phospholipids and cerebroside with unsaturated bonds
Osmium tetroxide[56]	−	Specific for unsaturated lipids

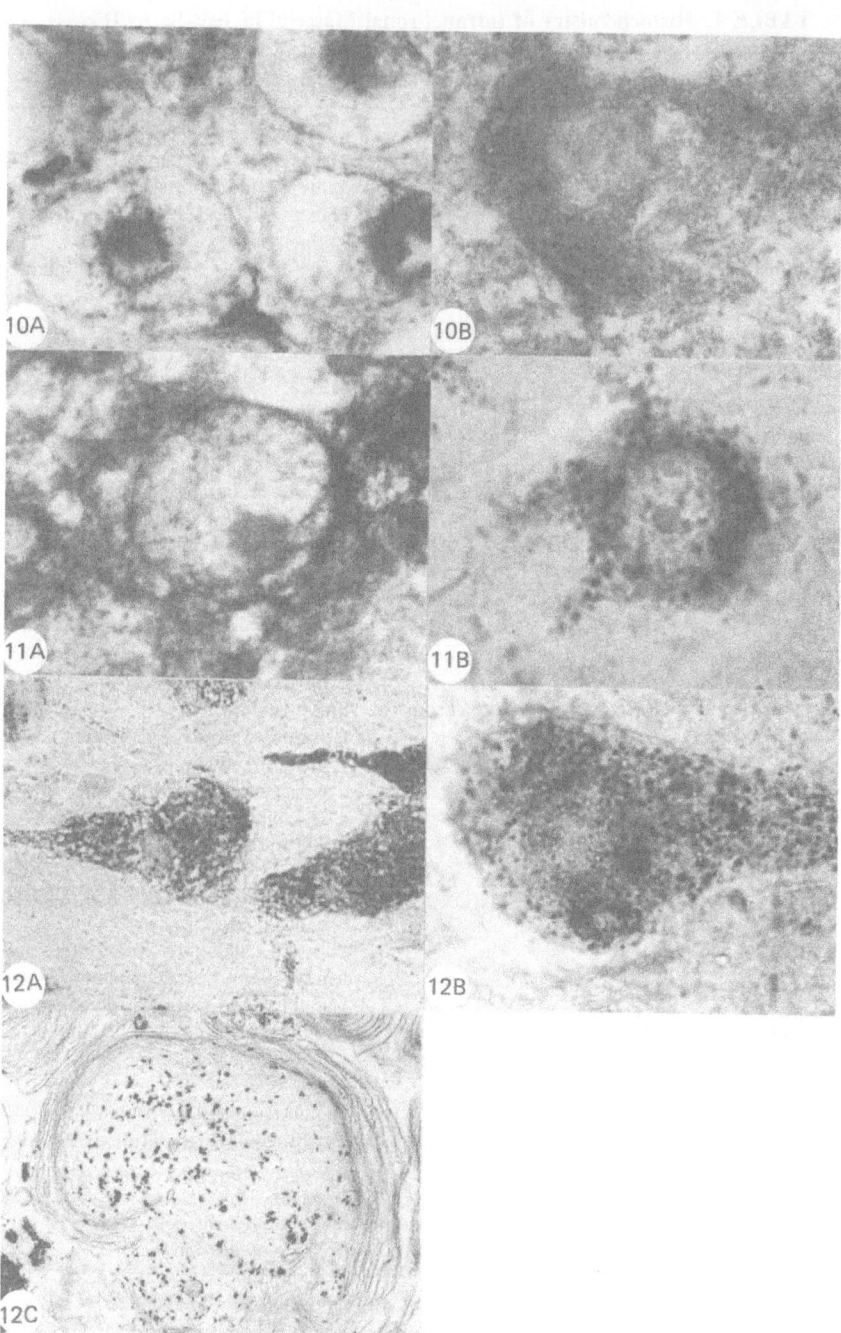

the presence of pentoses and hexoses. Because histochemical studies for proteins give a faintly positive or negative reaction with Millon's reagent, coupled tetrazonium, ninhydrin Schiff, and benzoylation methods,[56] it was suggested that there is a low concentration of protein in the intracytoplasmic deposits which becomes increasingly bound to the lipids during the progression of the disease.[8] The material shows a positive reaction in Alcian blue stains, and metachromasia with toluidine blue and acetic acid–cresyl violet stains on frozen sections.

Enzyme histochemical studies[11,12,20,34,47,48,57-61] show decreased activities of oxidative enzymes in the neurons, i.e., lactic dehydrogenase, malic dehydrogenase, diphosphopyridine nucleotide diaphorase (Figure 10), as well as of adenosine triphosphatase (Figure 11). The affected neurons also display a marked increase of acid phosphatase activity (Figure 12). The histochemical reactions are summarized in Table 2. The positive reaction in acid phosphatase preparations was originally interpreted to mark the presence of lysosomes.[62] The oxidative enzymes and adenosine triphosphatase are confined to the perinuclear zone and to the periphery of the cell, with sparsely distributed granules or rods in the swollen perikaryon.

The extent of these alterations in localization of activity, except for those of acid phosphatase activity, parallels the storage of lipid and suggests that the organelles associated with these enzymes are displaced to the periphery of the cell by the accumulating gangliosides. In general, the pattern of enzyme activity in neurons shows the unequal involvement of ganglion cells, which is shown to be more significantly involved in phylogenetically younger areas of the brain. Thus, the oxidative enzyme activities in medullary neurons, which are least involved by the disease process, show stained granules sparsely scattered throughout the cytoplasm, often concentrated around the eccentric nucleus. On the other hand, in the more involved cells of the cortex, this oxidative enzyme activity is confined to a

FIGURE 10. In preparations for diphosphopyridine nucleotide diaphorase, the neurons of a patient with TSD show reaction products in the perikarya (A), while the neuron of a control brain (B) displays diffuse distribution of enzyme activity within the cytoplasm and neuropil. The nucleus is pale. A, 960×; B, 1280×.

FIGURE 11. (A) Neuron in the medulla stained for adenosine triphosphatase exhibiting sparsely distributed activity within the ballooned out cytoplasm. (B) A neuron of a control brain shows diffusely staining cytoplasmic granules. A, 960×; B, 1280×.

FIGURE 12. (A) Acid phosphatase activity in neurons (A) of a Tay–Sachs patient is localized in granules evenly distributed throughout the cytoplasm and is not displaced by the stored lipids as in instances of oxidative enzymes. (B) A neuron of a control brain shows diffuse distribution of reaction granules scattered throughout the cytoplasm. (C) Electron microscopically, the reaction products are localized in a membranous cytoplasmic body. A, 500×; B, 1280×; C, 14,000×.

TABLE 2. Enzyme Histochemistry of Intraneuronal Material in Tay–Sachs Disease

| | | Tay–Sachs disease | | |
Methods	Reference	Early stage	Advanced stage	Normal range
Oxidative enzymes (LD, TPND, DPND, G6PD, MD, SD)^a	57	+	−	+ +	+ + +
Adenosine triphosphatase	57	+	−	+ +	+ + +
Acid phosphatase	57	+ +	+ + +	+	+ +

^{a} LD, lactic dehydrogenase; TPND, triphosphopyridine nucleotide diaphorase; DPND, diphosphopyridine nucleotide diaphorase; G6PD, glucose-6-phosphate dehydrogenase; MD, malic dehydrogenase; SD, succinic dehydrogenase.

narrow zone at the periphery of the cell and to the perinuclear region. These findings suggest that enzymatically intact organelles persist in the involved neurons, permitting them to carry on their metabolic function for an extended period of time though possibly at a decreased level of activity.

Electron Microscopy

The central and peripheral nervous systems of infants with TSD display neuronal and glial inclusions called membranous cytoplasmic bodies (MCBs)[63-69] (Figure 13) which measure 0.5–2.0 μm in diameter. They are composed of closely packed, concentrically arranged membranes, each measuring about 25 Å in thickness and showing in the center a homogeneous or finely granular zone. In addition to these inclusions, other compound bodies can be observed which consist of peripheral concentric layers surrounding an inner zone filled with slightly curved or straight membranes. A third form of cytosome consists of closely packed flat membranes (Figure

FIGURE 13. Electron microphotograph of portion of cortical neuron of a child with TSD. The cytoplasm is filled with large membranous cytoplasmic bodies (MCBs) which consist of concentric lamellar structures arranged around a heterogeneous granular core or around a core of flat horizontal membranes. 22,600×.

FIGURE 14. During the progression of TSD a mature membranous cytoplasmic body (A) develops from a fine granular material (B and C). The formation of the membranous cytoplasmic bodies can be traced to the cisternae of the endoplasmic reticulum (arrows) (D). A, 37,300×; B, 17,500×; C, 32,700×; D, 26,850×.

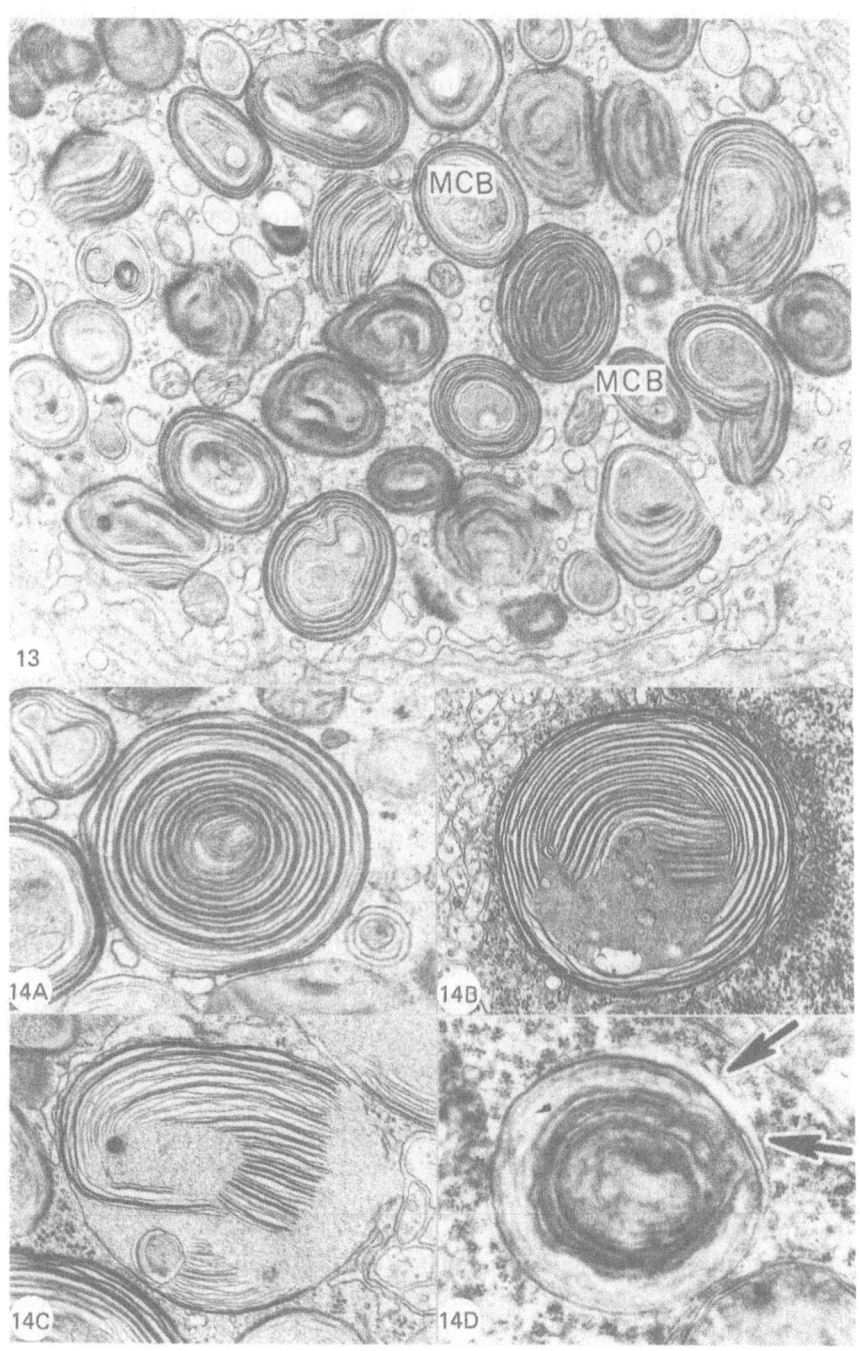

15). During the progression of the disease the mature MCBs develop from a fine, granular material (Figures 14A–14C). Histogenetically, their formation can be traced to the cisternae of the endoplasmic reticulum (Figure 14D), as was observed in a cerebral biopsy from a 14-week-old child with TSD.[1]

The alterations in astrocytes occurring during various stages of TSD indicate that the abnormal inclusions within the cytoplasm are due to an intrinsic metabolic disturbance rather than a result of phagocytosis of the abnormal product.[68] It seems, furthermore, that the astrocytic mitochondria and endoplasmic reticulum play an important role during the early phase of development of their inclusion bodies.[68]

In the autonomic nervous system the ganglion cells of the sympathetic chain and those of the plexus of the viscera contain a moderate number of inclusion bodies, which, in many instances, are different from the typical MCBs of the central nervous system.[70] The variegated picture of the cytoplasmic inclusions in different organs may be related to differences in the metabolic evolution of various cellular systems.

In the endocrine glands, occasional MCBs can be noted in both anterior and posterior lobes of the pituitary gland, as well as in the pineal gland.[3]

In the liver, both hepatocytes and Kupffer cells contain cytosomes which consist of often oval-shaped, membrane-bound bodies containing parallel membranes or concentrically arranged membranous structures.[11,12] Occasionally, hepatocytes show large cytoplasmic inclusions which are pleomorphic and consist of membranous structures mixed with a pale or dense material (Figure 16).

After the advent of prenatal diagnosis, the morphologic features of TSD at the fetal stage have been reported by several investigators.[71-74] In our own material of ten fetuses aborted during the 16th to 22nd weeks in which the diagnosis of TSD was made through amniocentesis and, in addition, in a fetus aborted by curretage at 12 weeks, it was possible to follow the morphogenesis of the cytoplasmic inclusions *in utero*. Between the 12th and 18th weeks the spinal cord and dorsal ganglia of the fetuses show abnormal inclusion bodies in the neuronal cytoplasm (Figure 17A). At 19–22 weeks of gestation, the TSD fetuses exhibit histologically normal development of the neurons in the cerebral cortex, brain stem, and cerebellum without any visible cytoplasmic vacuoles. On the other hand, the neurons in the anterior horn (Figure 17B) and of the dorsal ganglia (Figure 17C) contain many intracytoplasmic vacuoles. Ultrastructurally, during this period, the fetuses show occasional inclusion bodies within the cortical neurons of the cerebrum, brain stem, and cerebellum. They are bounded by a single membrane and contain granules and delicate parallel membranes

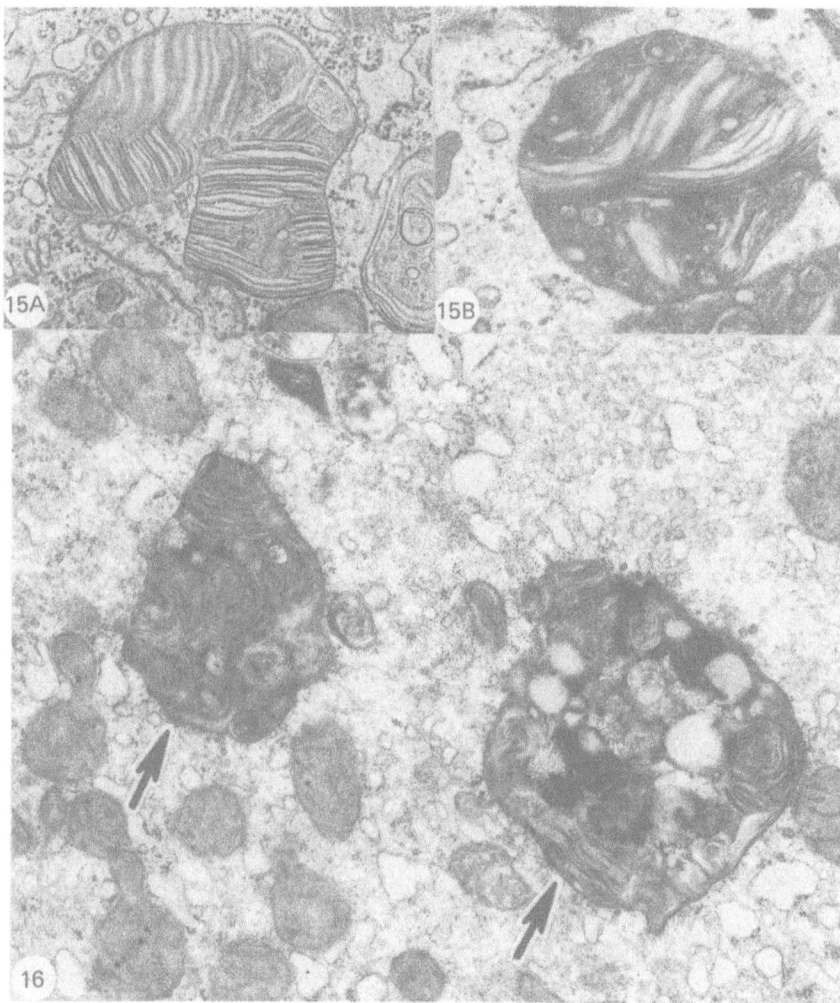

FIGURE 15. Some of the neuronal cytoplasmic inclusions in TSD are pleomorphic (A) or contain an electron-dense material mixed with membranous structures (B). A, 25,700×; B, 40,400×.

FIGURE 16. Some hepatocytes of TSD patients contain occasional large cytoplasmic inclusions (arrows) which are pleomorphic and consist of membranous structures mixed with an electron-dense or electron-lucent material. 12,300×.

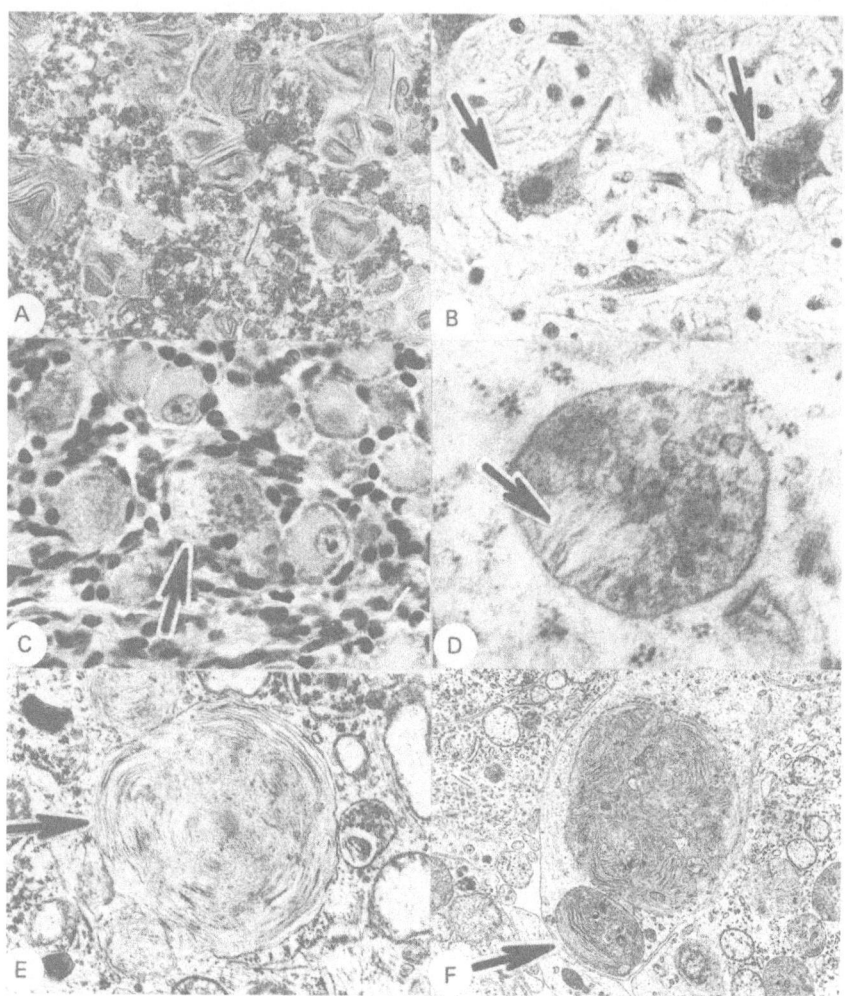

FIGURE 17. Portion of dorsal ganglion of a TSD fetus at 16 weeks of gestation (A) showing relatively preserved abnormal cytoplasmic inclusions, although the tissue was obtained three days after uterine infusion with saline solution. At 19 weeks of gestation, a TSD fetus shows many fine vacuoles (arrows) in the anterior horn cells (B) and in the neurons of a dorsal ganglion (C). Despite absence of neuronal vacuoles in the cerebral cortex by light microscopy of the 19-week-old fetus, ultrastructurally, the nerve cells show occasional inclusion bodies which are bounded by a single membrane and contain delicate membranes (arrow) mixed with varying-sized granules (D). The anterior horn cells of the spinal cord (E) and the ganglion cell layer of the retina (F) of a Tay–Sachs fetus at 22 weeks of gestation display inclusions with partially concentric membranes (arrows) mixed with electron-dense granules. A, 15,700×; B, 375×; C, 375×; D, 46,800×; E, 18,700×; F, 9,250×.

(Figure 17D). The neurons of the anterior horn of the spinal cord, the ganglion cells of the retina and the dorsal ganglia display partially membranous structures mixed with electron-dense granules (Figures 17E and 17F). In the dorsal and retinal ganglion cells the gradual evolution of the membranous structures can be traced from an electron-dense granular material to the cisternae of the endoplasmic reticulum.[74] This finding supports previous observations in postnatal TSD[1,68,70] in which this organelle was seen to play an important role during the formation of the MCBs.

In the neurons of the myenteric plexus occasional abnormal inclusions are present between the 16th and 22nd gestational weeks.[74]

In the endocrine system, the pituitary gland also shows sporadic cytoplasmic inclusions in both anterior and posterior lobes during the same gestational period.[74]

In acid phosphatase preparations, the membranous cytoplasmic bodies (Figure 18A) of a TSD fetus show no reaction product, while in the advanced stage of postnatal infantile TSD abundant reaction granules are present within the inclusions (Figure 18B). Similarly, the cisternae of the endoplasmic reticulum (Figure 18C) from the same fetus show absence of enzyme activity, although the Golgi complex (Figure 18D) displays intensive acid phosphatase activity.

Since acid phosphatase is a marker for lysosomes, the presence of reaction product in the advanced stage of the disease supports previous observations by light microscopy[57] and is interpreted to indicate that these inclusion bodies represent digestive structures of the residual body type which are lysosomal in nature and reflect the cellular effort to eliminate the accumulated material. On the other hand, the lack of enzyme activity in the cytoplasmic inclusions at the fetal stage suggests that the lysosomes have not yet developed at this early phase of life.

Sandhoff's Disease [$G_{M2}(0)$]

Although Sandhoff's disease[75-87] is clinically indistinguishable from TSD, morphologically abnormal cytoplasmic inclusion bodies are present in the central nervous system and viscera which are different from those of the other lipidoses.[85-87]

Gross Pathology

The gross appearance of the brain in Sandhoff's disease is similar to that of TSD. Its weight is markedly increased. The cerebral hemispheres are uniformly enlarged and firm, while the cerebellum is atrophic and rubbery.

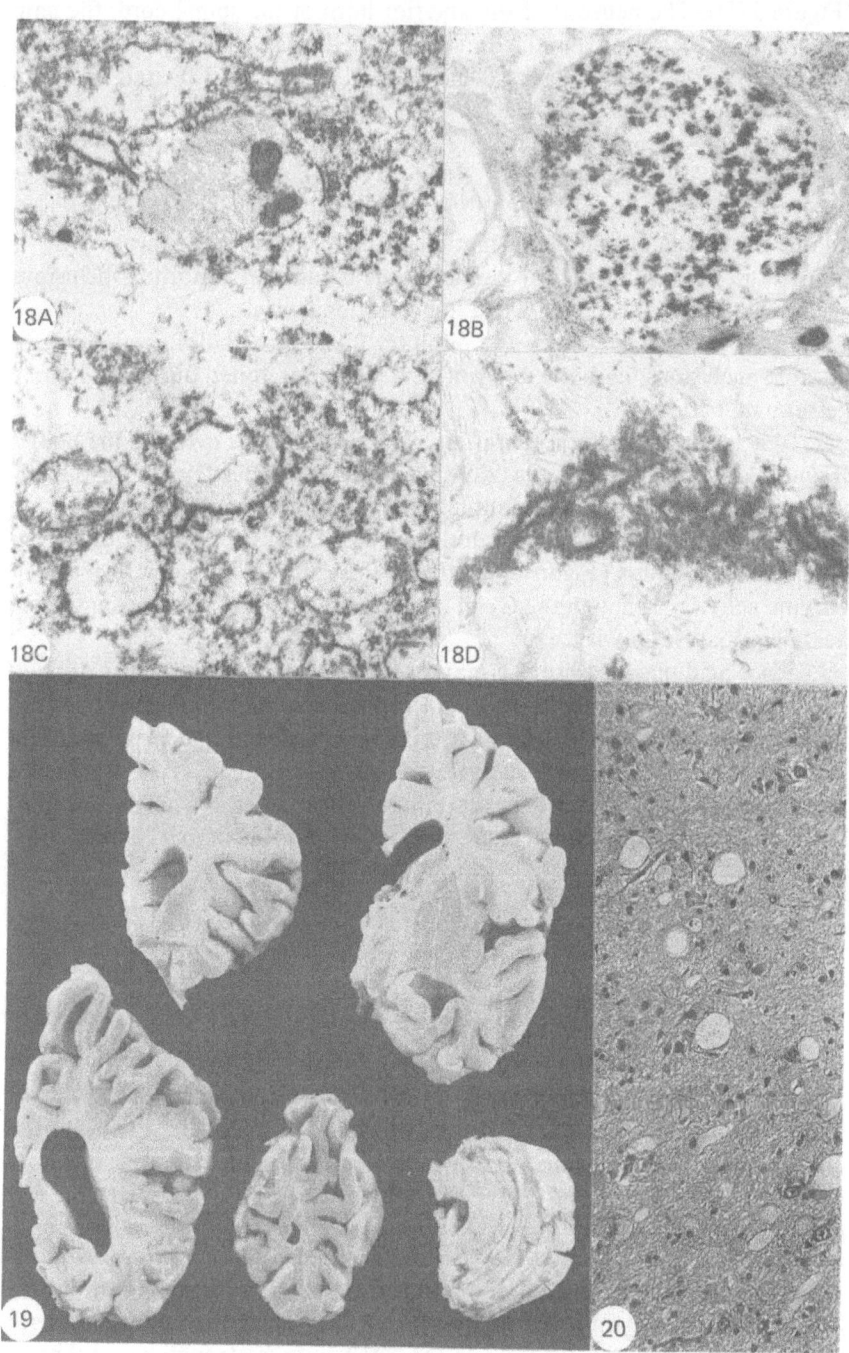

The optic nerves and chiasm are also atrophic. Sections of the cerebrum show attenuation of the cortices of all lobes and gray discoloration of the white matter. The ventricular system is not dilated. Sections of the cerebellum exhibit atrophic and pale folia of all lobules. There are occasional hepatomegaly and thickening of the endocardium, mitral, and tricuspid valves present.

Histopathology

The cerebral cortex shows varying degrees of neuronal loss and distortion of the cytoarchitecture. The remaining nerve cells are markedly swollen and contain numerous cytoplasmic vacuoles. The white matter exhibits diffuse demyelination, although the axons are relatively preserved. Both the cortex and white matter display marked astrocytosis and show the presence of macrophages containing a sudanophilic material. The neurons of the deep white matter and brain stem appear normal in number, although the neuronal cytoplasm is markedly distended and is filled with fine vacuoles.

The cerebellum reveals marked loss of the Purkinje and granular cells. They are replaced by proliferating reactive astrocytes and macrophages. There are also diffuse demyelination and severe gliosis in the cerebellar white matter, although the axons are preserved.

In the spinal cord, the neurons, at all levels, are distended by cytoplasmic vacuoles.

In the peripheral and autonomic nervous systems the ganglion cells show alterations which are similar to those of the central nervous system.

The involvement of the viscera varies from case to case. The liver shows fine vacuoles or granules in the hepatocytes and Kupffer cells, while the kidneys frequently contain similar vacuoles in glomeruli and epithelial cells of the collecting tubules, especially those of the loops of Henle. Cytoplasmic vacuoles are also observed in the acinar cells of the pancreas but are absent in the islets.[85]

FIGURE 18. In acid phosphatase preparations the membranous cytoplasmic bodies (A) of a TSD fetus show no reaction product, while in the advanced stage of postnatal infantile TSD abundant reaction granules are present within the inclusions (B). Similarly, the cisternae of the endoplasmic reticulum (C) from the same fetus show absence of enzyme activity although the Golgi complex (D) displays intensive acid phosphatase activity. A, 22,200×; B, 29,200×; C, 22,200×; D, 27,000×.

FIGURE 19. Coronal sections of the cerebrum and cerebellum of a six-year-old non-Jewish boy with generalized G_{M2}-gangliosidosis showing atrophic cortices and white matter of all lobes. (From Volk, B. W. et al.: Arch. Path., 87:393, 1969, with permission of the publisher.)

FIGURE 20. Portion of the cerebral cortex of the same child as Figure 19 displaying ballooned-out neuronal cytoplasm and processes. Hematoxylin-eosin stain, 125×.

Histochemistry

With Luxol fast blue stains, abnormal cytoplasmic granules are demonstrable in histiocytes in the spleen and lymph nodes, cardiac muscles, bronchial epithelium, endothelial cells, smooth muscle fibers of the arteries, fibroblasts, adrenal cortex, pituitary gland, and seminiferous tubules and germinal cells of the testis. The other histochemical features of these inclusions are similar to those of TSD.[80,85]

Electron Microscopy

Some of the neurons of the central, peripheral, and autonomic nervous systems contain typical MCBs.[77,80,82,85,87] However, many inclusions are pleomorphic and display a variety of structures which consist of a membranous material as well as of vesicles and granules. Similar cytoplasmic bodies are also observed in the viscera.[85-87]

Bernheimer–Seitelberger Disease [G_{M2}(A,B)]

Although this disease is a variant of G_{M2}-gangliosidosis,[88-97] the morphological features are different from those of TSD.

Gross Pathology

The weight of the brain is markedly decreased and the cerebral hemispheres are diffusely atrophic. Sections of the cerebrum and cerebellum show atrophy of the cortex and white matter of all lobes (Figure 19). The deep gray matter is pale and is relatively preserved. The entire ventricular system shows moderate dilatation resulting from the parenchymal atrophy. The liver and spleen are reduced in weight; otherwise the organs are not remarkable.

Histopathology

The cerebral and cerebellar cortices show ballooning of the neuronal cytoplasm (Figure 20) due to accumulation of numerous vacuoles. The white matter exhibits moderate demyelination but the axons are relatively preserved. The neurons in the deep gray matter, brain stem, spinal cord, dorsal, and somatic ganglia similarly contain intracytoplasmic vacuoles. The spinal tracts and peripheral nerves appear normal.

No visible intracytoplasmic vesicles are present in the viscera.

Histochemistry

The cytoplasmic vacuoles give reactions which are similar to those in TSD.

Electron Microscopy

The neurons in the central and autonomic nervous systems are filled with pleomorphic lipid bodies (Figure 21A) which consist of both parallel and concentrically arranged membranes. Some of them are similar to the MCBs of TSD. In some instances the inclusions contain an electron-dense material which is intermingled with membranous lamellae (Figure 21B).

The liver shows occasional cytoplasmic inclusions in the hepatocytes consisting of membranous lamellar structures (Figure 22).

G_{M1}-Gangliosidoses

Norman–Landing Disease [$G_{M1}(0)$] and Derry's Disease [$G_{M1}(A)$]

The central nervous system changes are similar in both groups.[98-132]

Gross Pathology

The brain is reduced in weight and increased in consistency. Sections of the cerebrum and cerebellum show atrophic cortices and the white matter is pale. The deep gray matter is not remarkable, while the brain stem frequently displays atrophy of the cerebral peduncles, the basilar portion of the pons, and the pyramids. The ventricular system is dilated. The spinal cord often shows tannish discoloration in both lateral portions of the white matter.

In contrast to the identical neuropathological changes, the viscera show significantly different features in both types. In Norman–Landing disease hepatosplenomegaly and skeletal changes are similar to those of Hurler's disease, while in Derry's disease the viscera appear normal.

Histopathology

The subarachnoid space contains foamy histiocytes. The neurons of all cortices and deep gray matter display cytoplasmic swelling resembling that

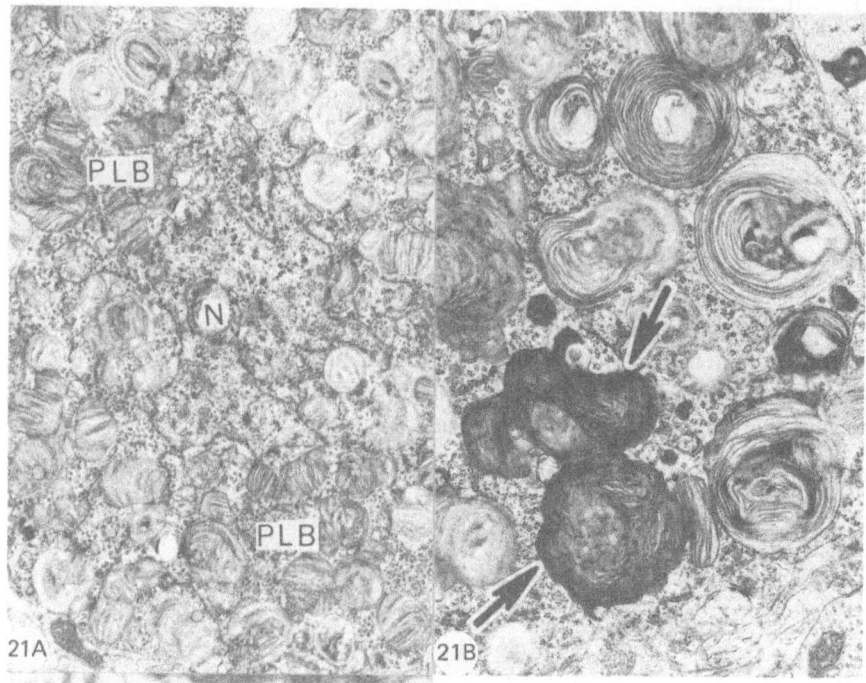

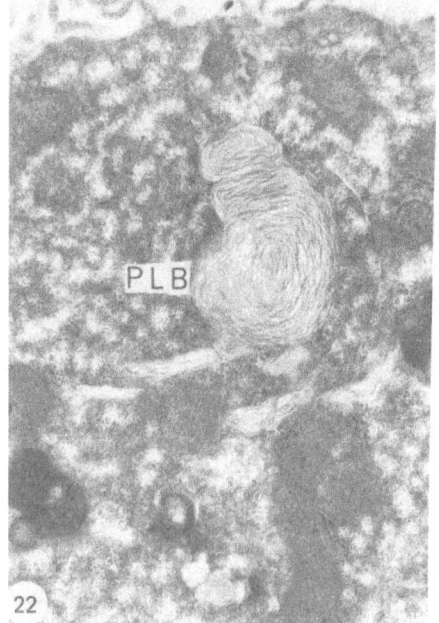

FIGURE 21. Electron microphotograph of a cerebral neuron of the same child as Figure 19 exhibiting pleomorphic lipid bodies (PLB) containing parallel or concentrically arranged membranes (A). Some of the PLBs contain membranous structures mixed with an amorphous electron-dense material (arrows) (B). N, nucleus. A, 7150×; B, 8250×.

FIGURE 22. Hepatocytes of the same boy as Figure 19 containing pleomorphic lipid body and an electron-dense material. 18,700×. (From Volk, B. W., *et al: Arch. Path.*, *87*:393, 1969, with permission of the publisher.)

seen in TSD. The cerebral and cerebellar white matter shows varying degrees of demyelination and axonal loss with concomitant astrocytosis and an increase of macrophages. There are varying degrees of axonal and myelin loss in the corticospinal tracts in the brain stem and spinal cord.

Although both types show different gross alterations, both display many foamy histiocytes in various organs, particularly in the lymph nodes, spleen, bone marrow, lungs, thymus, lamina propria of the intestines, liver, and the interlobular septa, acina, and ductular cells of the pancreas. In addition to the presence of histiocytes, the hepatocytes, the glomerular epithelium, and the loops of Henle also show numerous fine vacuoles.

Histochemistry

Although slight variations of histochemical reactions are observed in the cytoplasmic vacuoles in different organs, the bulk of the material is tinctorially essentially similar to that of TSD.

Electron Microscopy

Both types of G_{M1}-gangliosidosis show similar intraneuronal inclusion bodies (Figure 23) which measure 0.5–3.0 μm in diameter and exhibit considerable pleomorphism. Most of them consist of concentrically arranged lamellae surrounding an inner amorphic core, while others are composed of parallel membranes similar to the "zebra bodies"[104] seen in mucopolysaccharidosis. These consist of membranous structures mixed with an amorphous or granular material. Occasionally, some of them are round and resemble the MCBs of TSD. The neuronal processes also contain pleomorphic inclusions. The astrocytes and capillary endothelial cells frequently are filled with a dense amorphous material mixed with membranous lamellae.

The liver contains membrane-bound inclusions in both the hepatocytes (Figure 24) and Kupffer cells, which consist of an electron-lucent material and fine granules. The kidneys also show similar cytoplasmic bodies in epithelial cells and mesangial cells of the glomeruli (Figure 25A) as well as in the tubular epithelium of the loop of Henle, particularly in the proximal convoluted tubules (Figure 25B).[105,107,110,111,118,121,122,131]

Similar changes in endothelial cells of the interstitial vessels, smooth muscles of arterioles, and peripheral nerves are also present.[122]

Other investigators[129] observed alterations in the cardiac muscles as well as in capillary endothelium and nerve fibers of the heart which consisted of large vacuoles containing a granular or flocculent material.

The morphologic alterations at the fetal stage of G_{M1}-gangliosidosis

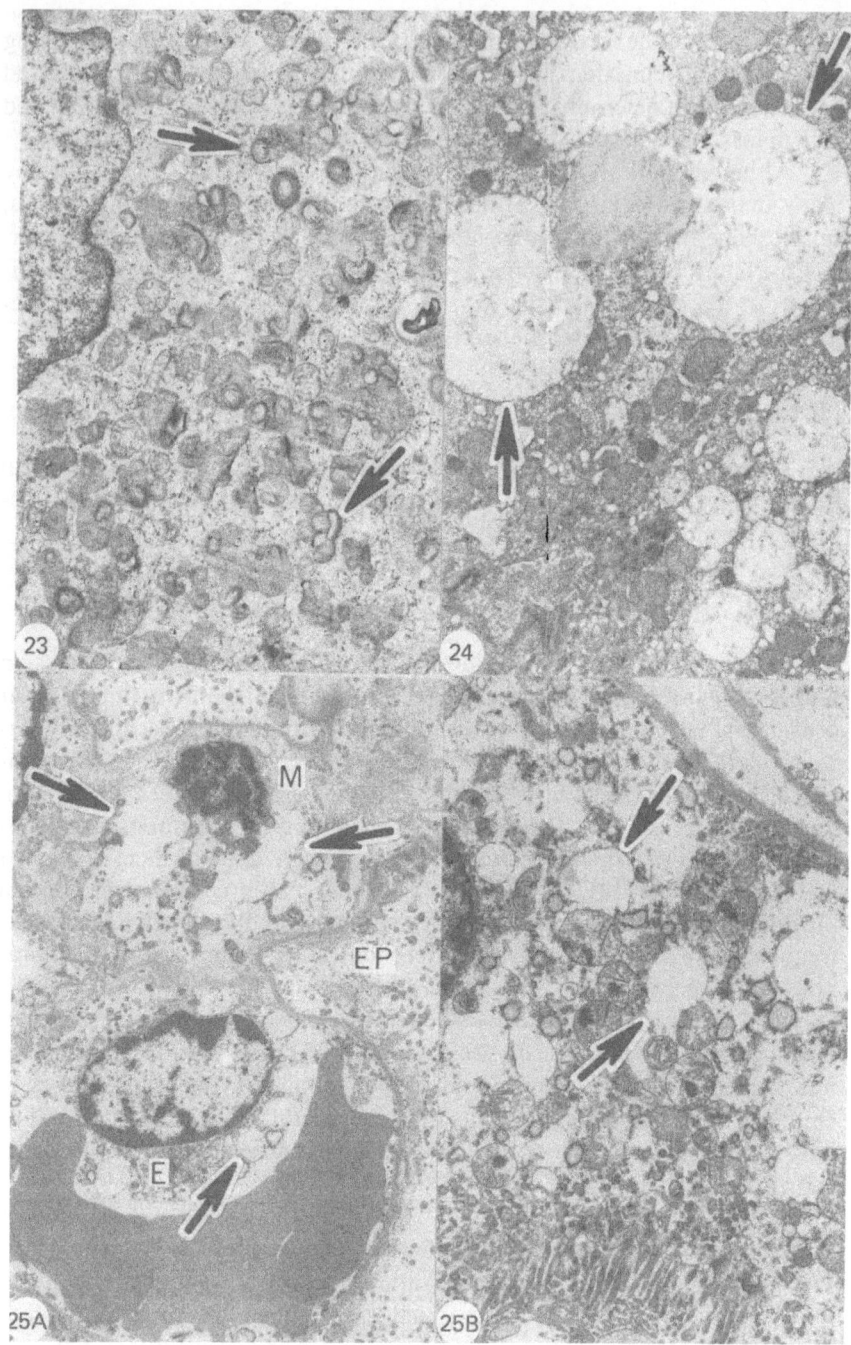

have been reported by several investigators.[73,133,134] A 17-week-old fetus showed neuronal vacuoles in the brain, hepatocytes, glomerular epithelial cells, renal tubular cells, exocrine cells of the pancreas, adrenal cortical cells, endothelial cells of all organs, and lymphocytes[133] and two midterm fetuses exhibited intracytoplasmic inclusions in the anterior horn cells of the spinal cord, liver, kidney, and myocardium.[73,134]

G_{M3}-Gangliosidosis

Two cases of G_{M3}-gangliosidosis have been reported so far.[135,136] The first case was that of a 29-month-old non-Jewish boy whose brain was fixed in formalin for about six years. Because of the storage in formalin, the original amount of G_{M3}-ganglioside accumulated in the brain was uncertain.[135] The morphological aspects of this case were reported by Jørgensen et al. as a "case of Niemann–Pick disease."[137] The central and autonomic nervous systems showed marked distention of neurons which contained cytoplasmic fine vacuoles exhibiting the histochemical characteristics of sphingomyelin or acid glycolipids. Similar foamy cells were also observed in the liver, spleen, bone marrow, thymus, several glands, and connective tissue of small vessels.

The second case was that of a 3½-month-old non-Jewish boy.[136] The brain showed spongy changes in the cortex and subcortical white matter. Ultrastructurally, the vacuoles visualized by optical microscope were seen to be due to swelling of the astrocytic cytoplasmic and separation of myelin lamellae.[138] These changes resembled those observed in cases of spongy degeneration of the central nervous system (van Bogaert and Bertrand type).[139] The brain showed no cytoplasmic inclusion bodies.[138]

FIGURE 23. A cerebral biopsy from an infant with variant A G_{M1}-gangliosidosis. A portion of a neuron shows numerous pleomorphic lipid bodies containing various membranous structures (arrows) as well as a homogeneous, electron-dense material. 8400×.

FIGURE 24. Portion of a hepatocyte from a child with variant 0 G_{M1}-gangliosidosis showing electron-lucent vacuoles (arrows) varying in size and containing sparse electron-dense granules. 4000×. Courtesy of Dr. H. B. Neustein and Dr. B. H. Landing, Los Angeles, Calif.

FIGURES 25A and B: (A) Portion of kidney from a child with variant 0 G_{M1}-gangliosidosis exhibiting vacuoles of varying sizes and shapes (arrows) in epithelial cells (EP) and mesangial cells (M) of a glomerulus as well as in (B) an epithelial cell of a proximal convoluted tubule. E, endothelial cells. A, 3500×; B, 5000×. Courtesy of Dr. H. B. Neustein and Dr. B. H. Landing, Los Angeles, Calif.

References

1. Adachi, M., Torii, J., Schneck, L., and Volk, B. W., Fine structure of early Tay–Sachs disease, in: *Sphingolipids, Sphingolipidoses and Allied Disorders*, B. W. Volk and S. M. Aronson, eds., Plenum Press, New York, pp. 1–13 (1972).
2. Globus, J. H., Amaurotic family idiocy, *J. Mt. Sinai Hosp. N.Y.* 9:451 (1942).
3. Adachi, M., Volk, B. W., Schneck, L., and Relkin, R., Ultrastructural alterations of endocrine glands in Tay–Sachs disease, *Am. J. Clin. Pathol.* 57:557 (1972).
4. Davison, C. and Jacobson, S. A., Generalized lipidosis in a case of amaurotic familial idiocy, *Am. J. Dis. Child.* 52:345 (1936).
5. Brouwer, B., The spleen, the liver and the brain, *Proc. R. Soc. Med.* 29:579 (1936).
6. Marburg, O., Studies on the pathology and pathogenesis of amaurotic family idiocy, *Am. J. Ment. Defic.* 46:312 (1942).
7. Turban, H., Über einen Fall familiärer amaurotischer Idiotie vom Typ Tay–Sachs, Thesis, Freiburg (1944).
8. Diezel, P. B., Histochemical study of primary lipidoses, in: *Cerebral Lipidoses. A Symposium*, L. van Bogaert, J. N. Cumings, and A. Lowenthal, eds., Blackwell, Oxford, pp. 11–31 (1957).
9. Fischer, R., Über Tay–Sachs'sche amaurotische Idiotie mit Organbeteiligung, Thesis, Frankfurt (1955).
10. Norman, R. M., Tingey, A. H., Newman, C. G. H., and Ward, S. P., Tay–Sachs disease with visceral involvement and its relation to gargoylism, *Arch. Dis. Child.* 39:634 (1964).
11. Volk, B. W. and Wallace, B. J., The liver in lipidosis. An electron microscopic and histochemical study, *Am. J. Pathol.* 49:203 (1966).
12. Wallace, B. J., Lazarus, S. S., and Volk, B. W., Electron microscopic and histochemical studies of viscera in lipidoses, in: *Inborn Disorders of Sphingolipid Metabolism*, S. M. Aronson and B. W. Volk, eds., Pergamon Press, New York, pp. 107–120 (1967).
13. Spiegel-Adolf, M., Baird, H. W., Coleman, H. S., and Szekely, E. G., Vacuolized blood lymphocytes in the lipidoses and other central nervous system diseases with special reference to histochemical studies, in: *Cerebral Sphingolipidoses: A Symposium on Tay–Sachs Disease and Allied Disorders*, S. M. Aronson and B. W. Volk, eds., Academic Press, New York, pp. 129–140 (1962).
14. Spiegel-Adolf, M., Baird, H. W., Kollias, D., and Szekely, E. G., Cerebrospinal fluid, serum and blood investigations in amaurotic family idiocy, *Am. J. Dis. Child.* 97:676 (1959).
15. Eeg-Olofsson, O., Kristensson, K., Sourander, P., and Svennerholm, L., Tay–Sachs disease. A generalized metabolic disorder, *Acta Paediatr. Scand.* 55:546 (1966).
16. Lazarus, S. S., Vethemany, V. G., Schneck, L., and Volk, B. W., Fine structure and histochemistry of peripheral blood cells in Niemann–Pick disease, *Lab. Invest.* 17:155 (1967).
17. Landing, B. H. and Freiman, D. G., Histochemical studies on the cerebral lipidoses and other cellular metabolic disorders, *Am. J. Pathol.* 33:1 (1957).
18. Diezel, P. B., Histochemische Untersuchungen an primären Lipoidosen: Amaurotische Idiotie, Gargoylismus, Niemann–Picksche Krankheit, Gauchersche Krankheit, mit besonderer Berücksichtigung des Zentralnervensystems, *Virchows Arch. A.* 326:89 (1954).
19. Diezel, P. B., Histochemischer Nachweis des Gangliosids in Ganglien und Gliazellen bei amaurotischer Idiotie und Isolierung der lipoidspeichernden Zellen nach der Methode von M. Behrens, *Dtsch. Z. Nervenheilkd.* 171:344 (1954).
20. Diezel, P. B., *Die Stoffwechselstörungen der Sphingolipoide*, Springer-Verlag, Berlin (1957).

21. Seitelberger, F., Eine unbekannte Form von infantiler Lipoidspeicher-Krankheit des Gehirns, *Proc. 1st Int. Congr. Neuropathol.* **3**:323 (1952).

22. Wildi, E., Contribution à l'étude anatomo-pathologique et chimique de la maladie de Tay-Sachs, Thèse No. 1978, Faculte de Médecine, Genève (1950).

23. Favarger, P. and Wildi, E., Chemical analysis and histochemical examination of an atypical case of Tay-Sachs disease, in: *Cerebral Lipidoses. A Symposium*, L. van Bogaert, J. N. Cumings, and A. Lowenthal, eds., Blackwell, Oxford, pp. 146–158 (1957).

24. Wolman, M., Histochemical study of the brain in an atypical case of amaurotic idiocy, *Acta Neuropathol.* **1**:73 (1961).

25. Jervis, G. A., Hallervorden-Spatz disease associated with amaurotic idiocy, *J. Neuropathol. Exp. Neurol.* **11**:4 (1952).

26. Feyrter, F., Zur Frage der Tay-Sachs-Schafferschen amaurotischen Idiotie, *Virchows Arch. A* **304**:481 (1939).

27. Hellström, B., Ivemark, B., and Zetterström, B., Atypisk cerebromaculär degeneration, *Nord. Medicin* **60**:1782 (1958).

28. Wolman, M., A histochemical study of various forms of cerebral lipidoses, *J. Clin. Pathol.* **15**:324 (1962).

29. Edgar, G. W. F. and Donker, C. H. M., Influence of lipid solvents on sphingolipids (sphingomyelins, cerebrosides, gangliosides) in tissue sections. With reference to the histochemistry of demyelination and lipidoses, *Acta Neurol. Psychiatr.* **57**:451 (1957).

30. Shanklin, W. M., Issidorides, M., and Salem, M., Histochemistry of the cerebral cortex from a case of amaurotic family idiocy, *J. Neuropathol. Exp. Neurol.* **21**:284 (1962).

31. Guminska, M., Pietrzykowa, B., Stefanko, S., and Sszybowska, M., Przypadek choroby Tay-Sachs'a w swietle badan klinicznych histologicznych i chemicznych, *Patol. Pol.* **12**:449 (1961).

32. Stefanko, S., Guminska, M., and Pietrzykowa, B., Histochemische und chemische Veränderungen im Gehirn bei einem Fall von familiärer amaurotischer Idiotie, *Schweiz. Arch. Neurol. Neurochir. Psychiatr.* **90**:295 (1962).

33. Nakai, H. and Landing, B. H., Suggested use of rectal biopsy in the diagnosis of neural lipidoses, *Pediatrics* **26**:225 (1960).

34. Franceschetti, A., Wildi, E., and Klein, D., Examen anatomo-clinique d'un cas d'idiotie amaurotique infantile (Tay-Sachs), *Acta Genet.* **5**:343 (1955).

35. Hurst, E. W., A study of the lipoids in neuronic degeneration and in amaurotic family idiocy, *Brain* **48**:1 (1925).

36. Diezel, P. B., Lipidoses of the central nervous system, in: *Modern Scientific Aspects of Neurology*, J. N. Cumings, ed., Edward Arnold Ltd., London, pp. 98–145 (1960).

37. Wolman, M., Histochemical study of the brain in an atypical case of amaurotic idiocy, *Acta Neuropathol.* **1**:73 (1961).

38. Aronson, S. M. and Volk, B. W., Pathogenesis of white matter changes in Tay-Sachs disease, in: *Cerebral Sphingolipidoses: A Symposium on Tay-Sachs Disease and Allied Disorders*, S. M. Aronson and B. W. Volk, eds., Academic Press, New York, pp. 15–28 (1962).

39. Jervis, G., Harris, R. C., and Menkes, J. H., Cerebral lipidosis of unclear nature, in: *Cerebral Sphingolipidoses: A Symposium on Tay-Sachs Disease and Allied Disorders*, S. M. Aronson and B. W. Volk, eds., Academic Press, New York, pp. 101–118 (1962).

40. Norman, R. M. and Tingey, A. H., Sudanophilic leucodystrophy and Pelizaeus-Merzbacher disease, in: *Brain Lipids and Lipoproteins and the Leucodystrophies*, J. Folch-Pi and H. Bauer, eds., Elsevier, Amsterdam, pp. 169–186 (1963).

41. Shanklin, W. M. and Salam, M., A comparison of the histochemistry of the cerebral cortex from siblings with gargoylism and Tay-Sachs disease, *Acta Neuroveg.* **25**:297 (1963).

42. Schob, F., Pathologische Anatomie der Idiotie, in: *Handbuch der Geisteskrankheiten*, O. Bumke, ed., Springer-Verlag, Berlin, p. 972 (1930).

43. Von Santha, K., Über drei reine von Niemann–Pickscher Krankheit verschonte Fälle der infantil-amaurotischen Idiotie, *Arch. Psychiatr. Nervenkr.* **93**:675 (1931).

44. Aronson, S. M., Volk, B. W., and Epstein, N., Morphologic evolution of amaurotic family idiocy. The protracted phase of the disease, *Am. J. Pathol.* **31**:609 (1955).

45. Adams, G. W. M., Cerebral storage diseases, in: *Neurohistochemistry*, G. W. M. Adams, ed., Elsevier, Amsterdam, pp. 488–517 (1965).

46. Wolman, M., II. The lipidoses, in: *Handbuch der Histochemie*, Gustav Fischer Verlag, Stuttgart, *Vol. 5, Lipides, Part 2, Histochemistry and Lipids in Pathology*, pp. 172–307 (1964).

47. Volk, B. W., Pathologic anatomy, in: *Tay–Sachs Disease*, B. W. Volk, ed., Grune & Stratton, New York, pp. 36–67 (1964).

48. Volk, B. W., Schneck, L., and Adachi, M., Clinic, pathology and biochemistry of Tay–Sachs disease, in: *Handbook of Clinical Neurology*, P. J. Vinken and G. W. Bruyn, eds., North-Holland, Amsterdam, Vol. 10, Leucodystrophies and Poliodystrophies, pp. 385–426 (1970).

49. Adams, C. W. M., VIII. The modified PAS method for cerebroside and protein-bound ganglioside, in: *Neurohistochemistry*, C. W. M. Adams, ed., Elsevier, Amsterdam, p. 58 (1965).

50. Kaufman, C. and Lehmann, E., Sind die in der histologischen Technik gebräuchlichen Fettdifferenzierungsmethoden spezifisch? *Virchow Arch. A* **261**:623 (1926).

51. Baker, J. R., Histochemical recognition of lipine, *Q. J. Microsc. Sci.* **87**:441 (1946).

52. Baker, J. R., Further remarks on the histochemical recognition of lipine, *Q. J. Microsc. Sci.* **88**:463 (1947).

53. Menschik, Z., Nile blue histochemical method for phospholipids. *Stain Technol.* **28**:13 (1953).

54. Weber, A. F., Phillips, M. G., and Bell, J. T., An improved method for the Schultz cholesterol test, *J. Histochem. Cytochem.* **4**:308 (1956).

55. Feigin, I., A method for the histochemical differentiation of cholesterol and its esters, *J. Biophys. Biochem. Cytol.* **2**:213 (1956).

56. Pearse, A. G. E., *Histochemistry. Theoretical and Applied*, Little, Brown & Co., Boston, Vol. 1 (1968).

57. Lazarus, S. S., Wallace, B. J., and Volk, B. W., Neuronal enzyme alterations in Tay–Sachs disease, *Am. J. Pathol.* **41**:579 (1962).

58. Koenig, H., McDonald, T., and Nellhaus, G., Morphological and histochemical studies of neurolipidosis by light and electron microscopy, *J. Neuropathol. Exp. Neurol.* **23**:191 (1964) (Abstract).

59. Friede, R. L. and Allen, R. J., Enzyme histochemical studies of Tay–Sachs disease, *J. Neuropathol. Exp. Neurol.* **23**:619 (1964).

60. Wallace, B. J., Volk, B. W. and Lazarus, S. S., Fine structural localization of acid phosphatase activity in neurons of Tay–Sachs disease, *J. Neuropathol. Exp. Neurol.* **23**:676 (1964).

61. Wallace, B. J., Volk, B. W., Schneck, L., and Kaplan, H., Fine structural localization of two hydrolytic enzymes in the cerebellum of children with lipidoses, *J. Neuropathol. Exp. Neurol.* **25**:76 (1966).

62. De Duve, C., Pressman, B. C., Gianetto, R., Wattiaux, R., and Applemans, F., Tissue fractionation studies. 6. Intracellular distribution patterns of enzymes in rat-liver tissue, *Biochem. J.* **60**:604 (1955).

63. Terry, R. D. and Korey, S. R., Membranous cytoplasmic granules in infantile amaurotic idiocy, *Nature (London)* **188**:1000 (1960).

64. Terry, R. D., Korey, S. R., and Weiss, M., Electron microscopy of the cerebrum in Tay–Sachs disease, in: *Cerebral Sphingolipidoses: A Symposium on Tay–Sachs Disease and Allied Disorders,* S. M. Aronson and B. W. Volk, eds., Academic Press, New York, pp. 49–56 (1962).

65. Terry, R. D. and Weiss, M., Studies in Tay–Sachs disease. II. Ultrastructure of the cerebrum, *J. Neuropathol. Exp. Neurol.* **22:**18 (1963).

66. Wallace, B. J., Schneck, L., Kaplan, H., and Volk, B. W., Fine structure of the cerebellum of children with lipidoses, *Arch. Pathol.* **80:**466 (1965).

67. Terry, R. D., Electron microscopy of selected neurolipidoses, in: *Handbook of Clinical Neurology,* P. J. Vinken and G. W. Bruyn, eds., North-Holland, Amsterdam, Vol. 10, Leudodystrophies and poliodystrophies, pp. 362–384 (1970).

68. Adachi, M., Torii, J., Karvounis, P. C., and Volk, B. W., Alterations of astrocytic organelles in various lipidoses and allied diseases, *Acta Neuropathol.* **18:**74 (1971).

69. Volk, B. W., Adachi, M., and Schneck, L., The gangliosidoses, in: *Progress in Neuropathology,* H. M. Zimmerman, ed., Grune & Stratton, New York, pp. 232–254 (1971).

70. Adachi, M., Volk, B. W., Schneck, L., and Torii, J., Fine structure of the myenteric plexus in various lipidoses, *Arch. Pathol.* **87:**228 (1969).

71. Adachi, M., Torii, J., Schneck, L., and Volk, B. W., The fine structure of fetal Tay–Sachs disease, *Arch. Pathol.* **91:**48 (1971).

72. O'Brien, J. S., Okada, S., Fillerup, D. L., Veath, M. L., Adornato, B., Brenner, P. H., and Leroy, J. G., Tay–Sachs disease: Prenatal diagnosis, *Science* **172:**61 (1971).

73. Percy, A. K., McCormick, U. M., Kaback, M. M., and Herndon, R. M., Ultrastructural manifestations of G_{M1} and G_{M2} gangliosidosis in fetal tissues, *Arch. Neurol.* **28:**417 (1973).

74. Adachi, M., Schneck, L., and Volk, B. W., Ultrastructural studies of eight cases of fetal Tay–Sachs disease, *Lab. Invest.* **30:**102 (1974).

75. Sandhoff, K., Andreae, U., and Jatzkewitz, H., Deficient hexosaminidase activity in an exceptional case of Tay–Sachs disease with additional storage of kidney globoside in visceral organs, *Life Sci.* **7:**283 (1968).

76. Sandhoff, K., Andreae, U., and Jatzkewitz, H., Deficient hexosaminidase activity in an exceptional case of Tay–Sachs disease with additional storage of kidney globoside in visceral organs, *Pathol. Eur.* **3:**278 (1968).

77. Pilz, H., Müller, D., Sandhoff, K., and ter Meulen, V., Tay–Sachssche Krankheit mit Hexosaminidase-Defekt. Klinische, morphologische und biochemische Befunde bei einem Fall mit viszeraler Speicherung von Nierenglobosid, *Dtsch. Med. Wochenschr.* **93:**1833 (1968).

78. Sandhoff, K., Variation of beta-*N*-acetyl-hexosaminidase pattern in Tay–Sachs disease, *FEBS Lett.* **4:**351 (1969).

79. Sandhoff, K., Jatzkewitz, H., and Peters, G., Die infantile amaurotische Idiotie und verwandte Formen also Ganglioside-Speicherkrankheiten, *Naturwissenschaften* **56:**356 (1969).

80. Suzuki, Y., Jacob, J. C., Suzuki, K., Kutty, K. M., and Suzuki, K., G_{M2}-Gangliosidosis with total hexosaminidase deficiency. *Neurology* **21:**313 (1971).

81. O'Brien, J. S., Okada, S., Ho, M. W., Fillerup, D. L., Veath, M. L., and Adams, K., Ganglioside storage disease, in: *Lipid Storage Diseases: Enzymatic Defects and Clinical Implications,* J. Bernsohn and H. J. Grossman, eds., Academic Press, New York, p. 225 (1971).

82. Desnick, R. J., Snyder, P. D., Desnick, S. J., Krivit, W., and Sharp, H. L., Sandhoff's disease: Ultrastructural and biochemical studies, in: *Sphingolipids, Sphingolipidoses and Allied Disorders,* B. W. Volk and S. M. Aronson, eds., Plenum Press, New York, pp. 351–371 (1972).

83. Okada, S., McCrea, M., and O'Brien, J. S., Sandhoff's disease (G_{M2}-gangliosidosis type 2): Clinical, chemical and enzyme studies in five patients, *Pediatr. Res.* **6**:606 (1972).

84. Krivit, W., Desnick, R. J., Lee, J., Moller, J., Wright, F., Sweeley, C. C., Snyder, P. D., and Sharp, H. L., Generalized accumulation of neutral glycosphingolipids with G_{M2}-ganglioside accumulation in the brain. Sandhoff's disease (variant of Tay–Sachs disease), *Am. J. Med.* **52**:763 (1972).

85. Dolman, C. L., Chang, E., and Duke, R. J., Pathologic findings in Sandhoff's disease, *Arch. Pathol.* **96**:272 (1973).

86. Sharp, H. L. and Desnick, R. J., Sandhoff's disease: Diagnosis and evaluation by percutaneous liver biopsy, *Gastroententerology* **60**:752 (1971).

87. Fontaine, G., Resibois, A., Tondeur, M., Jonniaux, G., Farriaux, J. P., Voet, W., Maillard, E., and Loeb, H., Gangliosidosis with total hexosaminidase deficiency: Clinical, biochemical and ultrastructural studies and comparison with conventional cases of Tay–Sachs disease, *Acta Neuropathol.* **23**:118 (1973).

88. Bernheimer, H. and Seitelberger, F., Über das Verhalten der Ganglioside im Gehirn bei 2 Fällen von Spätinfantiler Amaurotischer Idiotie, *Wien Klin. Wochenschr.* **80**:163 (1968).

89. Volk, B. W., Adachi, M., Schneck, L., Saifer, A., and Kleinberg, W., G_5-Ganglioside variant of systemic late infantile lipidosis. Generalized gangliosidosis, *Arch. Pathol.* **87**:393 (1969).

90. Klibansky, C., Saifer, A., Feldman, N. I., Schneck, L., and Volk, B. W., Cerebral lipids in a case of systemic G_{M2}-gangliosidosis of a late infantile type, *J. Neurochem.* **17**:339 (1970).

91. Schneck, L., Friedland, J., Pourfar, M., Saifer, A., and Volk, B. W., Hexosaminidase activities in a case of systemic G_{M2}-gangliosidosis of late infantile type, *Proc. Soc. Exp. Biol. Med.* **133**:997 (1970).

92. Suzuki, K., Suzuki, K., Rapin, I., Suzuki, Y., and Ishii, N., Juvenile G_{M2}-gangliosidosis: Clinical variant of Tay–Sachs disease or a new disease, *Neurology* **20**:190 (1970).

93. Suzuki, Y. and Suzuki, K., Partial deficiency of hexosaminidase component A in juvenile G_{M2}-gangliosidosis, *Neurology* **20**:848 (1970).

94. Young, E. P., Ellis, R. B., Lake, B. d., and Patrick, A. D., Tay–Sachs disease and related disorders. Fractionation of brain N-acetyl-beta-hexosaminidase, *FEBS Lett.* **9**:1 (1970).

95. Okada, S., Veath, M. L., and O'Brien, J. S., Juvenile G_{M2}-gangliosidosis: Partial deficiency of hexosaminidase A, *J. Pediatr.* **77**:1063 (1970).

96. Buxton, P., Cumings, J. N., Ellis, R. B., Lake, B. D., Mair, W. G. P., Roberts, J. R., and Young, E. P., A case of G_{M2}-gangliosidosis of late onset, *J. Neurol. Neurosurg. Psychiatr.* **35**:685 (1972).

97. Brett, E. M., Ellis, R. B., Hass, L., Ikonne, J. U., Lake, B. D., Patrick, A. D., and Stephens, R., Late onset G_{M2}-gangliosidosis. Clinical, pathological and biochemical studies on 8 patients, *Arch. Dis. Child.* **48**:775 (1973).

98. Norman, R. M., Urich, H., Tingey, A. H., and Goodbody, R. A., Tay–Sachs disease with visceral involvement and its relationship to Niemann–Pick disease, *J. Pathol. Bacteriol.* **78**:409 (1959).

99. Craig, J. M., Clarke, J. T., and Banker, B. Q., A metabolic neurovisceral disorder with the accumulation of an unidentified substance: A variant of Hurler's syndrome? *Am. J. Dis. Child.* **98**:577 (1959).

100. Landing, B. H. and Rubinstein, J. H., Biopsy diagnosis of neurologic diseases in children with emphasis on the lipidoses, in: *Cerebral Sphingolipidoses: A Symposium on Tay–Sachs Disease and Allied Disorders*, S. M. Aronson and B. W. Volk, eds., Academic Press, New York, pp. 1–13 (1962).

101. Sanfilippo, S. J., Yunis, J., and Worthen, H. G., An unusual storage disease resembling the Hunter–Hurler syndrome, *Am. J. Dis. Child.* **104**:553 (1962).

102. Landing, B. H., Silverman, F. N., Craig, J. M., Jacoby, M. D., Lahey, M. E., and Chadwick, D. L., Familial neurovisceral lipidosis, *Am. J. Dis. Child.* **108**:503 (1964).
103. O'Brien, J. S., Stern, M. B., Landing, B. H., O'Brien, J. K., and Donnell, G. N., Generalized gangliosidosis. Another inborn error of ganglioside metabolism? *Am. J. Dis. Child.* **109**:338 (1965).
104. Gonatas, N. K. and Gonatas, J., Ultrastructural and biochemical observations on a case of systemic late infantile lipidosis and its relationship to Tay–Sachs disease and gargoylism, *J. Neuropathol. Exp. Neurol.* **24**:318 (1965).
105. Scott, C. R., Lagunoff, D., and Trump, B. F., Familial neurovisceral lipidosis, *J. Pediatr.* **71**:357 (1967).
106. Attal, C., Farkas-Bargeton, E., Edgar, G. W. F., Pham-Huu-Trung, M. T., Girard, F., and Mozziconacci, P., Idiotie amaurotique infantile avec surcharge viscérale, *Ann. Pédiat.* **14**:457 (1967).
107. Sacrez, R., Juif, J. G., Gigonnet, J. M., and Gruner, J. E., La maladie de Landing, ou idiotie amaurotique infantile précoce avec gangliosidose généralisée de type G_{M1}, *Pédiatrie* **22**:143 (1967).
108. Okada, S. and O'Brien, J. S., Generalized gangliosidosis: Beta-galactosidase deficiency, *Science* **160**:1002 (1968).
109. Dacremont, G. and Kint, J. A., G_{M1}-ganglioside accumulation and beta-galactosidase deficiency in a case of G_{M1}-gangliosidosis (Landing's disease), *Clin. Chim. Acta* **21**:421 (1968).
110. Derry, D. M., Fawcett, J. S., Andermann, F., and Wolfe, L. S., Late infantile systemic lipidosis. Major monosialogangliosidosis: Delineation of two types, *Neurology* **18**:340 (1968).
111. Seringe, P., Plainfosse, B., Lautmann, F., Loriloux, J., Calamy, G., Berry, J. B., and Watchi, J. M., Gangliosidose généralisée du type Norman–Landing. A G_{M1}-étude a propos d'un cas diagnostique du vivant du malade, *Ann. Pédiatr.* **15**:165 (1968).
112. Suzuki, K., Suzuki, K., and Chen, G. C., Morphological, histochemical and biochemical studies on a case of systemic late infantile lipidosis (generalized gangliosidosis), *J. Neuropathol. Exp. Neurol.* **27**:15 (1968).
113. Schneck, L., Volk, B. W., and Saifer, A., The gangliosidoses, *Am. J. Med.* **46**:245 (1969).
114. Suzuki, K., Suzuki, K., and Kamoshita, S., Chemical pathology of G_{M1}-gangliosidosis (generalized gangliosidosis), *J. Neuropathol. Exp. Neurol.* **28**:25 (1969).
115. O'Brien, J. S., Generalized gangliosidosis. The clinical delineation of birth defects, *Birth Defects Orig. Art. Ser.*, **5**:190 (1969).
116. O'Brien, J. S., Generalized gangliosidosis, *J. Pediatr.* **75**:167 (1969).
117. Hooft, C., Senesael, L., Delbeke, M. J., Dacremont, G., and Kint, J., The G_{M1}-gangliosidosis (Landing's disease), *Eur. Neurol.* **2**:225 (1969).
118. Hubain, P., Adam, E., Dewelle, A., Druez, G., Farriaux, J. P., and Dupont, A., Étude d'une observation de gangliosidose à G_{M1}, *Helv. Paediatr. Acta* **24**:37 (1969).
119. MacBrinn, M. C., Okada, S., Ho, M. W., Hu, C. C., and O'Brien, J. S., Generalized gangliosidosis. Impaired cleavage of galactose from a mucopolysaccharide and a glycoprotein, *Science* **163**:946 (1969).
120. Wolfe, L. S., Callahan, J., Fawcett, J. S., Andermann, F., and Scriver, C. R., G_{M1}-Gangliosidosis without chondrodystrophy or visceromegaly. β-galactosidase deficiency with gangliosidosis and the excessive excretion of keratin sulphate, *Neurology* **20**:23 (1970).
121. Themann, H., Diekmann, L., and v. Bassewitz, D. B., Die Feinstruktur der menschlichen Leber bei Generalisierter Gangliosidose F_{M1}, *Beitr. pathol. Anat. allg. Pathol.* **140**:194 (1970).

122. Takebayashi, S., v. Bassewitz, D. B., and Themann, H., Feinstrukturelle Veränderungen der Niere bei generalisierter Gangliosidose G_{M1}, *Virchows Arch. B.* **5**:301 (1970).
123. Suzuki, Y., Crocker, A. C̆., and Suzuki, K̆., G_{M1}-gangliosidosis. Correlation of clinical and biochemical data, *Arch. Neurol.* **24**:58 (1971).
124. Hooft, C., Vlietinck, G., Dacremont, G., and Kint, A., G_{M1}-gangliosidosis type II, *Eur. Neurol.* **4**:1 (1970).
125. Emery, J. M., Green, W. R., Wyllie, M. B., and Howell, R. R., G_{M1}-gangliosidosis: Ocular and pathological manifestations, *Arch. Ophthal. Mol.* **85**:177 (1971).
126. Hadley, R. N. and Hagstrom, J. W. C., Cardiac lesions in a patient with familial neurovisceral lipidosis (generalized gangliosidosis), *Am. J. Clin. Pathol.* **55**:237 (1971).
127. Patton, V. M. and Dekaban, A. S., G_{M1}-gangliosidosis and juvenile cerebral lipidosis: Clinical, histochemical and chemical study. *Arch. Neurol.* **24**:529 (1971).
128. Goldberg, M. F., Cotlier, E., Fichenscher, L. G., Kenyon, K., Enat, R., and Borowsky, S. A., Macular cherry-red spot, corneal clouding and galactosidase deficiency: Clinical, biochemical and electron microscopic study of a new autosomal recessive storage disease, *Arch. Intern. Med.* **128**:387 (1971).
129. Backwinkel, K.-P., v. Bassewitz, D. B., Diekmann, L., and Themann, H., Ultrastructure of heart muscle in generalized gangliosidosis G_{M1}, *Z. Kinderheilk* **110**:104 (1971).
130. O'Brien, J. S., G_{M1}-gangliosidosis, in: *The Metabolic Basis of Inherited Disease,* J. B. Stanbury, J. B. Wyngaarden, and D. S. Fredrickson, eds., McGraw-Hill, New York, pp. 636–662 (1972).
131. Nihei, K., Abe, T., Kamoshita, S., and Suzuki, M., An autopsy case of generalized gangliosidosis, *Clin. Neurol.* **12**:329 (1972).
132. Taori, G. M., Basu, D. K., Chandi, S., Raman, P. T., Abraham, J., Leelavathy, R., and Job, C. K., G_{M1}-gangliosidosis, *J. Neurol. Sci.* **21**:77 (1974).
133. Lowden, J. A., Cutz, E., Conen, P. E., Rudd, N., and Doran, T. A., Prenatal diagnosis of G_{M1}-gangliosidosis, *New Engl. J. Med.* **288**:255 (1973).
134. Kaback, M. M., Sloan, H. R., Sonneborn, M., Herndon, R. M., and Percy, A. K., G_{M1}-gangliosidosis type I: *In utero* detection and fetal manifestations, *J. Pediatr.* **82**:1037 (1973).
135. Pilz, H., Sandhoff, K., and Jatzketwitz, H., A disorder of ganglioside metabolism with storage of ceramide lactoside, monosialoceramide lactoside and Tay–Sachs ganglioside in brain, *J. Neurochem.* **13**:1273 (1966).
136. Max, S. R., Maclaren, N. K., Brady, R. O., Fishman, P., Tallman, J., Garcia, J. H., Cornblath, M., Tanaka, J., Viloria, J. E., and Kamijyo, Y., G_{M3} gangliosidosis: A new lipid storage disease with a defect in ganglioside biosynthesis, presented at the 50th Annual Meeting of the American Association of Neuropathology, Boston, Mass., June 1974.
137. Jørgensen, L., Blacksted, T. W., Harkmark, W., and Steen, J. A., Niemann–Pick disease: Report of a case with histochemical evidence of neural storage of acid glycolipids, *Acta Neuropathol.* **4**:90 (1964).
138. Garcia, J. H., personal communication
139. Adachi, M., Schneck, L., Cara, J., and Volk, B. W., Spongy degeneration of the central nervous system (van Bogaert and Bertrand type; Canavan's disease). A review, *Human Pathol.* **4**:331 (1973).

EPIDEMIOLOGY*

STANLEY M. ARONSON

Quantitative appraisals of genetically determined diseases such as the gangliosidoses are only accurate to the degree to which the affected populations under study are genotypically homogeneous. It is certainly apparent that any genetic survey which includes the inadvertent pooling of phenotypically similar, but genetically different, disorders can lead to misleading conclusions.

The identification of a particular storage disease in earlier published surveys was based upon such gross clinical features as the age of onset, the presence or absence of hepatosplenomegaly, blindness or macular degeneration, and the duration of survival. As a result of these indefinite and frequently subjective clinical characteristics, the likelihood of grouping medically heterogeneous disorders became a major epidemiological risk. Cases were at times recorded which were, by the crude criteria available, intermediate between two diseases and were designated variously as instances of late onset of one disorder or precocious onset of another. When unorthodox cases were examined, awkward designations such as Tay–Sachs disease with visceral involvement, pseudo-Hurler's disease, juvenile Tay–Sachs disease, and juvenile amaurotic idiocy were frequently employed. It became apparent that such terms as idiocy or Tay–Sachs disease were sometimes employed to define a disease of ganglioside metabolism and at other times to denote a generic grouping subsuming most lipid storage diseases associated with blindness.

---

* Dedicated to the memory of Dr. Melissa L. Richter.

STANLEY ARONSON. Brown University, Miriam Hospital, Providence, Rhode Island.

Recognition of certain pathologic characteristics increased the degree of reliability in distinguishing the various forms of gangliosidosis, particularly when certain techniques became available. The development of ultrastructural capabilities in the last two decades, has provided a major morphologic tool for a more precise characterization of sphingolipid storage disorders by revealing that the stored cytoplasmic lipid assumes the form of small, numerous, membrane-bound structures, and further, that the morphology of these abnormal organelles is almost pathognomonic for each of the lipidoses.

Still a higher level of diagnostic refinement was achieved when the storage material was biochemically defined. Beginning with Klenk's pioneer efforts, it became apparent that Tay–Sachs disease (TSD) was distinguishable from the other classical lipidoses (e.g., Niemann–Pick and Gaucher's disease) by virtue of the progressive intracellular incorporation of a water-soluble glycolipid referred to as a ganglioside.[1] More detailed studies, particularly by means of chromatographic techniques, disclosed that the gangliosides represented a family of related substances rather than a structurally single compound. Application of these more refined analytic procedures has led to the recognition that there is more than one form of gangliosidosis.

In the last decade, still further resolution of these clinically similar disorders was achieved by recognition that the basic biochemical anomaly underlying each of these disorders consisted of an absence or notable deficiency of a specific lysosomal glycohydrolase.

The original gangliosidosis, Tay–Sachs disease, has now been joined by four other disorders (Table 1), all inherited as autosomal recessive traits, all commencing in infancy and early childhood, and all characterized clinically by unremitting central nervous system deterioration and pathologically by the continuing storage of ganglioside material within the neurons and occasionally nonneural cells. Each of these disorders of ganglioside metabolism appears to be genotypically discrete since there are no published reports suggesting two varieties of gangliosidosis in the same family constellation.

Other than TSD, the currently identified forms of gangliosidosis are each very rare. Thousands of cases of TSD have been identified in the last few decades.

Much of the data incorporated in this chapter are derived from a case registry of the cerebral sphingolipidoses which was begun at the Isaac Albert Research Institute in 1954 as a repository for accumulating demographic, genetic, and epidemiological information pertinent to these disorders.[2]

TABLE 1. Biochemically Defined Gangliosidoses

Classification	Eponym	Mode of inheritance	Approximate gene frequency
[G_{M1} (0)]	Norman–Landing	Autosomal recessive	<0.005
[G_{M1} (A)]	Derry	Autosomal recessive	<0.001
[G_{M2} (B)]	Tay–Sachs	Autosomal recessive	0.03 (Jews)
			<0.003 (non-Jews)
[G_{M2} (0)]	Sandhoff	Autosomal recessive	<0.003
[G_{M2} (AB)]	Bernheimer–Seitelberger	Autosomal recessive	<0.001

Mode of Inheritance

Analysis of Sibship Data

A total of 380 cases of clinically verified TSD [G_{M2} (B)] derived from 306 families contained within the Registry noted above were considered. The diagnosis in a significant number of these 380 cases was further substantiated by histopathological examination.

The familial character of this disease was clearly evident when reviewing these sibships. For example, 27.5% of the 224 families with two or more offspring contained two or more cases of TSD. The clinical components of the disorder were totally absent in the parents of children with TSD, in accordance with the recessive nature of the trait. More recent serum hexosaminidase studies in the parents of patients with TSD have shown concentrations intermediate between the normal range and the severely depressed range characteristic of the homozygous state, thus further suggesting the recessive heterozygous condition of the parents.

A factorial evaluation of collected TSD sibships is another means for the quantitative verification of the recessive characteristic of the disease.

In an autosomal recessive disease with complete penetrance, one-fourth of all offspring should be recessive homozygotes while three-fourths are either heterozygotes or normal homozygotes. Through expansion of the binomial expression $(q + 3p)^n$, where q represents the frequency of TSD, $3p$ indicates the normal phenotypes, and n is equal to the number of children within the sibships, the probability of disease frequency in sibships of any size may be theoretically calculated. If the *observed* frequency of disease in sibships of varying size closely approximates these *calculated* rates, one may then conclude that the hereditary mode of the disease is compatible with that of a recessive transmitted trait.

For example, in families of three children, this binomial expression is expanded to

$$q^3 + 9q^2p + 27qp^2 + 27p^3$$

This expression may be interpreted as follows: in the 64 three-child families constituting this expansion 1 family (q^3) will have all three children with the disease, 9 families ($9q^2p$) will have two of three children afflicted, 27 families ($27\,qp^2$) will have one of three children afflicted, and 27 families ($27p^3$) will have no children clinically affected. Thus, of 192 sibs (in the 64 sibships) 48 should theoretically be affected, an incidence of 25%, which is in conformity with a recessive Mendelian ratio. Obviously, though, the 27

TSD families $(27p^3)$ without clinically evident TSD in the offspring would not ordinarily be detected in those population surveys which identify TSD families exclusively by virtue of their production of a child with the disease. Those families without TSD children would therefore completely elude any statistical compilation. It becomes necessary then to alter the disease-frequency expectations for these populations in order to acknowledge the failure to detect those families in whom the parents are carriers but in whom the offspring fail to show the disturbance. These 27 hypothetical families $(27p^3)$ must therefore be subtracted from the 64 sibships, thus leaving 37 three-child families (111 children), of which 58 are affected with TSD [truncated frequency $(58/111)$ = 43.2%]. Calculations of a similar nature for families with two or more children will result in the calculated percentages expressed in column D of Table 2. These calculated percentages of affected children diminish as the size of the sibship increases, and the frequencies asymptotically verge upon the Mendelian frequency of 25% as the sibship size approaches infinity. When the two sets of frequencies (i.e., columns E and F) are sufficiently close, this may be taken to indicate that a recessive mode of transmission is the likeliest explanation for the quantitative dispersion of the disease. In the case of these 306 TSD families, 364.4 cases were expected and 380 cases were actually observed.

Of the other forms of ganglioside storage disease, only $[G_{M1} (0)]$-gangliosidosis has been identified in adequate numbers of cases to even warrant this form of sibship analysis. Again, the data would suggest a recessive mechanism of trait transmission. Nineteen cases have been verified in 14 families. A total of 18 cases were anticipated while 19 instances were observed (Table 2).

Sex Frequency

Earlier surveys (Table 3) regarding TSD indicated a predominance of the disease in female infants.[3,4] In the 36 years of his experience with the disease, Sachs noted that 76% of his 23 cases were female.[5] Slome, in a comprehensive review article incorporating all published cases up to 1933, also remarked upon a moderate preponderance of cases in the female.[3] Other series, however, have noted a male majority in their cases, including the present compilation (Table 4), indicating 206 cases in males and 174 cases in females. There were, however, more unaffected males than females in those 306 sibships and the frequency of disease in males (55.8%) did not differ appreciably from the encountered disease frequency in the females (53.7%).

TABLE 2. Observed and Calculated Frequency of $[G_{M2}(B)]$ (TSD) and $[G_{M1}(0)]$ under the Autosomal Recessive Hypothesis

A, Size of sibship	B, Number of families TSD	C, Total number of children (A × B)	D, % Children with TSD, expected	E, Number of children with TSD, expected (C × D/100)	F, Number of children with TSD, observed	G, Number of families $[G_{M1}(0)]$	H, Total number of children (A × G)	I, Number of children with $[G_{M1}(0)]$ expected (H × D/100)	J, Number of children with $[G_{M1}(0)]$ observed
1	82	82	100.0	82.0	82	4	4	4	4
2	112	224	57.1	127.9	135	3	6	3.4	4
3	81	243	43.2	105.2	105	3	9	3.9	4
4	18	72	36.5	26.3	25	2	8	2.9	2
5	9	45	32.8	14.8	19	1	5	1.6	2
6	2	12	30.4	3.6	7	0	0	0	0
7	0	0	28.8	—	0	0	0	0	0
8	1	8	27.7	2.2	3	1	8	2.2	3
9	1	9	26.9	2.4	4	0	0	0	0
Total	306	695		364.4	380	19	40	18.0	19.0

TABLE 3. Male : Female Frequencies in Various Collected Series of Cases of TSD

	Male		Female	
Source	Total number of sibs	Number with TSD	Total number of sibs	Number with TSD
Slome[3]	140	49	174	63
Goldschmidt *et al.*[4]	30	17	49	32
Kozinn *et al.*[12]	?	34	?	24
Present series[14]	369	206	326	174
Total		306 (51%)		293 (49%)

Table 3 shows the sex frequency in the various collected series of cases of TSD in the available literature. Of the 599 cases thus identified, 306 (51%) were males and 293 (49%) were females, suggesting that the earlier reports of sex predominance may represent bias in data collection.

Of the 18 published cases of $[G_{M1} (0)]$-gangliosidosis, 7 were females and 11 were males.[6] In the case of the other gangliosidoses, the numbers of cases are far too inadequate to render any judgment concerning the sex frequency.

TABLE 4. Male–Female Distribution in 306 Tay–Sachs Disease Sibships[a]

Family size	Affected		Unaffected	
	Male	Female	Male	Female
1	44	38	0	0
2	70	65	46	43
3	63	42	70	68
4	12	13	24	23
5	11	8	12	14
6	5	2	4	1
7	0	0	0	0
8	0	3	4	1
9	1	3	3	2
Total	206	174	163	152
		380		315

[a] Total sibship population = 695, total TSD cases = 380 (54.7%).

Birth Order

While birth rank is apparently not a phenomenon of biological significance in terms of the risk of TSD, a review of the data in Table 5 brings to light the predictable observation that the birth of an affected child, regardless of order, generally signals a family decision to avoid further conception. This voluntary truncation of fertility results in obviously higher frequencies of TSD in the terminal births of sibships of varying sizes.

One may calculate the anticipated frequency of TSD in the last offsprings of these families. In one particular analysis of 242 TSD families,[7] 148.7 cases of TSD were expected while 196 were actually recorded, probably indicating the bias introduced by the conscious decision to forego further pregnancies.

The sibship size in the currently considered series of TSD families varies, up to 9 children. The average number of children in the 306 families is 2.27. The ages of the parents at the time when children with TSD were born have shown no unusual variation from normal distribution of parenthood age in the United States.

Table 6 summarizes data regarding birth order, disease frequency, and religion as it pertains to a series of 25 cases of Niemann–Pick disease, a disorder of sphingolipid metabolism bearing some clinical and histopathological similarities to TSD.

Multiple Births

Twin births were recorded in seven of the 687 TSD family term pregnancies. Additional instances of twin births in TSD families, from

TABLE 5. Effect of Birth Rank Among Jewish TSD Cases in Families of Sibship Size of Two or More

Sibship size	Birth rank								Total number of cases
	1	2	3	4	5	6	7	8	
2	28	65							93
3	16	15	35						66
4	4	2	4	7					17
5	1	1			3				5
6									
7	1			1		1	1		4
8						1	1	1	3
Total	50	83	39	8	3	2	2	1	188

TABLE 6. Niemann–Pick Disease: Data Regarding Birth Order, Disease Frequency, and Religion

Family No.	Registry No.[a]	Religion	Birth order 1	2	3	4	Number of abortions (spontaneous)	Number of affected (NPD)	Total viable offspring
1	1	Jewish	F	(M)=(M)[b]			?	2	3
2	40	Jewish	(F)				0	1	1
3	50	Jewish	M	(M)			0	1	2
4	83	Jewish	(F)	(F)			0	2	2
5	104	Jewish	(M)	M	(F)		0	2	3
6	169	Jewish	(F)				0	1	1
7	181	Jewish	(M)				1	1	1
8	241	Jewish	(M)	M			0	1	1
9	257	Jewish	F		(M)		0	1	3
10	267	Jewish	(F)				1	1	1
11	295	Jewish	(M)				1	1	1
12	313	Jewish	(M)	F			0	1	2
13	317	Jewish	(M)				0	1	1
14	328	Non-Jewish	(M)				1	1	1
15	329	Non-Jewish	M	F	(F)		1	1	3
16	334	Jewish	(M)				0	1	1
17	340	Non-Jewish	(M)	(F)			0	2	2
18	347	Jewish	(M)				0	1	1
19	379	Jewish	(M)				0	1	1
20	381	Non-Jewish	(M)	(M)	F	F[c]	1	2	4
Total							5	25	35
Ratio[d]			16/20	6/10	3/4	0/1			

[a] Numbers signify Sphingolipidosis Registry number.
[b] Twin birth; parentheses indicates affected child.
[c] Newborn; too young to determine whether affected.
[d] Numerator = total number affected in birth order; denominator = total number in birth order.

TABLE 7. Twin Births in Tay–Sachs Disease Families

No.	Source[a]	Birth order	Sex[b]
1	Reg. No. 38	2	F – (M)
2	Reg. No. 55	2	M – (M)
3	Reg. No. 206	2	F – (M)
4	Reg. No. 209	2	M – (F)
5	Reg. No. 232	8	M – F
6	Reg. No. 245	2	F – (M)
7	Reg. No. M-25	1	(M) – (M)
8	Reg. No. 322	1	(F) – (F)
9	Ref. No. 8	3	F – F
10	Ref. No. 9	4	(M) – (M)
11	Ref. No. 10	7	F – (M)
12	Ref. No. 11	2	F – (F)

[a] Reg. No. = Registry case number, Ref. No. = Reference number.
[b] Parentheses signify an affected child.

published sources, are also incorporated in Table 7. One of the two twin children was affected with TSD in seven sets of twins; in three sets of twins, both offspring were affected; and in two sets, neither was affected. Only twin numbers 7, 8, 9, and 10 in Table 7 are likely to be monozygotic since the others showed a lack of concordancy in either the factor of sex or the presence or absence of TSD. This ratio of 4:12 is in accordance with the usual observation that monozygosis is generally encountered in about one-third of twins.

Twins have not been encountered in publications concerning the other forms of gangliosidosis.

Gene and Carrier Frequencies

The frequency of the gene responsible for TSD may be estimated by extrapolative techniques, by direct ascertainment means, or, in more current times, by direct determination of the serum levels of the lysosomal enzyme, Hex A.

Estimates Based on Disease Frequency

The number of cases of TSD recorded per unit time (in a defined population), related to the total number of births (for the same time span and group), should provide the basic information necessary to determine the frequency of the disease and the frequency of the gene in the general population under scrutiny. This, of course, requires that all infants homozygous for the trait under inquiry shall indeed develop the disease (i.e., that the disease is fully penetrant) and that all cases of TSD, or other gangliosidoses, be fully recognized and recorded during life.

In terms only of a particular trait such as TSD, three varieties of genotype may characterize a generation of a defined population: patients with TSD (recessive homozygotes), carriers (heterozygotes), and normals (dominant homozygotes). Within this population, the frequency of the gene for TSD may be expressed as q and its normal allele p, such that $q + p = 1$.

The ratios of these three possible genotypes within a particular population are therefore determined by the Hardy–Weinberg equilibrium which is $q^2:2pq:p^2$. It is obvious that the ratio of patients to carriers is $q^2:2pq$. In extremely rare diseases (i.e., where the value of p begins to approximate 1), this ratio may be simplified to $q:2$ (i.e., the carrier frequency is approximately twice the gene frequency). Thus, if the incidence of a particular autosomal recessive disorder in a defined population is recorded to be 1 case per 1000 births (i.e., $q^2 = 0.001$), then the gene frequency $q = 0.032$, the carrier frequency $(2pq) = 0.062$, and therefore the ratio of patients to carriers is about $1:62$. If there were 1 case per 5000 births (i.e., $q^2 = 0.0002$) then the gene frequency $q = 0.014$ and the carrier frequency $(2pq) = 0.028$ and the ratio of patients to carriers is $1:140$. The more rare the gene in a specified population, the greater will be the ratio of abnormal homozygotes (patients) to carriers.

Since 1952 there have been a number of comprehensive case surveys attempting to determine the gene and carrier frequencies for TSD. Slightly varied ascertainment techniques have been employed. Goldschmidt et al.[4] have reviewed the death registry of the Central Statistical Bureau of Israel, Kozinn and associates[12] studied the death certificates in New York City for a 12-year period, and Myrianthopoulos[13] reviewed the death certificates of the Bureau of Vital Statistics of the United States, particularly the rubrics for mental deficiency. Despite these slightly modified data bases and despite the fact that different geographical areas were surveyed, there is a surprising uniformity in the estimated gene frequencies within these various surveys (Table 8) within both Jewish and non-Jewish populations of the United States and Israel. The carrier rate among Jews in the United States, as indicated in the accompanying table, varies between 2.2% and 3.0%. The three independently conducted estimates of the gene frequency among non-Jews in the United States cluster around 0.3%.

If these approximate magnitudes of gene frequency are accepted, it now becomes possible to approximate the number of TSD-gene carriers in the present population of the United States (Table 9). About 792,000 het-

TABLE 8. Estimation of Gene Frequency for Tay–Sachs Disease by Case Ascertainment in Jews and Non-Jews

Source	Location	Years surveyed	Number of cases of TSD	Estimated number of births	Incidence of TSD, q^2	TSD gene frequency q	Carrier frequency, $2pq$
Jews							
Goldschmidt et al.[4]	Israel	1948–1952	31	153,200	0.00020	0.014	0.028
Kozinn et al.[12]	New York City	1944–1955	58	450,000	0.00012	0.011	0.022
Myrianthopoulos[13]	United States	1952–1955	56	352,000	0.00016	0.013	0.025
Present series[14]	New York City	1951–1960	86	380,000	0.00023	0.015	0.030
Non-Jews							
Kozinn et al.[12]	New York City	1944–1955	3	1,350,000	0.0000022	0.0015	0.003
Myrianthopoulos[13]	United States	1952–1955	27	15,460,000	0.0000017	0.0013	0.0026
Present series[14]	New York City	1951–1960	3	1,150,000	0.0000026	0.0016	0.0032

TABLE 9. Estimated Number of Carriers of Tay–Sachs Disease According to Religion

Area	Religion	Population	Carrier frequency	Estimated number of carriers
New York City	Non-Jewish	6,000,000	0.003	18,000
New York City	Jewish	1,750,000	0.03	52,500
United States	Non-Jewish	205,000,000	0.003	615,000
United States	Jewish	5,900,000	0.03	177,000

erozygotes are projected, the majority of whom (78%) are non-Jews. Thus, while the majority of TSD genes are found in the non-Jewish genetic pool, the dilution of the gene in that population is far greater and hence the risk of TSD homozygosity is appreciably smaller than in the Jewish population.

Carrier frequency for the TSD trait is 10-fold higher in the Jewish than non-Jewish population, and the incidence of TSD is 100-fold higher in the Jewish population of the United States. TSD appears approximately once in every 4000 Jewish births and once in every 400,000 non-Jewish births. O'Brien and colleagues estimate that about 52 new cases of TSD will be born per year in the United States and about 300 cases per year in the world population.[15]

Evidence will be reviewed later regarding still further nonrandom frequencies of this gene within subgroups of the Jewish and non-Jewish population.

Estimates Based on Frequency of TSD in First Cousins

There is an alternate method for the inferential determination of gene frequency based upon the number of TSD cases in the first cousins of probands.

The probability that the parent (aunt or uncle) related to the proband is a carrier is 0.5 since this parent is a sib of a known carrier (the parent of a child with TSD). The probability of the carrier state ($2pq$) in the parent unrelated to the proband is unknown but presumed to equal the carrier rate of the ethnic group from which he or she is derived. The risk of TSD in any single birth from parents, both of whom are carriers, is 0.25. The risk of TSD therefore in a first cousin (C) related to a population of TSD probands may then be expressed as follows:

$$C = (0.5)(2pq)(0.25)$$

or

$$2pq = 8C$$

Four cases of TSD were found among 1047 first cousins of the Jewish TSD index cases ($C = 0.0038$). Applying this to the equation above

$$2pq = 8(0.0038) = 0.003$$
$$q = 0.015$$

These heterozygote and gene frequency values for the United States Jewish population are in close accordance with the estimates reached by direct ascertainment procedures summarized in Table 8.

Estimates Based on Serum Hexosaminidase Concentrations

It has been shown in recent years that the essential enzymatic deficit in TSD is represented by the functional absence of N-acetyl-β-D-hexosamini-dase A, an acid hydrolase which functions normally in converting G_{M2}-ganglioside into G_{M3}-ganglioside through the cleavage of the terminal N-acetylgalactosamine residue of the former.[16-18] Two components of this hydrolase have been identified (Hex A and Hex B).[19] The combined hexosaminidase activity can be measured fluorometrically by its action upon a number of synthetic substrates. Since Hex A undergoes virtually complete denaturation by heating at 50°C for 3–4 hours (while the B fraction remains unaffected by this procedure), a determination of the separate fractional activities thus becomes possible. Alternatively, an acrylamide gel electrophoretic separation has been employed.[18]

Numerous laboratories have found that serum assay for Hex A is of great utility in detecting heterozygotes within TSD families and high-risk populations.[20]

It has been pointed out that TSD is the first recessive genetic disorder amenable to effective community screening efforts.[20] If properly designed and implemented, such a screening program can prevent the occurrence of this invariably fatal and untreatable disease of infancy. Three factors have made this feasible. First, the disease occurs in an ethnically well-defined population (arising one hundred times more frequently in Jewish children of East European ancestry); second, a deficiency of Hex A in serum is a proven and reliable genetic marker of the carrier state and the test is simple, essentially inexpensive, and reproducible; and third, should a pregnancy arise in a marriage partnership composed of two carriers, that techniques are now available to determine the presence or absence of TSD in the evolving fetus. Through the process of amniocentesis and the subsequent laboratory cultivation of amniotic fluid cells, it is now possible to infer the genetic status of the fetus with regard to TSD (i.e., whether the fetus is a normal homozygote, a carrier, or an abnormal homozygote). If the fetus is deemed to have TSD by biochemical criteria, the parents may then choose to terminate the pregnancy. Both biochemical and ultrastructural studies of those fetuses aborted have verified the predictive accuracy of this sequence of procedures.[21,22] Adachi and colleagues have performed a hexosaminidase analysis of cultured amniotic cells derived from 27 pregnancies with a high risk for TSD. An absence of Hex A was recorded in seven cases, and in all seven the pregnancies were terminated.[22] The prenatal diagnosis of TSD was confirmed in all cases by the ultrastructural demonstration of abnormal cytoplasmic bodies.

The first major community screening effort for the detection of TSD carriers was accomplished with the Jewish communities of Baltimore and Washington by Kaback and Zeiger.[20] A total of 1359 adults were tested, with a genotypic assignment of carrier state in 43 (frequency = 0.0316). These figures are in close accordance with those estimates derived from ascertainment techniques (see Table 8).

[$G_{\overline{M2}}$ (0)]-gangliosidosis (Sandhoff's disease) is characterized biochemically by the intracellular storage of G_{M2}-ganglioside and globoside, as well as by the absence of Hex A and Hex B within both tissues and biological fluids of the body. In the experience of O'Brien et al., biochemically identified cases of this disorder have been confined to the non-Jewish population.[15] The distribution of cases, otherwise, appears to be pan-ethnic with no evident clustering of cases in any particular population.

Observers have failed to identify any clinical characteristics which would serve to distinguish TSD from Sandhoff's disease. It has been suggested even that the incidence of Sandhoff's disease in the non-Jewish population may actually equal the incidence of TSD in the Jewish population. It is quite likely that a significant fraction of non-Jewish TSD cases, in previous surveys, may actually have been instances of Sandhoff's disease. O'Brien and colleagues have observed that in nine non-Jewish families, ostensibly with TSD, hexosaminidase assays indicated Sandhoff's disease in four.[23] No effort has been undertaken, as yet, to survey a defined population for carriers of the Sandhoff form of gangliosidosis.

Juvenile G_{M2}-gangliosidosis [Bernheimer–Seitelberger disease (A,B)] is a very rare disorder, characterized by a partial deficit in Hex A activity. While considerably less than normal, the activity of this enzyme is clearly higher than the activity measured in the serum of patients with TSD. Quantitative methods alone are not presently adequate to distinguish the obligatory heterozygotes of juvenile G_{M2}-gangliosidosis from similar heterozygotes of TSD.

The G_{M1}-gangliosidoses, characterized by a deficiency of β-galactosidase can, in theory, be detectable in the laboratory both in homozygote and heterozygote status. No population surveys have been undertaken as yet to determine the quantitative distribution of this abnormal trait, and gene frequencies are inferred by extrapolating from the number of cases of encountered generalized gangliosidosis.

Ethnologic Characteristics

Religion

Virtually from the time of its original description TSD has been preeminent among those genetically transmitted disorders which are closely identified with one religious group or another. The three contributions of Tay in 1881, 1884, and 1892 were largely ophthalmologic commentaries and did not specify the religion of the four young patients which formed the basis of his inaugural studies.[24-26] It was later found, however, that these patients were indeed of Jewish extraction. The first cases described by Sachs were New York City infants of Jewish extraction,[11,27] as were the first patients described by Kingdon.[28] Sachs' review paper of 1896 indeed commented upon the association of this disease with children of Jewish ancestry.[27] The association appeared so compelling, indeed, that Sachs stated in 1910, "the infantile form invariably occurs among Hebrews and among them only."[29] Falkenheim, however, had noted previously that 4 of his 36 cases, collated from various European sources, were children of presumed non-Jewish origin.[8] His report, however, was brief, the diagnostic criteria were not clarified, and indeed the clinical and geneological details concerning the four presumably non-Jewish patients were not given in this 1901 report. Some isolated case publications regarding TSD made occasional mention of the disorder in non-Jews but the reports were vague and without autopsy substantiation.

In 1914 Cockayne and Attlee published the first widely accepted report of TSD in a non-Jewish infant.[30] In 1916, Tarr noted a case of amaurotic family idiocy (TSD) in a child of Syrian background.[31] Both of these reports were well documented and both included details of macular degeneration. The detailed histories faithfully followed the usual clinical evolution ascribed to TSD.

The last notions of complete religious selectivity were effectively dispelled when a case of non-Jewish TSD was reported in 1931 with autopsy verification.[32]

Over 150 cases of TSD in non-Jewish infants have now appeared in the medical literature, such children derived from every continent and arising in almost all ethnically and religiously defined populations. Since it is claimed that Sandhoff's disease cannot be differentiated clinically from TSD (although each is genotypically discrete), there is no way of assessing how many cases of non-Jewish TSD actually represent instances of Sandhoff's disease. The experience of O'Brien and colleagues using the hexosaminidase procedure on serum suggests that a substantial fraction of non-Jewish TSD cases, perhaps as much as half, are instances of Sandhoff's gangliosidosis.[23]

On the other hand, no cases of G_{M2}-gangliosidosis, other than $[G_{M2}$ (B)] (TSD), have been identified in children of Jewish extraction. It has been noted previously that the highest known incidence of TSD occurs among Jews, particularly those resident to, or emigrating from, the northeastern regions of Europe, and, before it was biochemically recognized that a substantial number of non-Jewish TSD cases were in reality Sandhoff's disease, that the ethnic differences in gene frequency were ones of degree. This view, of course, is not modified by the existence of a genetically distinct form of G_{M2}-gangliosidosis seemingly confined to non-Jewish children, except that the magnitude of difference in gene frequency between these ethnic groups is even greater than was formerly predicted.

In the absence of comprehensive hexosaminidase and galactosaminidase surveys of various populations, it is not possible to determine the gene or disease frequency of the various gangliosidoses. If the assumption is made that a child fulfilling the clinical criteria for TSD represents the genotype of either $[G_{M2}$ (B)]- or $[G_{M2}$ (0)]-gangliosidosis, then some gene-frequency projections for certain ethnic groups may still be accepted with caution.

A gross approximation of gene frequency may be achieved through knowledge of the consanguinity rates in the parents of affected children. This consanguinity rate is an inverse function of the gene frequency within the index population, and Dahlberg[33] has suggested the following equation:

$$q = \frac{C(1 - k)}{16k - 15c - Ck}$$

where c equals the first-cousin marriage rate prevailing in a regional population, k equals the first-cousin marriage rate in parents of children with an identified recessively transmitted disease, and q equals the gene frequency of the disease under inquiry. It is undoubtedly hazardous to assume that the rates of consanguinity noted in families described in medical publications necessarily represent the consanguinity rates for the unreported cases in the region.

Nevertheless, if one makes these assumptions, the high rate of consanguinity in the published reports of Chinese and Japanese TSD families suggests that the gene frequency in the Far East must be extremely low, perhaps in the order of 0.0001. There are still further dangers in making the unwarranted assumption of a uniform gene frequency within major ethnic groups. When procedures for the biochemical recognition of heterozygotes became available, the data frequently disclosed highly uneven carrier frequencies in ostensibly uniform populations.

There have been instances, of course, when geographically determined non-Jewish enclaves may show clusters of TSD cases. Studies of certain Swiss communities, by Hanhart, have disclosed a significant number of TSD cases in certain isolated valleys of Switzerland.[34]

Table 10 lists the religious affiliations recorded in various studies of TSD, including years studied and areas surveyed.

The estimates of religion are no more accurate than the memories of the families contributing such information to these investigations. In the questionnaires employed by the Sphingolipidosis Registry,[2] only three generations have been explored and no statements were subjected to independent verification. Table 11 lists the religious affiliations of the grandfathers in 283 TSD sibships.

The factor of intermarriage obscures any attempts in the direction of assigning a precise gene frequency based upon religious lineage rather than religious affiliation. For example, the intermarriage rate for German Jews during the first decade of the twentieth century was recorded as 26.6 per 100 endogamous matings.[36] The offspring of these unions were undoubtedly raised in one of the two faiths but the percent assigned to each is not readily known. An unknown number of "non-Jewish" cases of TSD may therefore

TABLE 10. Religion of Children with Tay–Sachs Disease as Noted in Published Series

Series	Source	Years surveyed	Area surveyed	Percent Jewish[a]
A	Slome[3]	1884 1933	Summary of published cases	85.8
B	Ktenides[35]	1933–1954	Summary of published cases	60.2
C	Goldschmidt et al.[4]	1948–1952	Israel	100.0
D	Kozinn et al.[12]	1944–1955	New York City	94.8
E	Myrianthopoulos[13]	1954–1957	United States	67.5
F	Present series[14]	1951–1970	United States, principally New York City	85.7

[a] The percentages regarding religion are not precisely comparable. Series A and B determined percent of cases assignable to each religion, while series C, D, E, and F determined percent of families.

TABLE 11. Religion of Children with Tay–Sachs Disease (283 Sibships)

Religion of grandparents	Number of sibships	%
All Jewish	233 ⎫	
¾ Jewish	8 ⎬	85.7
½ Jewish	3 ⎭	
¼ Jewish	3 ⎫	
All non-Jewish[a]	36 ⎭	14.3

[a] Two families in this group each described a Jewish ancestor more than three generations prior to the proband.

be descended in part from a Jewish ancestor who converted to another religion.

The initial questionnaire submitted by the parents of a particular child with TSD clearly indicated a non-Jewish maternal and paternal ancestry extending back over three generations. About a year later, the family volunteered further information regarding the child's maternal great-great-grandmother who was born in Denmark and who was alleged to be Jewish. This information prompted still further geneologic investigation which uncovered the fact that this Jewish great-great-grandmother had married a second time (to a Jewish male) and that a Jewish great-great-grandchild, born in New York City and also afflicted with TSD, was derived from the lineage of this second marriage. It is probable that this Danish forbearer was a contributor of the TSD gene to both the Jewish family living in New York City and to the non-Jewish family living in a small midwestern rural community.

TSD in Still Further Ethnic Populations

No cases of TSD have been noted in Eskimo, Melanesian, Micronesian, or Polynesian populations. It is possible that the current lack of extensive medical records or diagnostic resources among isolated peoples such as those in Oceania prevents us from having any knowledge of the true prevalence of TSD in these peoples. Only a sustained screening program employing tests such as the concentration of serum hexosaminidase would provide this information.

Documented cases of TSD (or Sandhoff's disease) have now been reliably identified in non-Jewish infants in Switzerland, France, Belgium, The British Isles, Germany, Italy, Scandinavia, Spain, Poland, Russia, as well as many other European countries.[7,37] Cases have also been noted in Asia and Africa.

The geographical origins of 152 non-Jewish grandparents (cases registered in the Sphingolipidosis Registry) are recorded in Table 12. It is interesting to note that a majority of those grandparents born in Europe did not come from the northeastern regions which typify the Jewish ancestry of TSD cases. Again it must be cautioned that an unknown but probably substantial number of non-Jewish "TSD" forbearers were indeed carriers of the gene for Sandhoff's disease.

Among the verified cases of TSD in individuals of non-Jewish background were two American Negro families.[37] Autopsy examination of these children disclosed the classical histopathological and histochemical features of TSD. Elevated concentration of ganglioside was demonstrated in the brain tissue of one case in which this was measured. The clinical presentation of these children was regarded as quite classical and included the

TABLE 12. Tay–Sachs Disease: Places of Birth of 152 Non-Jewish Grandparents

United States			
Michigan	14	New Hampshire	2
Pennsylvania	13	Ohio	2
Massachusetts	12	Tennessee	2
New York	12	Kentucky	2
Indiana	6	Maryland	2
Utah	5	West Virginia	2
Virginia	4	New Mexico	1
South Carolina	4	Oklahoma	1
Connecticut	3	New Jersey	1
Texas	3	Hawaii	1
Nebraska	3	Illinois	1
Kansas	2	Minnesota	1
North Carolina	2	Vermont	1
Rhode Island	2	District of Columbia	1
Other			
Canada	11	Yugoslavia	2
Italy	7	France	2
England	5	Eire	2
Azores	4	Czechoslovakia	1
Greece	4	Germany	1
Hungary	4	Guatemala	1
Russia	2	Lithuania	1

recognition of cherry-red spots. Still other cases of TSD have been identified in children of Black background.

Demography of Jewish TSD Ancestors

Sachs noted the disproportionately high frequency of TSD in offspring of Jews from northeastern Europe. Such immigrants, admittedly, constituted the vast bulk of the New York City population during the early decades of the twentieth century. Further collection of information however tended to strengthen Sachs' intuitive impressions.

The Jewish population of the world is by no means a homogeneous group. Social anthropologists have segregated the world Jewish population into three major but loosely defined divisions: the Ashkenazic Jews, recently derived from eastern Europe; the Sephardic Jews, residents to or derived from the southwestern and levantine areas of Europe and neighboring northwestern Africa; and the Oriental Jewish, from enclaves of Yemen, the Middle East, and southern Asia. The geographic dispersal of the original Hebraic Semites was a continuing process which was accelerated during certain historic moments.

Based largely upon Biblical citation, Groen expressed the view that the constitutional separation between the Ashkenazic and Sephardic Jewry is not a contemporary phenomenon but a reality which extended back in time to at least the fifth century B.C. [38] He expressed the view that there was little intermarriage between the Hebraic populations of the Kingdom of Israel and the Kingdom of Judea, following the partition of the unified nation after the death of King Solomon. It is presumed that many of the Jews involuntarily exiled to the Babylonian region, and representing the remote ancestors of the Ashkenazic Jews, returned to the area of Judea after their Mesopotamian liberation by Cyrus in the year 538 B.C. The Kingdom of Israel, on the other hand, was conquered by the Assyrians, and a majority of the captured Israelites were dispersed to the upper Syrian regions. It is possible that some of these displaced Israelites represent an unknown fraction of the lineage later referred to as the Sephardic Jews. Some of the upper Mesopotamian enclaves may also constitute the ancestral source of the contemporary Kurdistan Jewish groups. During the Hellenic era, Jewish colonies were established in Asia Minor, the Balkans, and even Crimea.

Between the years 62 and 135 A.D. following the destruction of The Second Temple by Titus and the subsequent unsuccessful revolt of Bar Kochba, most of the Judean Jews were involuntarily dispersed throughout the western Roman provinces of Europe, concentrating eventually in the

Rhine Valley. The westward movement of the Jews still remaining in the Babylonian region represented a more voluntary diaspora and coincided with Muslim expansion through North Africa and eventually the Iberian Peninsula, these movements occurring largely between the years 500 and 700 A.D. The further exile of the Sephardic Jews from Spain and Portugal, commencing during the latter part of the fifteenth century, spread these peoples to the Low Countries, southern France, Italy, Greece, Turkey, and the North African territories bordering upon the Mediterranean Sea.

A third, and the numerically smallest, group of Jews continued their lives in the Near East, forming the nuclei of the Yemenite, Iraqi, Kurdistan, and other Oriental Jewish enclaves.

Historic circumstances have therefore separated these major groups for over twenty centuries, although some intermingling has resumed in recent times, particularly in the United States and Israel. It must be assumed, therefore, that the gene constitution of these present-day Jewish groups represents to but a minor degree the heritage common to the original Jewish population, prior to the Assyrian and Babylonian dispersals, and, to a far greater degree, the genetic contributions of intermarriage with resident non-Jewish peoples and the effects of continuing selective pressures which rendered survival advantage of certain genotypes over others.

A survey of randomly published cases clearly indicates that the frequency of TSD is highest in the Ashkenazic Jews, intermediate in Sephardic Jews, and low in Oriental Jews.

Israel is presently populated largely by first- and second-generation Jewish immigrants from scattered areas of the world, predominantly Europe, and intermixed with a small population of original Middle East Jews. Goldschmidt and her associates have conducted careful surveys of TSD in Israel in order to ascertain the approximate gene frequency in the various Jewish ethnic subgroups mentioned above. Only cases confirmed by an ophthalmological examination and/or autopsy examination were accepted. These investigators calculated a gene frequency for TSD which was 20 times higher in the Ashkenazic (29 cases in 85,000 births) than non-Ashkenazic (Mediterranean and Sephardic) Jews (2 cases in 77,000 births). They were unable to find any cases of TSD in children from Yemenite, Iraqi, or Persian Jewish populations during their five-year period of ascertainment; nor have other investigators ever noted cases in these Oriental Jewish groups. No cases of TSD have ever been described in the small Near Eastern colonies of Samaritans ("original" Jews).

This observation, namely that the gene of TSD occurs with much higher frequency among the descendants of Ashkenazic Jews than Sephardic or Oriental Jews, has been repeatedly asserted. All major retrospective surveys concerned with this disease have noted the paucity of cases in Jews of Sephardic or Near East origin and indeed have suggested that the gene frequency in these two populations is of the same magnitude as the TSD gene frequency in the non-Jewish population of Western Europe.

An effort was then made to determine whether or not the gene for TSD is distributed randomly among the entire Ashkenazic community. These studies were undertaken prior to the development of the Hex A procedure for the detection of TSD heterozygosis and consisted of studies designed to determine the demographic origins of the Jewish grandparents of verified TSD cases. Appropriate control populations were sampled as well. It was noted that grandparents born in Germany or other West European countries were less frequent in the TSD-grandparent group than in the control group. It became further evident that particular northeastern European communities contributed a significantly larger proportion to the TSD-grandparent population than to the control population (Table 13). From this, it was cautiously inferred that the TSD gene frequency was higher in Jewish immigrants born in the Northeast Polish–Russian provinces of Kovno, Grodno, Suwalki, Latvia, and neighboring Byelorussia.

Interestingly, the forbearers of Jewish children with Niemann–Pick disease (NPD) also seem to have issued from these same contiguous territories bordering upon the Baltic Sea (Table 14). In contrast to this, the ancestry of patients with familial dysautonomia (Reilly–Day syndrome, RDS), an inherited disease encountered predominantly in Jewish children, was derived largely from the Jewish populations within the more southerly areas of eastern Europe, particularly the Balkan provinces of Bukovina, Rumania, eastern Hungary, Moldavia, and the neighboring Polish–Russian

TABLE 13. Tay–Sachs Disease: Places of Birth of 820 Grandparents of Jewish Children

Region	Percent of TSD grandparents	Percent of control grandparents[a]
Baltic provinces	12.6	5.3
Northeast Poland	13.4	7.8
Central Poland; Byelorussia	19.1	13.7
South Poland; Galicia	12.3	11.2
Ukraine; Rumania; Moldavia	14.1	14.9
Russia, other	13.4	13.2
Hungary; Czechoslovakia	6.8	5.4
Germany; West Europe	3.8	8.0
North America	4.4	20.3

[a] Based on sample of 2576 Jewish families without known cases of TSD.

TABLE 14. Niemann–Pick Disease: Places of Birth of Grandparents

Family No.	Registry No.	Maternal		Paternal	
		Grandmother	Grandfather	Grandmother	Grandfather
Jewish cases					
1	1	Lithuania	Lithuania	Lithuania	Lithuania
2	40	Poland-Russia	Pennsylvania	Missouri	Pennsylvania
3	50	Turkey	Illinois	Lithuania	Lithuania
4	83	New York	Vilno	Byelorussia	Rumania
5	104	Lithuania	Russia	Lithuania	Lithuania
6	169	Poland	Latvia	Latvia	Poland
7	181	Poland	Poland	Poland	Poland
8	241	Ukraine	Poland	Latvia	Ukraine
9	257	Ukraine	Grodno	Vilno	Grodno
10	267	New York	Rumania	New York	Germany
11	295	New York	New York	Poland	Russia
12	313	Russia	Russia	Unknown	Russia
13	317	New York	New York	New York	New York
16	334	New York	New York	New York	New York
18	347	Latvia	Vilno	Lithuania	Lithuania
19	379	Suwalki	Byelorussia	Ukraine	Byelorussia
Non-Jewish cases					
14	328	Oregon	Minnesota	Minnesota	Illinois
15	329	Pennsylvania	Pennsylvania	Pennsylvania	Pennsylvania
17	340	Illinois	Illinois	Illinois	Illinois
20	381	Ohio	Missouri	Kentucky	Kentucky

area of Krakow and Lwow (Galicia). Considerable and often reciprocal differences thus appear to prevail between the demographic profiles of the ancestors of these hereditary diseases (TSD, NPD, and RDS). The ancestors of the two sphingolipid storage disorders (TSD and NPD) emigrated predominantly from Lithuanian and adjacent territories, while the RDS progenitors appeared to stem principally from the Galician, Balkan, and Ukrainian Jewish settlements.[39] In an attempt to find a rational explanation for these nonrandom distributions, it was noted that significant parallels existed between the skewed geographic distribution of the TSD, NPD, and RDS group on the one hand, and the linguistic and cultural discontinuities which characterize Ashkenazic Jewry on the other hand. In fact, the locations of significant breaks in the distribution of inferred heterozygotes seem to correspond to the very locations of some of the important Yiddish language and culture boundaries. We would expect to find that the historical events underlying the linguistic and cultural differentiation of central and eastern European Jewry (including such factors as the chronology of settlements and the degrees of contact or isolation among geographically discrete communities) would also aid in explaining the existing heterogeneity of inherited neurological disease frequencies.

The genetic diversity of the Jewish population is further substantiated by anthropologic observations. Nathan and Haas have studied skeletons from the Judean desert attributed to periods from the second century B.C. to the second century A.D.[40] They noted wide variations in skull dimensions (both dolichocephalic and brachycephalic), suggesting considerable physical heterogeneity. It appears that some of these anthropometric differences persist to contemporary times. Sephardic Jews are predominantly dolichomesocephalic while the Ashkenazic Jews are mostly brachycephalic. In answer to the rhetorical question as to whether the Jews were *ever* a genetically homogeneous group, Dr. Milton Alter[41] has referred to Chapter XII, Verse 37 in Exodus which discusses the departure of the Jews from Egypt some 5000 years ago, ". . . and the *mixed multitude* went out also with them."

The death of each child with an autosomal recessive defect removes two lethal genes from the genetic pool and, if no other factors are operative, then the frequency of such lethal traits tend to diminish with time. The preservation or even increase in the frequency of a lethal trait in successive generations of a particular populations requires that some explanation be invoked. The major mechanisms regarded as capable of producing augmented frequencies of a lethal gene include the following: (1) differential breeding patterns, (2) genetic drift, (3) differential mutation rates, (4) differential fertility of the heterozygotes, and (5) a combination of any of these mechanisms. Differential breeding patterns, involving such forces as intermarriage with genetically different peoples and close inbreeding, does not appear instrumental since there is no evidence that TSD was present to any appreciable degree in the non-Jewish Lithuanian, Polish, or Russian populations. Furthermore, the consanguinity rates in the Jewish populations at highest risk for TSD are not abnormally high. For example, in a series of 83 TSD families, the first-cousin marriage rate among parents of afflicted infants was but 1.78%, while the first-cousin marriage rate among the Ashkenazic population ranged between 1 and 2%. Consanguinity in the Sephardic and Oriental communities, on the other hand, ranges from 7 to 29%, and yet in these populations, the frequency of the gene for TSD is quite low.

Genetic drift might be a seriously considered mechanism if it could be demonstrated that the Jewish communities of eastern Europe were indeed composed of very small marriageable populations without social contact with neighboring communities. There is, however, sufficient historic information to suggest a fertile intercommunication between the various East European Jewish communities.

The likelihood of a differential mutation rate is most improbable. The rate needed to account for the enhanced frequency of the TSD gene in the Jewish population would require about one mutation per 6000 gametes per generation (in Jews), and one mutation per 500,000 gametes per generation (in non-Jews), a most unlikely biological phenomenon. Current information suggests rather that mutation rates of specific loci tend to be constant.

The possibility of heterozygote advantage was then explored.[42]

Evidence for Heterozygote Advantage

Heterozygote advantage would indeed provide an adequate explanation for the selective increase of the TSD gene in the Northeast European Jewish communities if it could be shown that the otherwise-healthy carriers of this trait were more fertile than members of the neighboring Jewish population homozygously normal for TSD. If such were so, TSD heterozygotes would thus be able to transmit the mutant gene of TSD in greater numbers to the successive generations than would an equivalent number of coreligionists possessing the normal alleles.

The magnitude of this selective advantage required by carriers in order to maintain the frequency of the lethal TSD gene at the high level currently noted among the Ashkenazic Jewish population is given by the formula

$$S = \frac{q}{1 - q}$$

where S equals the selection coefficient against the normal homozygote. Substituting the estimated frequency of the TSD gene among Ashkenazic Jews (0.014),

$$S = \frac{0.014}{1 - 0.014} = 0.0142$$

and the fitness of the three genotypes, therefore, is

$$TT = 1 - S = 0.9858$$
$$Tt = 1$$
$$tt = 0$$

which signifies that a selective advantage of about 1.4% on the part of the TSD heterozygote is adequate to maintain the gene at equilibrium despite its mass elimination via the death of TSD homozygotes.

Since selective heterozygote advantage is ultimately expressed as a function of relative reproductive fitness, studies were undertaken to determine the relative fertility of the heterozygous carriers of the TSD gene when compared with an appropriate control population presumed not to be carriers of this gene. The unit of fertility in this study was determined as a live birth surviving to reproductive age (21 years).

As a result of these studies it became evident that consistent differences in fertility between TSD and controlled sibships emerged. Table 15 indicates the ratio of adjusted fertilities of TSD grandparents and controls. Both groups were of Jewish heritage and were born in the same decade. The observed differences in fertility were of the approximately current magnitude and in the same direction, and were therefore deemed compatible with the hypothesis that the TSD carrier has a selective biological advantage over the presumed homozygous normal. The statistical evidence for this assumption was not regarded as decisive.

Naylor, in reviewing fertility data on TSD grandparents, explored the magnitude of selective advantage necessary to raise the TSD gene from 0.0013 at the end of the first century A.D. (coincident with the onset of forced emigration of the Judean Jews to Europe) through approximately 50 generations to the late nineteenth century, when TSD was recognized as occurring chiefly among Ashkenazic Jews with a gene frequency on the order of 0.013–0.015.[43] Naylor's arithmetic calculations suggested that a selective advantage of about 4.5% would be adequate under these assumptions in order to raise the gene frequency to its present level. This is not very different from the overall advantage noted in the Table 15.

These studies, while suggesting that the presence of the TSD allele confers some biological advantage to its carrier, does not however offer any explanation for the selectively enhanced fertility of these heterozygotes.

Shaw and Smith have recently reanalyzed the epidemiological data

TABLE 15. Ratio of Adjusted Fertilities of Jewish TSD Grandparents and Jewish Controls

Population studied	TSD	Controls	Ratio
US Born			
Total siblings	1010.30	1007.22	1.0031
Siblings surviving to age 21	991.25	953.70	1.0394
Non-US Born			
Total siblings	235.85	211.34	1.1160
Siblings surviving to age 21	221.91	191.00	1.1618

TABLE 16. Distribution of TSD Grandparents and TBC Patients in Three North–South Geographic Groups[a]

Geographic group	TSD		TSD : control ratio	TBC		TSD : TBC ratio	Controls	
	Number	%		Number	%		Number	%
Northern[b]	281	45.5	1.5	324	22.1	2.0	560	33.4
Central[c]	182	29.4	0.9	269	18.4	1.6	507	30.3
Southern[d]	155	25.1	0.7	873	59.5	0.4	608	36.3
Total	618	100.0		1466	100.0		1675	100.0

[a] $X_2^2 = 221.1$, $p < 0.0005$.
[b] Baltic provinces, Northwest Poland, Vilno, and Byelorussia.
[c] Central, Southeast Poland, Galicia, Ukraine.
[d] Southern Balkan regions.

among Jewish children with TSD and have surmised that the frequency of this gene may indeed be increasing.[44] In any case, such suggestions provide further incentive for efforts to identify the selective force which might have been operative among the East European Ashkenazic communities in the areas where the antecedents of the TSD cases lived for many generations.

The most reasonable factor in attempting to explain differential survival is to attribute biological fitness in the heterozygote to resistance to some adverse agent (such as an infectious disease) conferred by the TSD gene heterozygosis. In reviewing the questionnaires of families with TSD patients, incorporated in the Sphingolipidosis Registry, the records of 306 grandparents who had died were reviewed. The usual distribution of cardio-vascular, cerebrovascular, and neoplastic diseases were recorded. What was surprising was the virtual absence of deaths ascribed to tuberculosis, a disease which was quite prevalent in northeastern Europe.

In an attempt to test the hypothesis of TSD heterozygote resistance to tuberculosis, the records of large numbers of Jewish patients with tuberculosis were reviewed particularly in terms of the places of birth of these patients.[45] Table 16 summarizes the distribution of TSD grandparents, tuberculosis patients and a control series, by region of origin. In essence, the studies showed that the frequency of tuberculosis was almost three times higher in the southeastern European Jewish population (where the TSD frequency was the lowest) and lowest in the northern region (where the TSD frequency was the highest). These results are at least consistent with the hypothesis of some resistance to tuberculosis on the part of the Jewish TSD heterozygotes.

References

1. Klenk, E., Über die Ganglioside, eine neue Gruppe von Zuckerhältigen Gehirnlipoiden, *Z. Physiol. Chem.* **273**:76 (1942).
2. Aronson, S. M., Myrianthopoulos, N. C., Schneck, L., and Volk, B. W., A sphingolipidosis registry, *Pathol. Eur.* **3**:487 (1968).
3. Slome, D., The genetic basis of amaurotic family idiocy, *J. Genet.* **27**:363 (1933).
4. Goldschmidt, E., Lenz, R., Merin, S., Ronen, A., and Ronen, I., Frequency of the Tay-Sachs gene in the Jewish communities of Israel, *Abstr. 25th Ann. Meet. Genet. Soc. Am. Aug. 27, 1956.* (1956).
5. Sachs, B., The hereditary factors operative in amaurotic family idiocy, in: *Heredity in Nervous and Mental Disease,* Hoeber, New York, p. 155 (1923).
6. O'Brien, J., Generalized gangliosidosis, *J. Pediatr.* **75**:167 (1969).
7. Aronson, S. M., Epidemiology, in: *Tay-Sachs Disease,* B. W. Volk, ed., Grune & Stratton, New York (1964).
8. Falkenheim, K., Ueber familiäre amaurotische Idiotie, *Jahrb. Kinderheilkd.* **54**:123 (1901).
9. Hymanson, A., Metabolism studies of amaurotic family idiocy, with clinical and pathological observations, *Arch. Pediatr.* **30**:825 (1913).
10. Herrman, C., A case of amaurotic family idiocy in one of twins, *Arch. Pediatr.* **32**:902 (1915).
11. Sachs, B., On arrested cerebral development with special reference to its cortical pathology, *J. Nerv. Ment. Dis.* **14**:541 (1887).
12. Kozinn, P. J., Wiener, H., and Cohen, P., Infantile amaurotic family idiocy, *J. Pediatr.* **51**:58 (1957).
13. Myrianthopoulos, N. C., Some epidemiologic and genetic aspects of Tay-Sachs disease, in: *Cerebral Sphingolipidoses: A Symposium on Tay-Sachs Disease and Allied Disorders,* S. M. Aronson and B. W. Volk, eds., Academic Press, New York, p. 359, (1962).
14. Aronson, S. M. and Myrianthopoulos, N. C., Epidemiology and genetics of the sphingolipidoses, in: *Handbook of Clinical Neurology,* P. J. Vinken and G. W. Bruyn, eds., North-Holland, Amsterdam Vol. 10, Chap. 24, (1970).
    Holland, Amsterdam Vol. 10, Chap. 24, (1970).
15. O'Brien, J. S., Okada, S., Ho, M. W., Fillerup, D. L., Veath, M. L., Adams, K. Ganglioside storage diseases, *Fed. Proc. Fed. Am. Soc. Exp. Biol.* **30**:956 (1971).
16. Okada, S. and O'Brien, J. S., Tay-Sachs disease: Generalized absence of beta-D-N-acetylhexosaminidase component, *Science* **165**:698 (1969).
17. Kolodny, E. H., Brady, R. O., and Volk, B. W., Demonstration of an alteration of ganglioside metabolism in Tay-Sachs disease, *Biochem. Biophys. Res. Commun.* **37**:526 (1969).
18. Friedland, J., Schneck, L., Saifer, A., Pourfar, M., and Volk, B. W., Identification of Tay-Sachs disease carriers by acrylamide gel electrophoresis, *Clin. Chim. Acta* **28**:397 (1970).
19. Robinson, D. and Stirling, J., *N*-Acetyl-beta-glucosaminidase in human spleen, *Biochem. J.* **107**:321 (1968).
20. Kaback, M. M. and Zieger, R. S., Heterozygote detection in Tay-Sachs disease: A prototype community screening program for the prevention of recessive genetic disorders, in: *Sphingolipids, Sphingolipidoses and Allied Disorders,* B. W. Volk and S. M. Aronson, eds., Plenum Press, New York (1972).

21. Schneck, L., Friedland, J., Valenti, C., Adachi, M., Amsterdam, D., and Volk, B. W., Prenatal diagnosis of Tay–Sachs disease, *Lancet* 1:582 (1970).
22. Adachi, M., Schneck, L., and Volk, B. W., Ultrastructural studies of eight cases of fetal Tay–Sachs disease, *Lab. Invest.* 30:102 (1974).
23. O'Brien, J. S., Ho, M. W., Okada, S., Zielke, K., Veath, M., and Tennant, L., Sphingolipidoses: Detection of heterozygotes and homozygotes, in: *Sphingolipids, Sphingolipidoses and Allied Disorders*, B. W. Volk and S. M. Aronson, eds., Plenum Press, New York (1972).
24. Tay, W., Symmetrical changes in the region of the yellow spot in each eye of an infant, *Trans. Ophthalmol. Soc. U.K.* 1:55 (1881).
25. Tay, W., A third instance in the same family of symmetrical changes in the region of the yellow spot in each eye of an infant, closely resembling those of embolism, *Trans. Ophthalmol. Soc. U.K.* 4:158 (1884).
26. Tay, W., A fourth instance of symmetrical changes in the yellow spot region of an infant, closely resembling those of embolism, *Trans. Ophthalmol. Soc. U.K.* 12:125 (1892).
27. Sachs, B., A family form of idiocy, generally fatal, associated with early blindness, *J. Nerv. Ment. Dis.* 21:475 (1896).
28. Kingdon, E. C., A rare fatal disease of infancy, with symmetrical changes at the macula lutea, *Trans. Ophthalmol. Soc. U.K.* 12:126 (1892).
29. Sachs, B., quoted in: Davies, A. J., Report of two cases of amaurotic familial idiocy in infants of non-Jewish parentage, *J. Am. Inst. Homeopathy,* 21:830 (1928).
30. Cockayne, E. A. and Attlee, J., Amaurotic family idiocy in an English child, *Proc. Roy. Soc. Med. Ophthalmol. Sec.* 8:65 (1914).
31. Tarr, E. M., A case of amaurotic family idiocy of non-Jewish parentage, *Louisville Month. J. Med.* 22:353 (1916).
32. Gear, J. N., Jr., Infantile amaurotic family idiocy with report of a case in a child of non-Jewish parentage, *South. Med. J.* 23:324 (1930).
33. Dahlberg, G., On rare defects in human populations with particular regard to inbreeding and isolate effects, *Proc. Roy. Soc. Edinburgh* 58:213 (1938).
34. Hanhart, E., Über 27 Sippen mit infantiler amaurotischer Idiotie (Tay–Sachs), *Acta Genet. Med. Gemellol.* 3:331 (1954).
35. Ktenides, M., Au subjet de l'hérédité de l'idiotie amaurotique infantile (Tay–Sachs), Thesis No. 2264, L'Université de Genève (1954).
36. Engelman, U. Z., *The Rise of the Jew in the Western World,* Behrman Publishers, New York, pp. 187–201 (1944).
37. Aronson, S. M., Valsamis, M. P., and Volk, B. W., Infantile amaurotic family idiocy. Occurrence, genetic considerations and pathophysiology in the non-Jewish infant, *Pediatrics* 26:229 (1960).
38. Groen, J., Gaucher's disease. Hereditary transmission and racial distribution, *Arch. Intern. Med.* 113:543 (1964).
39. Aronson, S. M., Herzog, M., Brunt, P., McKusick, V., and Myrianthopoulos, N. C., Inherited neurologic diseases of Ashkenazic Jewry: Demographic data suggesting non-random gene frequencies, *Trans. Am. Neurol. Assoc.* 92:117 (1967).
40. Nathan, H. and Haas, H., Anthropological data on the Judean desert skeletons, in: *The Genetics of Migrant and Isolate Populations,* E. Goldschmidt, ed., Williams and Wilkins, Baltimore, Md. (1963).
41. Alter, M., In discussion of Reference 39.
42. Myrianthopoulos, N. C. and Aronson, S. M., Population dynamics of Tay–Sachs disease. I. Reproductive fitness and selection, *Am. J. Hum. Genet.* 18:313 (1966).

43. Naylor, A., In discussion of Reference 42.
44. Shaw, R. F. and Smith, A. P. Is Tay–Sachs disease increasing? *Nature (London)* **224:**1214 (1969).
45. Myrianthopoulos, N. C. and Aronson, S. M., Population dynamics of Tay–Sachs disease. II. What confers the selective advantage upon the Jewish heterozygote? in: *Sphingolipids, Sphingolipidoses and Allied Disorders,* B. W. Volk and S. M. Aronson, eds., Plenum Press, New York (1972).

CELL CULTURE STUDIES

DANIEL AMSTERDAM

Cultured cells can mirror and preserve the enzyme defect or defects that cause the individual to be afflicted. An enzyme present in multiple tissues of the body is readily accessible for study via peripheral blood and/or in biopsy of the skin or other tissues of the living individual. Enzymatic activity with diverse *in vivo* tissue distribution is, as a rule, found in the usual type of human cell culture—the diploid fibroblast. In addition to providing definitive diagnosis of the full-blown metabolic defect, cell culture can be used for diagnosis of the heterozygote state when enzyme function may be found to be intermediate between normal homozygote individuals and homozygote defectives. Maintenance of enzyme markers in culture also provide experimental models for the study of enzyme controls and effects at the cellular level in that cells derived from the affected human can be used rather than those from a more remote type of a cell system. That a single enzyme can exist in several, i.e., multimolecular, forms suggests that isoenzymes can cause different clinical diseases, or a spectrum of involvement within one disease group, or that the same clinical signs of an enzyme deficiency could result from multiple types of molecular defects. Thus, the patient's own defective enzyme frequently needs to be studied both qualitatively and quantitatively in order to understand and treat his disease effectively. The diagnosis of an enzymatic defect rests upon demonstration of de-

DANIEL AMSTERDAM. Isaac Albert Research Institute of the Kingsbrook Jewish Medical Center, Brooklyn, New York.

fective enzymatic activity. This demonstration is often only possible in cultured cells from the affected individual.

The Biology of Human Cells

Cell Types

Cells grown in the laboratory result in one of two types of cultures, depending on the origin of the tissue from which the cells were derived and the properties of the cultured cells themselves.[1] Heteronuclear cell lines originate from malignant tissues whose karyotypes exhibit considerable variation, even among cells of a single clone, and are presumably different from the donor's original karyotype. Lines appear to have an unlimited life span, are epithelioid in appearance, and grow in suspension or as monolayers. Homonuclear cell strains originate from nonneoplastic autopsy or biopsy material and are characterized by their fibroblastic morphology, stable karyotype, and limited lifetime. These and other differences are detailed in Table 1. Because homonuclear cells are endowed with a limited life expectancy and cannot withstand serial propagation for indeterminable periods of time, early-passage generations are stored in liquid-nitrogen refrigerators so as to preserve cells early in their life span so that they can be retrieved at any time for additional study. Cell strains can be grown only as monolayers on the surface of plastic or glass vessels. Although variation and

TABLE 1. Characteristics of Cell Lines and Cell Strains

Heteronuclear cell lines	Homonuclear cell strains
Originate usually from malignant tissue	Originate from biopsy material or autopsy material which is nonneoplastic
Karyotype inherently unstable and yields cytogenetic variants; exhibits considerable variation	Chromosomal karyotype exhibits little or no variation from cell to cell; karyotype like that of donor
Indefinite life span	Finite life span; 50 ± 10 generations
Epithelioid in appearance	Fibroblastic in appearance
Nonmotile	Motile
High plating efficiency on cloning	Low cloning efficiency; thought to result at least in part from the leakiness of the cells, i.e., the fact that they readily lose cellular metabolites to the medium
Grow as monolayers or suspension	Grow only as monolayers

modification of this cultural procedure is available, e.g., roller culture,[2,3] it still acts as a limiting factor in obtaining large yields of cell populations.

Human diploid fibroblasts in culture exhibit similarities to normal cellular aging *in vivo*.[4] Homonuclear cells have been delegated a finite life span of 50 ± 10 generations.[4] The cell's life expectancy in culture is determined by and inversely related to, the chronologic age of the donor and can be altered or modified by the pathological state of the individual or by the intervention of oncogenic agents.[5] The entire life span of serially propagated normal cells is divided into three phases: the primary growth phase (phase I) subsequent to explanation is characterized by slow initial proliferation. This is followed by eugonic, rapid growth (phase II). In the last stage (phase III) cells display decreased capacity for proliferation and granulation, and ultimately degenerate. It is during this terminal stage that the cell is susceptible to metabolic deregulation.

Growth support requirements of human cell cultures are not completely understood. Essentially, cells require a carbohydrate—usually glucose—a mixture of balanced salts, vitamins, cofactors, and amino acids. The sole nondefined component which is necessary to complete any basal medium is the protein adjuvant, horse, calf, or fetal calf serum. In many experimental procedures it is imperative to delimit one or more of the nutritive components and this is readily accomplished. However, because of the ill-defined nature of serum, problems can arise. Specifically, horse and bovine sera can contribute to the glycosphingolipid concentration of cells,[6] serve as a source of hexosaminidase enzymes,[7] and harbor potential viral contaminants. The contribution of glycosphingolipids can be eliminated by employing fetal calf serum;[6] thermolabile hexosaminidase A (Hex A) activity can be inactivated, and viral activity is not readily detectable.

Enzymes in Cultured Cells

The assay of enzymes in serial passages of fibroblasts resulting from the explant of organ or skin tissue or in amniotic fluid cell cultures poses questions as to the stability and constancy of enzymes in cultured cells. Since the growth of diploid cells is constantly modulated by the aging process, differences would be expected between cells in various growth phases, as well as between cell types.

As new cell growth is being established there is an initial lag (phase I) during which cellular adaptation occurs. It is during this lag phase that metabolic activity is profoundly affected by a great array of enzymatic activities.[8] Initially, enzymes are synthesized discontinually at periods in the cell cycle, producing characteristic step patterns similar to that for the macromolecular synthesis of biopolymers. Some cells produce a peak pattern, whereas others produce a step pattern which is related to the lability of the enzyme. If the enzyme is unstable, a peak pattern is usually produced followed by a general degradation.

Early work on the stability of enzymes in cultured cells indicated that the levels of various dehydrogenases and phosphatases in KB cells (a heteronuclear line) were stable over a three-day interval.[9] Although this is indicative of steady-state controls operating within the cell culture system, it did not take into account differences between cell types and variability that could result from serial propagation.

Isoenzymes have been used as a means of characterizing animal cell cultures. DeOca and co-workers[10] found that isoenzymes could be used to characterize and identify animal cell cultures derived from a variety of species. The particular enzymes studied were glucose-6-phosphate dehydrogenase and lactic acid dehydrogenase patterns of 86 animal cell lines using starch gel electrophoresis. From the data it was possible to construct a fingerprint identification chart which represented 20 out of 22 taxonomic groups. The relationship between this kind of fingerprint analysis of cells derived from species can be contrasted with the concept of isoenzymes of serum from individuals afflicted with various inborn errors of metabolism. Patterns of enzyme activity in relation to subculture are also characteristic of an enzyme. This is supported by Cristofalo et al.,[11] who demonstrated that acid phosphatase, alkaline phosphatase, and lactic dehydrogenase vary between cell types, and further, that enzyme activities for phosphatases, dehydrogenases, and transaminases fluctuate during the growth and aging of WI38 cells.[11,12] Other studies with diploid WI38 cells evidence temporally related changes on serial subcultivation in the relative amounts of a cathodal esterase, acid and alkaline phosphatase, glucosaminidase, and β-glucouronidase.[13,14] Fibroblasts cultured from galactosemic patients have been shown to have negligible enzyme activity initially, and after subculture the enzyme activity increased.[15] Cyclical changes in the activity of lactic dehydrogenase have also been noted.[8]

The degree of cell confluency in culture can affect enzyme activity. An increase in the activity of glucose-6-phosphate dehydrogenase,[8] glucouronidase,[16] hexosaminidase,[17] and a galactose transferase[15] have been noted as the culture accumulates a number of cells and becomes confluent. Additionally, the activity of certain glycolipids[18] increases as the culture reaches a state of confluency. Other factors contributing to cyclic variation in enzyme levels of cultured cells are the nutrient medium and the mode of culture.[19,20]

Thus, the detection of heterozygotes could easily be confused if cell cultures were compared at different stages of growth. When using somatic cells for diagnosis the investigator must be cognizant of the variability in enzymatic activity depending upon the origin of the cells, i.e., amniotic, fetal, or adult. Our own experience with cells derived from patients with G_{M2}-gangliosidoses has indicated that, although passage variations are observed in Hex A and Hex B levels, the homozygosity or heterozygosity is maintained within the accepted ranges.

Amniocentesis and Amniotic Cell Culture

The indications,[21,22] risks, techniques,[23,24] and applications of amniocentesis for prenatal diagnosis have been adequately discussed by others.[24-31]

Transabdominal amniocentesis is rapidly becoming, or has already been, accepted as an effective therapeutic modality for genetic counseling. More than 8000 transabdominal amniocenteses have been performed, and over 500 were completed between the 14th and 22nd week of pregnancy. The procedure, when performed under meticulous, aseptic conditions, appears to carry minimal risk for the mother and fetus. Although the incidence of complications of amniocentesis is less than 1%, the procedure should be reserved for specific indications and performed only by those with previous experience. Prior localization of the placenta by ultrasound (sonorgraph) or radioactive-isotope scan may be helpful in avoiding an anteriorly implanted placenta. The privacy of the fetus can be invaded by transabdominal amnioscopy, an experimental procedure utilizing fiber optics to sight the fetus. This would enable the obstetrician to visualize the fetus, sex it, or determine the presence or absence of major, external, congenital abnormalities, or both. The instrument, when appropriately modified, could sample fetal skin or blood for metabolic and enzymatic studies.

Antedating the development of techniques for obtaining and culturing fetal cells, the counsel frequently given to parents in previous decades consisted mainly of informing them that a genetically abnormal child would likely result, or advise them against future pregnancies. The only alternative was to accept another defective child. With the development of the cultural and biochemical techniques, options can be offered. In the case of the ganglioside storage diseases therapy is unavailable, and abortion represents an alternative in the guise of a veto power.

Mothers who are likely candidates for amniocentesis and are considered "high-risk" can be divided into several groups: those who are known to be carriers of abnormal genes or chromosomes, women who have been biochemically screened and represent the maternal half of a high-risk couple, women closely related to a person with a known chromosomal or metabolic disorder, mothers over 35 years of age, and women with a history of repeated abortion.

The Amniotic Fluid

The composition of amniotic fluid represents a dynamic balance which continually changes during development of the fetus. The amniotic fluid can be considered as a mixture composed of a solution in which are suspended undissolved solids. These solids may be organized, i.e., possess a cellular component, or unorganized. The unorganized, undissolved materials are substances derived from the products of conception, the fetus, the cord, the fetal surface of the placenta, or the amnion.

Viable cells in the fluid are derived from various tissues: epithelial cells from the urinary tract or respiratory tract, amniotic cells, or fibroblasts. The number of viable cells continually vary, as they are shed into the fluid during the course of fetal development. Hence, primary cultures obtained from the amniotic fluid must be passaged in order to obtain sufficient cells to detect chemical abnormalities.

Amniotic fluid removed during the second trimester may be examined before or after *in vitro* culture. The optimum time for consistent cell growth is during the 16th and 17th week of gestation. At this time 175–250 ml of amniotic fluid is present, and the withdrawal of 15–20 ml apparently produces no untoward effect on the fetus or mother. However, the time necessary to obtain a sufficient number of cells for prenatal diagnosis of metabolic diseases poses a problem because of the availability of current techniques. When fluid is withdrawn the material obtained in this direct manner can be used to determine the sex,[32] blood group,[33] and any chromosomal abnormality[34-36] of the fetal cells. Although chromosome studies can be completed in two weeks, three to six weeks may be required to grow a sufficient quantity of cells for biochemical determinations. As most amniocenteses are undertaken at 16–17 weeks of gestation, only a short span remains until the 22nd week of pregnancy, when therapeutic abortion becomes hazardous to the mother and occasionally ethically objectionable to the obstetrician. The diagnosis of the expression of any phenotypic genetic disorder is difficult and hazardous to execute for any biochemical assay on the small number of viable cells obtained directly from the amniocentesis procedure. Thus, it is necessary to culture cells obtained from the amniotic tap.

Initiation of Amniotic Fluid Culture

The procedural outline for antenatal detection using amnion cells is indicated in Figure 1. The diagnoses of cultured cells for any hereditary disorder is dependent upon the outcome of many variables.

The number of viable amniotic cells per cubic centimeter apparently increases between the 11th and the 34th week of pregnancy.[37] However, because of the possibility that a therapeutic abortion may be opted by the mother, the period providing the optimum condition for culture with a possibility of pregnancy interruption occurs between the 15th and 18th week of gestation. Many techniques have been described for the culture of

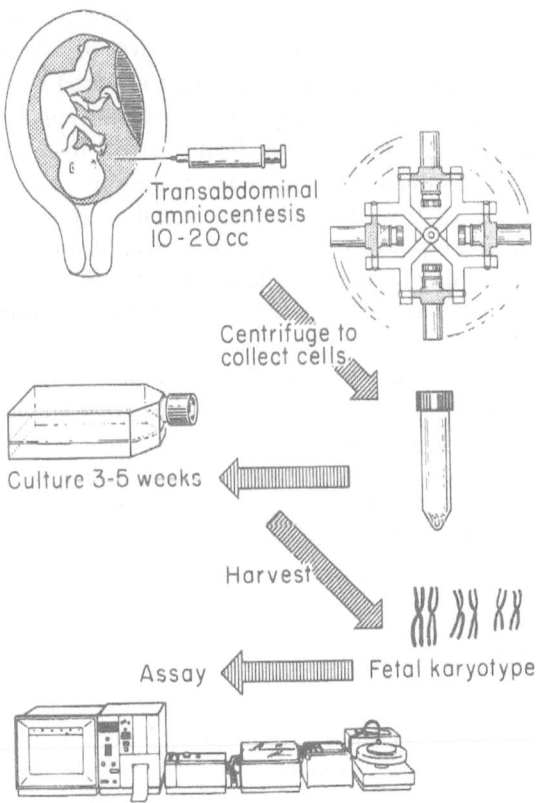

Transabdominal amniocentesis 10-20 cc

Centrifuge to collect cells

Culture 3-5 weeks

Harvest

Assay

Fetal karyotype

FIGURE 1. Antenatal diagnosis of genetic disease.

amniotic fluid cells,[38-42] including the using of amniotic fluid itself as the initial culture medium.[42] Fluids contaminated with maternal blood can pose difficulties in culture procedure and confuse fetal diagnosis, but techniques are available for eliminating the red blood cells.[43] During the early second trimester, the fetal cells shed into the amniotic fluid are mostly epithelial and fibroblastic in nature. On culture, however, the fibroblastic types survive. Cells obtained from the amniotic fluid can be categorized as cell homonuclear strains. The term "fibroblast-like" applied to those cells does not clearly assign any embryologic significance but rather refers to the appearance of the cells in culture as spindle-shaped units.

Problems relating to the culture of amniotic cells can pose potential sources of error in diagnoses. As noted above, a paucity of viable cells or contamination of cells with maternal blood will delay or confuse diagnosis. Prolonged subculture is undesirable as it may delay diagnosis and incur potential risks of contamination, mutation, or differential selection of cell types in the *in vitro* environment. The enzyme level of cells will vary with their passage and with the type of nutrients that are used by different laboratories. Cultures may become contaminated with mycoplasma or Gram-negative bacteria, and this not only may lead to errors in culture results, but the latter case will terminate and vitiate the procedure. Viral agents which do not immediately destroy the cells may significantly alter the enzyme activity. Some of these problems can be minimized if one employs storage techniques of the cultured amniotic cells in the early-passage generations so as to make them available for verification analyses or future investigations.[44] The storage of cells under liquid nitrogen can be established with little loss in viability as compared to prefreeze viability. The methodology is similar to that of established cell strains and lines and employs a cryoprotective compound like glycerol (see Appendix E).

All of the ganglioside storage diseases discussed in this work will be considered as metabolic disorders with a recognizable phenotype expressed in cultured fibroblasts, which means that one can obtain these cells either from the amniotic fluid culture or from skin-biopsy material.

Experience with Amniotic Fluid Cell Cultures

Experience in our laboratory with amniotic fluid cell cultures has been directed for the antenatal diagnosis of the sphingolipidoses, mainly Tay–Sachs disease. To date, we have attempted to culture 74 amniotic fluid cell specimens; approximately one-third were initiated in other laboratories and sent to us. The success rate for achieving a confluent cell population for enzyme analysis is depicted in Table 2. Of the 13 specimens which could not

TABLE 2. Amniotic Fluid Cell Cultures[a]

| | Basal culture medium | |
	Eagle's MEM	McCoy's
Number of fluids	48	26
Days in culture prior to harvest		
Range	7–56[b]	7–30
Mean	22	16
Successful cultures		
Number	35	25
%	77	96

[a] Unpublished data from this laboratory.
[b] 34 fluids remained in culture 7–34 days.

be harvested from MEM, 12 were lost due to contamination. The increased success ratio achieved with McCoy's medium also reflects greater experience gained during later studies when this medium was introduced. However, the average time in culture for strains cultured in Eagle's MEM was 22 days; this time was reduced to 16 days when McCoy's medium was utilized. Thus far, experience does not suggest any differences in achieving confluent cell yields between mothers at risk for the gangliosidoses as compared to others.

Other Cells from Antenates and Neonates

Cells obtained from the urines of infants less than two days old and those gestational ages ranging from 31 to 48 weeks can be cultured. Cells collected from older children failed to grow.[45] These cells can be used to achieve a cytogenetic screening of the developing fetus.[46] To the best of our knowledge none of these cultures have been used for enzymatic assays.

Enzymatic Defects

Tay–Sachs Disease [G_{M2} (B)]

Hexosaminidase components were first demonstrated by Robinson and Stirling.[47] Later, it was found that total β-galactosaminidase activities were elevated in brain tissue from patients with Tay–Sachs disease (TSD).[48]

Okada and O'Brien[49] then reported that of the two hexosaminidase moieties, Hex A and Hex B, which occur in human brain tissue, the Hex A component is absent in TSD. In TSD, Hex A cannot be detected in liver, brain, skin, kidney, leukocytes, serum, and cultured skin fibroblasts.[49] Yet, both Hex A and Hex B are present in these tissues in control subjects. Skin fibroblasts cultivated from heterozygotes have intermediate values of Hex A[17] (see also Chapter 3 in this volume). While both Hex A and Hex B are present in cultured amniotic-fluid cells obtained by amniocentesis from control subjects in the second trimester of pregnancy,[49] Hex A is absent or present in traces in the developing TSD fetus. This data was applied in the initial antenatal diagnosis.[50] The application of Hex A determination as a universal criterion for prenatal diagnosis has been challenged by a recent study which reported the absence of Hex A in the father of a TSD infant.[51]

Sandhoff's Disease [G_{M2} (0)]

Sandhoff *et al.*[48] documented deficiencies in β-D-N acetyl-galactosaminidase and β-D-N-acetylglucosaminidase in the brain and kidney of their patients. Furthermore, while there are deficiencies of both Hex A and B to the same extent, other lysosomal enzymes are present in either normal or increased amounts. The primary enzymatic deficit persists in cultured cells.[17] Because the specific activity of hexosaminidase varies with the confluence of the culture growth, the kinetics of enzyme activity must be considered in the detection of heterozygotes using skin-fibroblast cultures or in prenatal diagnosis using amniotic cell cultures.

Bernheimer–Seitelberger Disease [G_{M2} (A,B)]

O'Brien[52] and Suzuki[53] demonstrated a partial deficiency of Hex A in the [G_{M2} (A,B)] disorder. The deficiency is present in brain, liver, serum,[54] and cultured skin fibroblasts.[17] Diminished Hex A levels were found in the serum of the parents of patients,[54] and their values are within the range of individuals who are heterozygous for the TSD gene. Assay of the enzyme in cultured amniotic cells predicted a normal birth.

Norman–Landing Disease [G_{M1} (0)]

This storage disease entity was shown to be due to the accumulation of G_{M1}-ganglioside which is the result of a marked deficiency of a lysosomal β-

galactosidase that normally participates in its breakdown.[55] The diagnosis of Norman–Landing disease can be documented by β-galactosidase assay of leukocytes,[56] urine,[57] and skin biopsies.[58] The defect persists in cultured fibroblasts after many generations.[58] Heterozygotes exhibit β-galactosidase levels intermediate between homozygotes and controls.[56] Amniotic fluid cells obtained by amniocentesis display the enzyme activity. A β-galactosidase assay can be used to diagnose homozygotes prenatally and postnatally and to detect individuals heterozygous for the gene for this disease. The defect has been diagnosed *in utero*.[59,60]

Derry's Disease [G_{MI} (A)]

A marked deficiency of β-galactosidase, using synthetic substrates, has been found in tissues from patients with Derry's disease.[61] A β-galactosidase deficiency in this disorder is present in leukocytes, and assays of leukocytes from parents give intermediate values.[61,62] Cultured skin fibroblasts also demonstrate a profound deficiency of the enzyme after many passage generations.[58]

Histochemistry and Morphology

In much the same manner as tissues taken directly from the affected individual and stained for identifying various storage diseases, cultured cells can similarly be used (see Chapter 4 in this volume). Cells grown in monolayer culture may be accumulated directly on coverslips contained in Petri dishes. When a sufficient growth is obtained, the coverslips can be removed and stained for examination. The advantage of this procedure is that the cells cultivated on the coverslips are flat and do not require freezing, embedding, and sectioning.

Skin fibroblasts cultured from patients with a variety of storage diseases have been studied with the aid of the electron microscope.[63-65] Their common feature is that they display a variety of cytoplasmic inclusions, considered to be lysosomes which have retained substances due to a specific enzyme deficiency. Yet, although many of these storage disorders display identifiable cytoplasmic inclusions in the cultured cells, none have been demonstrated in the gangliosidoses. A sole exception was noted by Dawson *et al.*[7] as an unpublished finding for TSD fibroblasts. In these studies the investigators were cognizant that serial propagation of cells that have become senescent in culture may be accompanied by progressive increase in the number and size of lysosomes, which can exhibit profound alterations.[66,67]

Gangliosides in Cultured Cells

Gangliosides are recognized as significant and necessary components of brain.[68] It is also apparent that they are present in extraneural tissues, although in lesser quantities than found in brain.[69] There have been several reports of gangliosides in cultured cells. Human skin fibroblasts from normal subjects do not contain detectable amounts of G_{M1}- and G_{M2}-ganglioside.[6] The G_{M3}-ganglioside was detectable in all mammalian cells tested, including mouse 3T3 fibroblasts, (Swiss and Balb) BHK cells, a rat glial tumor, and mouse neuroblastoma lines. The G_{M1}- and G_{M2}-gangliosides were found in the Balb mouse 3T3 and the neuroblastoma cell lines.[6] Yogeeswaran et al.[70] confirmed the results with 3T3 cells. Prior to the report by Dawson and co-workers,[6] Hakomori and Murakami[71] detected in hamster fibroblasts the presence of a hematoside which decreased markedly in amount following transformation by polyoma virus. Gangliosides have also been reported in L cells grown in suspension,[72] a variety of cultured kidney cells,[73] in mouse cells transformed by SV40 and polyoma virus,[74,75] and in a rat hepatoma line.[76]

Although fibroblasts derived from patients afflicted with the gangliosidoses repeatedly express the enzymatic defect in culture, the heritable defect in degradation of these substances which results in their accumulation *in vivo* remains routinely undetectable *in vitro*.[7]

Culture of Neural Tissue

The mammalian brain is comprised of diverse cell populations with varied functions. In order to appreciate and understand these functions at the cellular and molecular levels, first, classes of cells types, and, then, individual cell types must be characterized. It would be of considerable aid in investigations of the ganglioside storage diseases, and indeed other diseases of the nervous system, if it were possible to isolate neurons in large numbers with reasonably intact processes and completely free of contamination.

Methods for the separation of neuronal from glial cells have been based either on microdissection techniques,[77] on explant cloning techniques, or on the dispersion of nervous tissue and subsequent isolation of cells by differential centrifugation.[78-81] Techniques for establishing brain-cell cultures capable of expressing differentiated functions have been developed.[82] However, the difficulty in separating glial cells and neurons has proved to be a major obstacle in the biochemical characterization of the components of the nervous system. Indeed, if neurons were cultivable in substantially

large numbers they would have to satisfy numerous morphologic and physiologic criteria of differentiated nervous-system functions (Table 3). The nervous system has been studied utilizing cells which were cloned in cell culture and adapted from a mouse-cell-line neuroblastoma shown to possess a major number of properties characteristic of the differentiated neuron.[83] Similarly, clonal lines of glial cells[84] and Schwann cells[85] have also been established and studied.

Although brain biopsies are no longer required in order to confirm or establish a clinical diagnosis of ganglioside storage disease, in former years it was frequently used. Assays for Hex A and Hex B have bypassed this approach.

The first work to report the propagation of cells from the brain of a TSD child was made by Batzdorf et al.[86] These investigators described cell types which grew from the explants and which were shown to accumulate ganglioside. Modification of the explant procedure was used by McKhann and co-workers[77] for culturing juvenile TSD brain. They used a disaggregation technique in which the cells were extruded with nylon mesh.

In work from this laboratory, cell types were grown which had not previously been described from explant procedures. We observed that within 12 days after planting the major outgrowth consisted mainly of macrophages. Infrequently, individual cells in the field exhibited glial-type extension processes (Figure 2). In other areas this cell type was seen as a minor component intermixed with fibroblastlike cellular elements. In these latter associations the macrophages appeared to be degenerative in that the cells were rounded and possessed little nuclear structure. Seven days after planting, the macrophages had degenerated; they rounded up, lost all evidence of

TABLE 3. Some Properties of Differentiated Neurons

Process formation	Neurohormone receptors
Neurites	Acetylcholine chemosensitivity
Neurofibrils (silver staining)	Localization of ACh^a receptors
	PGE$_1$^{a} chemosensitivity
Electrically excitable membranes	
Na$^+$, Ca^{2+} influx	Neurohormone degradation
K$^+$ efflux	AChE^a
Hyperpolarizing activation	COMT^a
Neurohormone synthesis	Miscellaneous
Acetylcholine (CAT)^a	Complex glycoproteins, glycolipids
Catecholamine (TH)^a	

^{a} Abbreviations: CAT, choline acetyltransferase; TH, tyrosine hydroxylase; ACh, acetylcholine; COMT, catechol-O-methyltransferase; AChE, acetylcholinesterase; PGE$_1$, prostaglandin E$_1$.

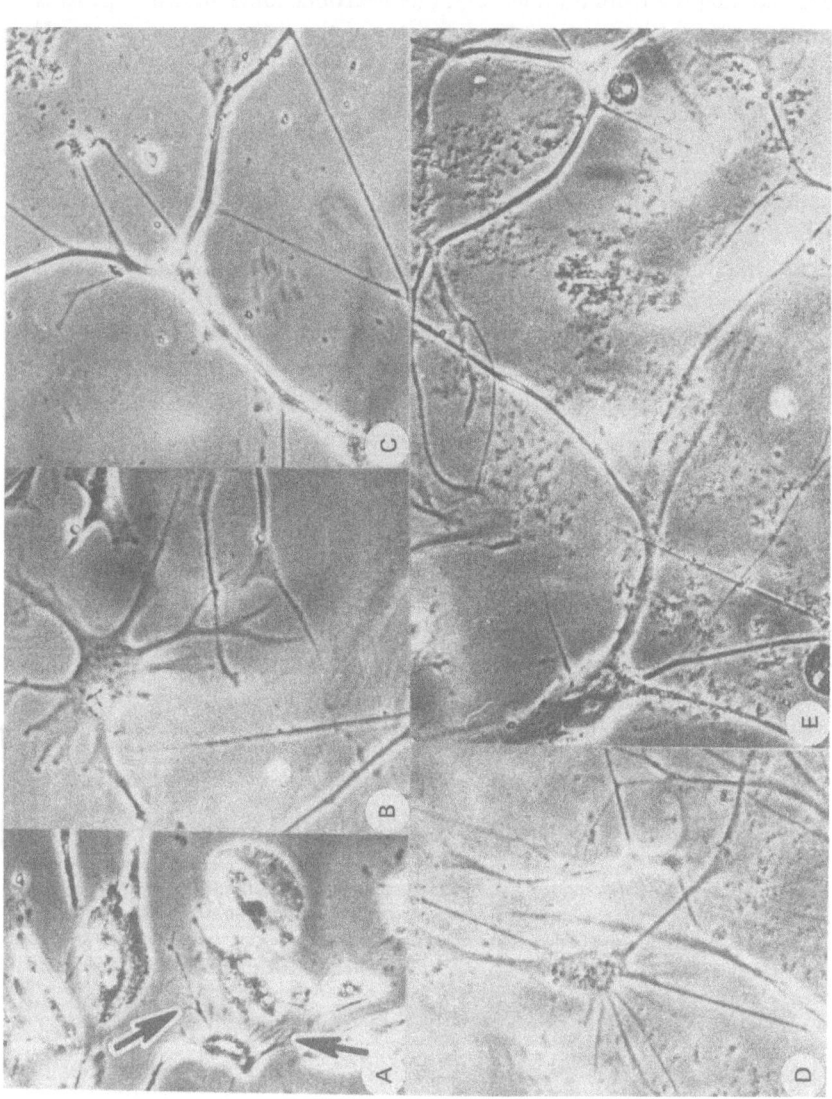

FIGURE 2. Explant culture of TSD brain biopsy. (A) macrophages 12 days after explantation, note neuritic processes (arrows); (B) protoplasmic astrocyte; (C) glial cell; (D) fibrous astrocyte, 27 days in culture; (E) neural cells, 32 days in culture. 300×

a nucleus, and were reduced to about one-half their original size; fibroblasts were still in evidence. Four weeks after tissue was explanted, new cell types appeared. Multispoked, astrocyticlike cells with a large, central, protoplasmic mass containing nuclei without distinct nucleoli were seen; other brain cell types were also noted at this time (Figure 2). Thirty-two days after planting, other glial cells were observed (Figures 2 and 3), with 11 protruding processes interlaced with other cell types. One week later (six weeks after explanting) only neural cell types which appeared to contain refractile material were observed. A fibrous astrocyte and a glial cell were included in this group (Figure 3).

Macrophages, which were the first cell types to appear, degenerated at about the third week of cell maintenance. Whether or not they gave rise to other glial elements is uncertain, or whether their senescence was required for the outgrowth of the glial elements is also questionable. Attempts to subculture any of these cell types failed.

The TSD Fibroblast as an Experimental Model

Enzyme Replacement

Currently, therapy is unavailable for any of the ganglioside storage diseases. Replacement of the deficient enzyme does not appear promising as a long-term solution, and we have discussed some of these problems in a recent review.[81] In our laboratory we have used TSD fibroblasts as a model for enzyme-replacement therapy.[87] Hex A was added exogenously to TSD cultures, however, no measurable incorporation of the enzyme into the cells was detected, as measured by activity against fluorogenic substrate or intracellular radioactivity of the ^{125}I-labeled enzyme.[87] Similarly, Tallman et al.[88] reported that Hex A added to control and TSD lysosomal preparations had no synergistic effect on G_{M2}-ganglioside hydrolysis. Porter et al.[89] observed that metachromatic leukodystrophy (MLD) cultured skin fibroblasts, pretreated with arylsulfatase A, metabolize sulfatide in a normal manner. These discordant results between the TSD and the MLD culture systems underscores the need for employing a specific culture model in each of the sphingolipidoses. A problem associated with effective enzyme modulation in lysosomal storage diseases is the alignment of the surface structural ordering of these enzymes within the lysosome. Liposomes entrapped with replacement enzyme could circumvent this kind of topological problem and the technique has been proposed for treating inherited enzyme deficiencies.[90] The use of liposomes as enzyme carriers has directed target component ap-

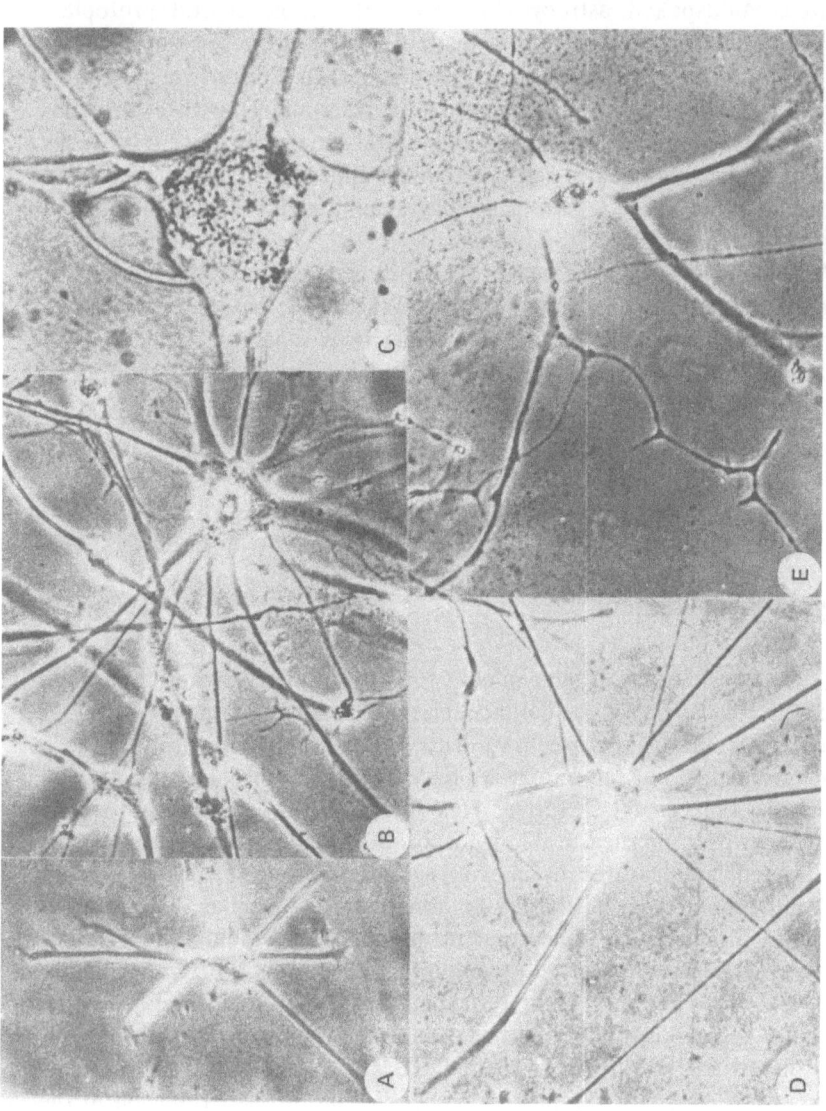

FIGURE 3. Explant culture of TSD brain biopsy. (A) glial cells, 32 days in culture, 300×; (B) fibrous astrocyte with interlaced glial cells, 32 days in culture, 300×; (C) astrocyte, 39 days after explantation, 1200×; (D) fibrous astrocyte, 39 days in culture, 300×; (E) glial cell, 39 days in culture, 300×. The latter three frames depict cells with refractile material, presumably G_{M2}-ganglioside.

plicability and bypasses the approaches which might provoke immunologic reactions or induce oncogenicity.

Genetic Studies

An alternative to enzyme replacement is the fusion of fibroblasts derived from the gangliosidoses and from normal cells mediated by Sendai virus,[91] or the co-cultivation of fibroblasts derived from the inheritable enzyme disorder with a cell containing the counterpart absent enzyme. Recently, we were able to successfully fuse TSD fibroblasts with Lesch–Nyhan (LN) cells, resulting in the expression of Hex A activity in the developing cell hybrids. The LN cells were prevented from proliferating by incorporating azaserine into the culture medium. Co-cultivation of cells derived from Sandhoff's disease with TSD cells failed to demonstrate either the Hex A or Hex B moiety in the resulting cell population.[92] However, hybridization of fibroblasts from TSD and Sandhoff's disease patients did result in detectable amounts of heat-labile Hex A when compared with assays on fusion of each of the parental cell strains.[93]

Hybridization between somatic cells *in vitro* has provided the basis for genetic analysis of these cells. In the past, human–mouse hybrids fused by Sendai virus have been used.[94] Somatic-cell hybrids provide an alternative system for linkage studies since human chromosomes, but not mouse chromosomes, are preferentially lost from proliferating hybrid cells. Linkage relationships of genes involved in the expression of Hex A and Hex B and linkage to genes from other enzyme markers have been studied. Results have led to opposing conclusions as to the partial[95] or independent segregation[96] of the two Hex forms, but both studies concur that genes coding for Hex A and Hex B are on separate chromosomes.

Another approach which does not appear to have immediate clinical application is the use of reconstructed cellular components.[97] Nuclei of normal cells can be exchanged for enzymatic-deficient nuclei. The reconstructed cell's metabolic apparatus could then be directed to deliver the proper genetic message.

Viral Susceptibility and Membrane Structure

Analysis of membrane-enclosed viruses and the events in viral assembly is important to an understanding of virus structure and replication, and it may also contribute to our knowledge of membrane structure and permeability. Certain viruses, notably SV5, have been shown to exhibit differential lytic capability based upon the ganglioside content of the membrane of the host cell which it infects. Klenk and Choppin[73] demonstrated that cells with high membrane ganglioside content are more sensitive to lysis than those cells with low ganglioside but high neutral glycolipids. The TSD cell strains derived from the central nervous system which accumulate G_{M2}-ganglioside were therefore postulated to be more susceptible to lysis than normal cells or TSD fibroblasts not derived from brain. Results of a recent study did not support this hypothesis.[98] SV5 is capable of infecting cells cultured from various TSD organs and from appropriate normal controls producing similar cytopathic results.

Conclusion and Prospectus

The heritable gangliosidoses have initiated research activity of far greater magnitude then one might expect from their relative rare occurrence. These investigations have been focused because genetic disorders afford the opportunity to merge biological concepts with the tools of biochemistry.

Clearly, for prenatal diagnoses, enzymatic assays are needed which would require less cellular material and could provide a more rapid result. Certainly, the time allotted for analysis is not as significant as the time it takes to obtain a sufficient quantity of cells for biochemical study. No less than the multiple risks inherent in such delays are the tensions created for the prospective parents and within the family. Single-cell analytic techniques will do doubt satisfy this condition.[99]

Although the heralded advances in genetic tinkering have yielded such elegant approaches as enzyme replacement and enzyme-entrapped carriers, virion messengers and macromolecule information intercalation, and somatic hybridization and cellular rearrangement, none have, as yet, mollified the clinical course of any of the ganglioside storage diseases.

Cell-surface phenomena of the mammalian membrane are manifest by hexosamine-containing macromolecules, specifically glycosphingolipids and glycoproteins. Numerous biologic properties have been ascribed to the role of these compounds at the surfaces of mammalian cells, e.g., blood group specificities, histocompatability antigens, tumor-specific antigenic activity which is responsible for the abnormal biologic behavior of tumor cells, and receptor sites for viruses. Because investigators have appreciated the importance of these cell-surface interactions, the existence of the gangliosidoses have achieved signal attention.

Cultured cells can provide an experimental tool for the investigation of the biological role of gangliosides. Since they play an important role in membrane recognition, manipulation of the culture medium or transformation of the cell by oncogenic viruses would permit one to correlate the changes in ganglioside patterns with changes in cell-contact inhibition, alteration in receptor sites of the plasma membrane, as well as changes in membrane permeability to various ions and water-soluble compounds. Cell culture models can also serve to identify control points in the regulation of positive and negative feedback systems in glycolipid and glycoprotein synthesis. The introduction of labeled gangliosides monitored by cytochemical as well as ultrastructural analysis should provide further insight into the evolution of the morphological changes that result in the disease state. Chromosomal linkage studies using somatic-cell hybridization is of obvious importance in understanding the genetic regulation of various disease entities. Finally, cell culture models provide a useful experimental system for evaluating the efficacy of enzyme replacement and enzyme induction in these heritable disorders.

References

1. Green, H. and Todaro, G. J., The mammalian cell as differentiated microorganism, *Annu. Rev. Microbiol.* **21**:573 (1967).
2. House, W. and Wildly, P., Large scale production of tissue cells and virus, *Lab. Pract.* **14**:594 (1965).
3. Taylor, G. C., Huey, N. J., Bramblett, G. H., and Moore, J. A., Production of monolayer cell cultures in roller bottles. A pilot study, *In Vitro* **2**:128 (1966).
4. Hayflick, L., The limited *in vitro* lifetime of human diploid cells strains, *Exp. Cell Res.* **37**:614 (1965).
5. Goldstein, S., The biology of aging, *N. Engl. J. Med.* **285**:1120 (1971).
6. Dawson, G., Matalon, R., and Dorfman, A., Glycosphingolipids of cultured human skin fibroblasts. I. Characterization and metabolism in normal fibroblasts, *J. Biol. Chem.* **247**:5944 (1972).
7. Dawson, G., Matalon, R., and Dorfman, A., Glycosphingolipids of cultured human skin fibroblasts. I. Characterization and metabolism in fibroblasts from patients with inborn errors of glycosphingolipid and mucopolysaccharide metabolism, *J. Biol. Chem.* **247**:5951 (1972).
8. DeMars, R., Some studies of enzymes in cultivated human cells, *Natl. Cancer Inst. Monogr.* **13**:181 (1964).
9. Yagil, G. and Feldman, M., The stability of some enzymes in cultured cells, *Exp. Cell Res.* **54**:29 (1969).
10. DeOca, F. M., Macy, M. L., and Shannon, J. E., Isoenzyme characterization of animal cell cultures, *Proc. Soc. Exp. Biol. Med.* **132**:462 (1969).
11. Cristofalo, V. J., Kabalyian, J. R., and Kritchevsky, D., Enzyme activities of some cultured human cells, *Proc. Soc. Exp. Biol. Med.* **126**:273 (1967).
12. Cristofalo, V. J., Animal cell cultures as a model system for the study of aging, *Adv. Gerontol. Res.* **4**:45 (1972).
13. Milisaukas, V. and Rose, N. R., Immunochemical quantitation of enzymes in human diploid cell line WI-38, *Exp. Cell Res.* **81**:279 (1973).

14. Turk, B. and Milo, G. E., An *in vitro* study of senescent events of human embryonic lung (WI-38) cells. 1. Changes in enzyme activities of cellular and membrane associated enzymes of untreated and cortisone acetate-treated cultures during senescence, *Arch. Biochem. Biophys.* **161**:46 (1974).

15. Russell, J. D., Variation of UDP Glu:α-D-gal-P-uridyl transferase activity during growth of cultured fibroblasts, in: *Galactosemia*, D. Y. Y. Hsia, ed., Thomas, Springfield Ill., pp. 204–212 (1969).

16. DeLuca, C. and Nitowsky, H. M., Variations in enzyme activities during the growth of mammalian cells *in vitro:* Lactate and glucose-6-phosphate dehydrogenases, *Biochim. Biophys. Acta* **89**:208 (1964).

17. Okada, S., Veath, M. L., Leroy, J., and O'Brien, J. S., Ganglioside G_{M2} storage diseases: Hexosaminidase deficiencies in cultured fibroblasts, *Am. J. Hum. Genet.* **23**:55 (1971).

18. Hakomori, S., Cell density-dependent changes of glycolipid concentrations in fibroblasts, and loss of this response in virus transformed cells, *Proc. Natl. Acad. Sci. U.S.A.* **67**:1741 (1970).

19. Cox, R. P., Regulation of alkaline phosphatase in skin fibroblast cultures from patients with mongolism, *Exp. Cell Res.* **37**:690 (1965).

20. DeLuca, C., Effects of mode of culture and nutrient medium on cyclic variations in enzyme activities of mammalian cells cultured *in vitro, Exp. Cell Res.* **43**:39 (1966).

21. Lubs, H. A. and Lubs, M. L. E., Indications for amniocentesis, in: *Antenatal Diagnosis*, A. Dorfman, ed., University of Chicago Press, Chicago, pp. 17–27 (1972).

22. Fried, K., Indications for amniocentesis, in: *Antenatal Diagnosis of Genetic Disease*, A. E. H. Emery, ed., Williams and Wilkins, Baltimore, pp. 4–10 (1973).

23. Jacobson, C. B., Techniques and risk of amniocentesis, in: *Antenatal Diagnosis*, A. Dorfman, ed., University of Chicago Press, Chicago, pp. 29–32 (1972).

24. Scrimgeour, J. B., Amniocentesis: Technique and complications, in: *Antenatal Diagnosis of Genetic Disease*, A. E. H. Emery, ed., Williams and Wilkins, Baltimore, pp. 11–39 (1973).

25. Jacobson, C. B. and Barter, R. H., Intrauterine diagnosis of genetic defects, *Am. J. Obstet. Gynecol.* **99**:796 (1967).

26. Nadler, H. L., Antenatal detection of hereditary disorders, *Pediatrics* **42**:912 (1968).

27. Nadler, H. L., Prenatal detection of genetic defects, *J. Pediatr.* **74**:132 (1969).

28. Nadler, H. L. and Gerbie, A. B., Role of amniocentesis in the intrauterine detection of genetic disorders, *New Engl. J. Med.* **282**:596 (1970).

29. Nadler, H. L., Prenatal detection of genetic disorders, in: *Advances in Human Genetics*, H. Harris and K. Hirschhorn, eds., Plenum Press, New York, Vol. 3, pp. 1–37 (1972).

30. Milunsky, A., *The Prenatal Diagnosis of Hereditary Disorders*, Thomas, Springfield, Ill. (1973).

31. Schneck, L., Amsterdam, D., and Volk, B. W., Antenatal diagnosis and therapeutic trends in sphingolipidoses, *J. Am. Med. Assoc.* **228**:615 (1974).

32. Nelson, M. M., Antenatal sex discrimination, in: *Antenatal Diagnosis of Genetic Disease*, A. E. H. Emery, ed., Williams and Wilkins, Baltimore, pp. 58–68 (1973).

33. Horger, E. O., III and Hutchinson, D. L., Diagnostic use of amniotic fluid, *J. Pediatr.* **75**:503 (1969).

34. Steele, M. W. and Breg, W. R. Jr., Chromosome analysis of human amniotic fluid cells, *Lancet* **1**:383 (1966).

35. Thiede, H. A., Creasman, W. T., and Metcalfe, S., Antenatal analysis of human chromosomes, *Am. J. Obstet. Gynecol.* **94**:589 (1966).

36. Nelson, M. M., Amniotic fluid cell culture and chromosome studies, in: *Antenatal Diagnosis of Genetic Disease*, A. E. H. Emery, ed., Williams and Wilkins, Baltimore, pp. 69–81 (1973).

37. Wahlstrom, J., Brosset, A., and Bartsch, F., Viability of amniotic cells at different stages of gestation, *Lancet* **2**:1037 (1970).

38. Valenti, C. and Kehaty, T., Culture of cells obtained by amniocentesis, *J. Lab. Clin. Med.* **73**:355 (1969).

39. Marchant, G. S., Evaluation of methods of amniotic fluid cell culture, *Am. J. Med. Technol.* **37**:391 (1971).

40. Cedergvist, L. L., Wennerstrom, C., Senterfit, L. B., Baldrige, P. B., and Rothe, D. J., Simplified method for the accelerated growth of amniotic fluid cell cultures, *Am. J. Obstet. Gynecol.* **116**:871 (1973).

41. Chitham, R. G., Quayle, S. J., and Hill, L., The selection of a method for the culture of cells from amniotic fluid, *J. Clin. Pathol.* **26**:721 (1973).

42. Gray, C., Davidson, R. G., and Cohen, M. M., A simplified technique for the culture of amniotic fluid cells, *J. Pediatr.* **79**:119 (1971).

43. Lee, C. L. Y., Gregson, N. M., and Walker, S., Eliminating red blood cells from amniotic fluid samples, *Lancet* **2**:316 (1970).

44. Greene, A. E., Trojl, L., Nichols, W. W., and Coriell, L. L., Amniocentesis cells: Culture, cryogenic storage, isozymes, and finite life *in vitro, In Vitro* **9**:156 (1973).

45. Sutherland, G. R. and Bain, A. D., Culture of cells from the urine of newborn children, *Nature (London)* **239**:231 (1972).

46. Sutherland, G. R., Grace, E., and Bain, A. D., Metaphase chromosomes from neonatal urine, *Humangenetik* **17**:273 (1973).

47. Robinson, D. and Stirling, J. L., *N*-Acetyl-β-glucosaminidases in human spleen, *Biochem. J.* **107**:321 (1968).

48. Sandhoff, K., Andreae, U., and Jatzkewitz, H., Deficient hexosaminidase activity in an exceptional case of Tay–Sachs disease with additional storage of kidney globoside in visceral organs, *Life Sci.* **7**:283 (1968).

49. Okada, S. and O'Brien, J. S., Tay–Sachs disease: Generalized absence of a beta-D-*N*-acetylhexosaminidase component, *Science* **165**:698 (1969).

50. Schneck, L., Valenti, C., Amsterdam, D., Friedland, J., Adachi, M., and Volk, B. W., Prenatal diagnosis of Tay–Sachs disease, *Lancet* **1**:582 (1970).

51. Navon, R., Padeh, B., and Adam, A., Apparent deficiency of hexosaminidase A in healthy members of a family with Tay–Sachs disease, *Am. J. Hum. Genet.* **25**:287 (1973).

52. O'Brien, J. S., Five gangliosides, *Lancet* **1**:805 (1969).

53. Suzuki, Y. and Suzuki, K., Partial deficiency of hexosaminidase component A in juvenile G_{M2}-gangliosidosis, *Neurology* **20**:848 (1970).

54. Okada, S., Veath, M. L., and O'Brien, J. S., Juvenile G_{M2} gangliosidosis: Partial deficiency of hexosaminidase A, *J. Pediatr.* **77**:1063 (1970).

55. Okada, S. and O'Brien, J. S., Generalized gangliosidosis; beta-galactosidase deficiency, *Science* **160**:1002 (1968).

56. Singer, H. S. and Schafer, I. A., White cell β-galactosidase activity, *New Engl. J. Med.* **282**:571 (1970).

57. Thomas, G. H., β-D-Galactosidase in human urine. Deficiency in generalized gangliosidosis, *J. Lab. Clin. Med.* **74**:725 (1969).

58. Sloan, H. R., Uhlendorf, B. W., Jacobson, C. B., and Frederickson, D. S., β-Galactosidase in tissue culture derived from human skin and bone marrow: Enzyme defect in G_{M1} gangliosidosis, *Pediatr. Res.* **3**:532 (1969).

59. Kaback, M. M., Sloan, H. R., Sonneborn, M., Herndon, R. M., and Percy, A. K., G_{M1} Gangliosidosis type I: *In utero* detection and fetal manifestations, *J. Pediatr.* **82**:1037 (1973).

60. Lowden, J. A., Cutz, E., Conen, P. E., Rudd, N., and Doran, T. A., Prenatal diagnosis of G_{M1}-gangliosidosis, *N. Engl. J. Med.* **288**:225 (1973).

61. Wolfe, L. S., Callahan, J., Fawcett, J. S., Andermann, F., and Scriver, C. R., G_{M1} gangliosidosis without chondrodystrophy or visceromegaly β-galactosidase deficiency with gangliosidosis and the excessive excretion of a keratin sulfate, *Neurology* **20**:23 (1970).

62. Kint, J. A., Dacremont, G., and Vlietinck, R., G_{M1} gangliosidosis type 2, *Lancet* **2**:108 (1969).

63. Hani, J., and Leroy, J., and O'Brien, S. S., Ultrastructure of cultured fibroblasts in I-cell disease, *Am. J. Dis. Child.* **122**:34 (1971).

64. Kamensky, E., Philippart, M., Cancilla, P., and Frommes, S. P., Cultured skin fibroblasts in storage disorders, *Am. J. Pathol.* **73**:59 (1973).

65. Rutsaert, J., Menu, R., and Resibois, A., Ultrastructure of sulfatide storage in normal and sulfatase-deficient fibroblasts *in vitro, Lab. Invest.* **29**:527 (1973).

66. Robbins, E., Levine, E. M., and Eagle, H., Morphologic changes accompanying senescence of cultured human diploid cells, *J. Exp. Med.* **131**:1211 (1970).

67. Coelho-Maciera, A., Garcia-Giralt, E., and Adrian, M., Changes in lysosomal associated structures in human fibroblasts kept in resting phase, *Proc. Soc. Exp. Biol. Med.* **138**:712 (1971).

68. Svennerholm, L., The gangliosides, *J. Lipid Res.* **5**:145 (1964).

69. Puro, K., Maury, P., and Huttunen, J. K., Qualitative and quantitative patterns of gangliosides in extraneural tissues, *Biochim. Biophys. Acta* **187**:230 (1969).

70. Yogesswaran, G., Sheinin, R., Wherrett, J. R., and Murray, R. K., Studies on the glycosphingolipids of normal and virally transformed 3T3 mouse fibroblasts, *J. Biol. Chem.* **247**:5146, (1972).

71. Hakomori, S. and Murakami, W. T., Glycolipids of hamster fibroblasts and derived malignant-transformed cell lines, *Proc. Natl. Acad. Sci. U.S.A.* **59**:254 (1968).

72. Weinstein, D. B., Marsh, J. B., Glick, M. C., and Warren, L., Membranes of animal cells. VI. The glycolipids of the L cell and its surface membrane, *J. Biol. Chem.* **245**:3928 (1970).

73. Klenk, H. D. and Choppin, P. W., Glycosphingolipids of plasma membranes of cultured cells in an enveloped virus (SV5) grown in these cells, *Proc. Natl. Acad. Sci. U.S.A.* **66**:57 (1970).

74. Mora, P. T., Brady, R. O., Bradley, R. M., and McFarland, V. W., Gangliosides in DNA virus transformed and spontaneously transformed tumorigenic mouse cell lines, *Proc. Natl. Acad. Sci. U.S.A.* **63**:1290 (1969).

75. Cumar, F. A., Brady, R. O., Kolodny, E. H., McFarland, V. W., and Mora, P. T., Enzymatic block in the synthesis of gangliosides in DNA virus-transformed tumorigenic mouse cell lines, *Proc. Natl. Acad. Sci. U.S.A.* **67**:757 (1970).

76. Brady, R. O., Borek, C., and Bradley, R. M., Composition and synthesis of gangliosides in rat hepatocyte and hepatoma cell lines, *J. Biol. Chem.* **244**:6552 (1969).

77. McKhann, G. M., Ho, W., Raiborn, C., and Varon, S., The isolation of neurons from normal and abnormal human cerebral cortex, *Arch. Neurol.* **20**:542 (1969).

78. Bocci, V., Enzyme and metabolic properties of isolated neurones, *Nature (London)* **212**:826 (1966).

79. Rose, S. P. R., Preparation of enriched fractions from cerebral cortex containing isolated, metabolically active neuronal and glial cells, *Biochem. J.* **102**:33 (1967).

80. Varon, S. and Raiborn, C. W., Jr., Dissociation, fractionation, and culture of embryonic brain cells, *Brain Res.* **12**:180 (1969).

81. Norton, W. T. and Poduslo, S. E., Neuronal soma and whole neuroglia of rat brain: A new isolation technique, *Science* **167**:1144 (1970).

82. Seeds, N. W., Differentiation of aggregating brain cell cultures, in: *Tissue Culture of the Nervous System*, G. Sato, ed., Plenum Press, New York, pp. 35–54 (1973).

83. Augusti-Tocco, G., Parisi, E., Zucco, F., Casola, L., and Romano, M., Biochemical characterization of a clonal line of neuroblastoma, in: *Tissue Culture of the Nervous System*, G. Sato, ed., Plenum Press, New York, pp. 87–106 (1973).

84. Pfeiffer, S. E., Clonal lines of glial cells, in: *Tissue Culture of the Nervous System*, G. Sato, ed., Plenum Press, New York, pp. 203–230 (1973).

85. Pfeiffer, S. E. and Wechsler, W., Biochemically differentiated neoplastic clone of Schwann cells, *Proc. Natl. Acad. Sci. U.S.A.* **69**:2885 (1972).

86. Batzdorf, U., Sarlieve, L. L., Gold, V. A., and Menkes, J. H., Tay–Sachs disease: Demonstration of the stored ganglioside in cultured cells from brain biopsy, *Arch. Neurol. (Chicago)* **20**:650 (1969).

87. Schneck, L., Amsterdam, D., Brooks, S. E., Rosenthal, A. L., and Volk, B. W., The Tay–Sachs disease fibroblast model: Failure to respond to exogenous hexosaminidase A, *Pediatrics* **52**:221 (1973).

88. Tallman, J. F., Johnson, W. G., and Brady, R. O., The metabolism of Tay–Sachs ganglioside: Catabolic studies with lysosomal enzymes from normal and Tay–Sachs brain tissue, *J. Clin. Invest.* **51**:2339 (1972).

89. Porter, M. T., Fluharty, A. L., and Kihara, H., Correction of abnormal cerebroside sulfate metabolism in cultured metachromatic leukodystrophy fibroblasts, *Science* **172**:1263 (1971).

90. Gregoriadis, G. and Buckland, R. A., Enzyme-containing liposomes alleviate a model for storage disease, *Nature (London)* **244**:170 (1973).

91. Harris, H. and Watkins, J. F., Hybrid cells derived from mouse and man: Artificial heterokaryons of mammalian cells from different species, *Nature (London)* **205**:640 (1965).

92. Kolodny, E. H., Milunsky, A., Sheng, G. S., G_{M2}-Gangliosidosis: Studies in cultured fibroblasts, *Birth Defects Orig. Art. Ser.* **9**:130 (1973).

93. Galjaard, H., Hoogeveen, A., deWit-Verbeek, H. A., Reuser, A. J. J., Keijzer, W., Westerveld, A., and Bootsma, D., Tay–Sachs and Sandhoff's Disease: Intergenic complementation after somatic cell hybridization. *Exp. Cell Res.* **87**:444 (1974).

94. Nabholz, M., Miggiano, V., and Bodmer, W., Genetic analysis with human–mouse somatic cell hybrids, *Nature (London)* **223**:358 (1969).

95. Lalley, P. A., Rattazzi, M. C., and Shows, T. B., Human β-D-N-acetyl-hexosaminidases A and B: Expression and linkage relationships in somatic cell hybrids, *Proc. Natl. Acad. Sci. U.S.A.* **71**:1569 (1974).

96. Gilbert, F., Kucherlapati, R., Creagan, R. P., Murnane, M. J., Darlington, G. J., and Ruddle, F. H., Tay–Sachs' and Sandhoff's Diseases: The assignment of genes for hexosaminidase A and B to individual human chromosomes. *Proc. Natl. Acad. Sci. U.S.A.* **72**:263 (1975).

97. Veomett, G., Prescott, D. M., Shay, J., and Porter, K. R., Reconstruction of mammalian cells from nuclear and cytoplasmic components separated by treatment with cytochalasin B, *Proc. Natl. Acad. Sci. U.S.A.* **71**:1999 (1974).

98. Brooks, S. E. and Amsterdam, D., Effects of EMC viral variants in human fetal cell cultures, *Fed. Proc. Fed. Am. Soc. Exp. Biol.* **33**:605 (1974).

99. Wudl, L., and Paigen, K., Enzyme measurements on single cells. *Science,* **184**:992 (1974).

Chapter 7

SPONTANEOUS GANGLIOSIDOSES IN ANIMALS

MASAZUMI ADACHI

G_{M2}-Gangliosidosis

During the past two decades, an increasing number of reports have appeared in the literature which have dealt with diseases considered to be the counterpart of human gangliosidoses. Thus for the first time, in 1953, Hagen[1] described clinical and pathological features of two cases of "amaurotic idiocy" in English setters. Histochemically, however, the cytoplasmic inclusion material seemed to be mainly phosphatides. Koppang[2] used animals for the same breeding stock of English setters and obtained, by planned mating, dogs of both sexes affected with the disease. Fourteen of them developed slowly progressive clinical signs at one year of age which consisted of incoordination and decreased vision. Later the dogs displayed various mental disturbances and died at about two years of age. He considered the clinical course to be similar to that seen in the juvenile form of familial amaurotic idiocy, but could not reach any conclusions regarding the genetic pattern of transmission. Grossly, the brain showed edematous leptomeninges and atrophic changes, especially in the cerebellum. Micro-

MASAZUMI ADACHI. Isaac Albert Research Institute of the Kingsbrook Jewish Medical Center and State University of New York, Downstate Medical Center, Brooklyn, New York.

scopically, the neurons of the brain exhibited a cytoplasmic granular material which displayed histochemical characteristics of glycolipids.

Ribelin and Kintner[3] reported a male dog which exhibited clinical and morphological features which they claimed resembled Tay–Sachs disease (TSD). The animal was a mixed fox terrier and cocker spaniel and remained in apparently good health until one year of age, at which time he began to bump into objects. On examination, the pupils responded to light very slowly. During the next several months, his vision became progressively impaired until he could no longer see. The pupils remained dilated. During the final months of life the animal became incoordinated and eventually developed paralysis of all limbs. Grossly, the brain and viscera were normal. Histologically, only the cerebellum and brain stem were examined. The cerebellar Purkinje and granular cells and the neurons in the brain stem were reduced in number. The remaining neurons were distended and contained multiple, fine vacuoles. Although no biochemical studies were performed, histochemically, the cytoplasmic material was thought to be a glycolipid.

Fankhauser[4] described a similar disease in a 17-month-old male golden spaniel and in a 4-year-old female springer spaniel. However, he was unable to identify the histochemical character of the intracytoplasmic material.

The animal model which most closely resembles human TSD was described by McGrath and associates.[5] Genetic study of these German shorthair pointers suggested that the disease is autosomal recessive. Clinically there was gradual acoustic deterioration. Later, the animals developed progressive incoordination, postural difficulties, impairment of vision, and psychic changes. Terminally, the dogs became convulsive and prostrated. The clinical course lasted approximately 11 months. Histologically, various degrees of distention of neurons were seen. They contained a cytoplasmic inclusion material showing positive reactions with PAS, Sudan black B, and Luxol fast blue stains, which was neither birefringent nor fluorescent. A similar material was also noted in neuronal dendrites, astrocytes, and macrophages. Ultrastructurally, the cytoplasmic inclusion bodies were 0.5–5.0 μm in diameter and were composed of trilaminar membranes measuring 50–60 Å in thickness and had a periodicity of 48–58 Å at points of membrane fusion.

Biochemical aspects of the German shorthair pointers were reported on by Gambetti and associates.[6] The cerebral gray matter showed a 3.6–4.0 times increase of lipid sialic acid. Further analysis disclosed G_{M2}-ganglioside which contained 60–65% of the total sialic acid. No significant variations were found in the other major constituents. In the liver, the level of sialic acid was three times higher than in controls. Thin-layer chromatograms showed a high amount of G_{M2}-ganglioside. Membranous cytoplasmic bodies, isolated from the cerebral cortex by ultracentrifugation, were found to have a lower density and protein content than similar bodies isolated from the tissues of patients with TSD. The total ganglioside content was 25–35% of the dry weight of the fraction, and 65–70% of the total sialic acid was present in G_{M2}-ganglioside. The activities of three glycosidases were measured using the p-nitrophenyl derivatives. In the brain, β-galactosidase activity was increased 1.6–2.5 times and β-N-acetylgalactosaminidase activity was increased 3–5 times, while β-glucosidase was normal. Unfortunately, no report was made on the percentage of Hexosaminidase A and B.

A similar disease in male German shorthair pointers, reported by Karbe and associates,[7-10] was characterized by progressive neurological impairment noted at six months of age. At that time, the dogs showed nervousness and decreased ability for training. The most striking clinical sign was progressive ataxia, which started at about 9–12 months of age. Some of the animals had occasional difficulty maintaining their balance and were forced to move sideways to prevent falling. Their appetites were good but their feeding manners were clumsy. In bright daylight they did not bump into subjects, but in dim light their vision was obviously impaired. However, most of the dogs never became totally blind. There were occasional seizures, and the animals died before the age of two years. The pedigree of the dogs indicated a recessive, sex-linked mode of hereditary transmission. Grossly, there were no obvious lesions, except for an increased amount of clear cerebrospinal fluid (CSF). The most striking histologic change was distention of the neuronal cytoplasm in the central nervous system, which was filled by multiple granules. The histochemical reactions of the intracytoplasmic material were similar to those of human TSD. The loss of neurons, accompanied by mild gliosis, was most apparent in the Purkinje and granular cells of the cerebellum. There were perivascular macrophages especially in the mesen- and telencephalon. Ultrastructurally, the neuronal cytoplasm contained concentrically arranged membranous structures which were identical with those of TSD. Biochemically, the total gangliosides in the cortex were five times as high as in controls, which was mainly caused by an accumulation of G_{M2}-ganglioside. In addition to this finding, G_{M3}-ganglioside, trihexosylceramide, and probably lactosylceramide were also increased when compared with normal controls. A deficiency of activity of a specific enzyme has not been demonstrated.

G_{M1}-Gangliosidosis

Kuruhara and Mochizuki[11] reported a hereditary neuronal disease in Siamese cats which had symptoms and histologic features resembling those of G_{M1}-gangliosidosis of man. Handa and Yamakawa[12] observed an increase of total gangliosides in the brain, liver, and spleen of Siamese cats and a marked augmentation of G_{M1}-gangliosidose in the brain. Despite the increased total gangliosides in the viscera, the chromatographic pattern of the visceral organs was almost normal. The sugar analysis of brain ganglioside indicated that the molar ratio of hexosamine, sialic acid, glucose, and galactose was $1.0:0.9:0.9:2.0$, which corresponded to that of G_{M1}-gangliosidosis. Glycosidase activities indicated a defect of β-galactosidase activity. Glycosidase activities for glucosyl- and galactosylceramide were unchanged.

Baker and associates[13] described clinical, pathological, genetic, and biochemical aspects of a male Siamese cat with G_{M1}-gangliosidosis. The animal developed normally until the age of four months, when he showed weakness and incoordination of his hind legs. General ataxia appeared and progressed until he was totally incapacitated at the age of six months, at which time euthanasia was performed. At necropsy, no gross lesions were found. Microscopically, the neurons in the central nervous system, as well as in the sympathetic system and retina, showed distention and loss of Nissl bodies. Frozen sections showed cytoplasmic inclusion granules which were strongly positive in PAS and Sudan black B stains. Increased numbers of glial cells were evident throughout the brain, and there was occasional neuronophagia. Lesions outside the nervous system were limited to the spleen, where a few macrophages showed a foamy, vacuolated cytoplasm. Biochemically, the total amount of gangliosides of the brain were more than twice normal. The quantity of G_{M1}-ganglioside was more than eight times normal, but the other gangliosides were present in nearly normal amounts. The activities of β-galactosidase in the brain and kidneys were approximately 15–20% less than those of normal cats. Activities of arylsulfatase A in both the brain and kidneys of the diseased animal were equal to or slightly higher than those in control animals. A pedigree of the cat's family disclosed that two sisters exhibited similar clinical signs. Unfortunately, neither of these cats was studied by necropsy. However, genetic studies strongly suggest that feline G_{M1}-gangliosidosis is inherited as an autosomal-recessive trait. Lack of significant visceral involvement and several other aspects of the feline disease more closely parallel the features of Derry's disease (G_{M1}-gangliosidosis, variant A) in the human.

Further details of biochemical and ultrastructural features of a Siamese cat were reported by Farrell and associates.[14] They observed that β-galactosidase activity with a pH optimum of 3.8 was found to be markedly reduced in the brain and kidneys; a second β-galactosidase activity with a pH optimum of 5.0 was present at normal levels in the kidneys. Certain physical differences were noted when the residual β-galactosidase activity was compared to the same activity of normal animals. The residual β-galactosidase activity from the affected cat was slightly more thermostable than that from the controls. The β-galactosidase activity from the normal cat brain had an apparent Michaelis' constant (K_m) of 2.32×10^{-6} M, whereas the β-galactosidase from the diseased cat brain showed an apparent K_m of 5.5×10^{-6} M. Galactono-(1 → 4)-lactone did not appear to inhibit the residual β-galactosidase activity from the affected cat, while the addition of this inhibitor to β-galactosidase activity of normal animals resulted in a 63% reduction of activity. These features suggested that the mutant residual β-galactosidase activity was due to structural alterations in the enzyme which would account for the reduction in measurable enzyme activity and the concomitant accumulation of G_{M1}-gangliosides. Ultrastructurally, the brain of the affected cat showed irregularly arranged aggregates of lamellae and random membranous structures scattered through the neuronal cytoplasm, without the regular "whorl" appearance seen in more mature membranous cytoplasmic bodies. The periodicity of the lamellae was 50–60 Å, which is identical to that found in G_{M1}-gangliosidosis and TSD in man.

Blakemore[15] also reported a cat with a similar disease which showed an increased amount of G_{M1}-ganglioside in the liver. Ultrastructurally, the brain displayed multilamellar inclusions similar to the membranous cytoplasmic bodies of human TSD. It, therefore, appears that from genetic, pathologic, biochemical, and enzymatic criteria, the Siamese cat is an appropriate model for its human counterpart.

Donnelly and associates[16,17] observed G_{M1}-gangliosidosis in Friesian calves. The first clinical signs occurred in the first months of life. The animals were slow to feed, dull, reluctant to move, and ataxic. Progression of the disease resulted in coma and death at six to nine months of age. Seven of the affected animals were studied by necropsy. In coronal sections of the cerebrum there was bulging of the cortical gray matter above the level of the white matter, with distinctive, linear, dark discoloration at the junction between the cortex and white matter. The visceral organs were grossly normal. Histologically, the neurons in the central and peripheral nervous systems were uniformly involved. They were ballooned out and contained vacuoles which showed histochemical reactions similar to those observed in cases of G_{M1}-gangliosidosis in man. Although the neurons were preserved in number, axonal swelling was frequently observed in the white matter of the cerebrum and cerebellum. Despite lack of gross changes, the lymph nodes and spleen contained swollen macrophages which displayed fine cytoplasmic vacuoles. Neurochemically, the brains of the affected calves showed markedly increased total gangliosides (a two to three times increase in the cortex and a six to ten times increase in the white matter) as compared with normal controls. G_{M1}-ganglioside was increased about two to three times in the gray and white matter. No abnormal accumulation of G_{M1}-ganglioside was noted in the liver and spleen. Preliminary studies[16] indicated a remarkable reduction in β-galactosidase activity in the central nervous system.

G_{M3}-Gangliosidosis

Bernheimer and Karbe[9] reported an instance of amaurotic idiocy in an English setter which was characterized by neuronal storage of granular material. The total gangliosides in the brain was 1.5 times higher than found in normal animals. This increase could only partly be ascribed to the accumulation of G_{M3}-ganglioside and was believed to be nonspecific.

Conclusion

In conclusion, there are increasing numbers of reports on lipidoses in various animal species. The Siamese cat, the most extensively studied animal, appears to be closely related to the human G_{M1}-gangliosidosis. Unfortunately, the animal model of G_{M2}-gangliosidosis, the German shorthair pointer has not, to this date, been analyzed for Hex A activity. It is anticipated that the use of these models will introduce a powerful new investigative approach to the pathogenesis of these diseases, especially in the prenatal state.

References

1. Hagen, L. O., Lipid dystrophic changes in the central nervous system in dogs, *Acta Pathol. Microbiol. Scand.* **33**:22 (1953).
2. Koppang, N., Familiäre Glykosphingolipoidose des Hundes (juvenile amaurotische Idiotie), *Ergebn. allg. Pathol. pathol. Anat.* **47**:1 (1966).
3. Ribelin, W. E. and Kintner, L. D., Lipodystrophy of the central nervous system in a dog. A disease with similarities to Tay–Sachs disease of man, *Cornell Vet.* **46**:532 (1956).
4. Fankhauser, R., Degenerative, lipoid-idiotische Erkrankung des Zentralnervensystems bei zwei Hunden, *Schweiz. Arch. Tierheilk.* **107**:73 (1965).
5. McGrath, J. T., Kelly, A. M., and Steinberg, S. A., Cerebral lipidosis in the dog, *J. Neuropathol. Exp. Neurol.* **27**:141 (1968).
6. Gambetti, L. A., Kelly, A. M. and Steinberg, S. A., Biochemical studies in a canine gangliosidosis, *J. Neuropathol. Exp. Neurol.* **29**:137 (1970).
7. Karbe, E., G_{M2}-gangliosidose und andere neuronale Lipodystrophien mit Amaurose beim Hund. Eine vergleichende histopathologische, histochemische, elektronenmikroskopische und biochemische Studie, *Arch. Exp. Veterinarmed.* **25**:1 (1971).

8. Karbe, E. and Schiefer, B., Familial amaurotic idiocy in male German shorthair pointers, *Pathol. Vet.* **4**:223 (1967).

9. Bernheimer, H. and Karbe, E., Morphologische und neurochemische Untersuchungen von zwei Formen der amaurotischen Idiotie des Hundes: Nachweis einer G_{M2}-Gangliosidose, *Acta Neuropathol.* **16**:243 (1970).

10. Karbe, E., G_{M2}-gangliosidoses (amaurotic idiocies) types I, II and III, *Am. J. Pathol.* **71**:151 (1973).

11. Kuruhara, Y. and Mochizuki, H., Feline case of cerebral lipidosis with similarities to Tay–Sachs disease, *Progr. Neurol. Sci.* **13**:260 (1969).

12. Handa, S. and Yamakawa, T., Biochemical studies in cat and human gangliosidosis, *J. Neurochem.* **18**:1275 (1971).

13. Baker, H. J., Lindsey, J. R., McKhann, G. M., and Farrell, D. F., Neuronal G_{M1}-gangliosidosis in a Siamese cat with beta-galactosidase deficiency, *Science* **174**:838 (1971).

14. Farrell, D. F., Baker, H. J., Herndon, R. M., Lindsey, J. R., and McKhann, G. M., Feline G_{M1}-gangliosidosis: Biochemican and ultrastructural comparisons with the disease in man, *J. Neuropathol. Exp. Neurol.* **32**:1 (1973).

15. Blakemore, W. F., G_{M1}-gangliosidosis in a cat, *J. Comp. Pathol.* **82**:179 (1972).

16. Donnelly, W. J. C., Sheahan, B. J., and Kelly, M., Beta-galactosidase deficiency in G_{M1}-gangliosidosis of Friesian calves, *Res. Vet. Sci.* **15**:139 (1973).

17. Donnelly, W. J. C., Sheahan, B. J., and Rogers, T. A., G_{M1}-gangliosidosis in Friesian calves, *J. Pathol.* **111**:173 (1973).

METHODOLOGY: SPHINGOLIPID ANALYSIS

LINDA M. HOFFMAN AND LARRY SCHNECK

Extraction of the Sample

Each tissue sample is weighed and then homogenized with 20 volumes of redistilled $CHCl_3$–CH_3OH (2:1, vol/vol) in a blender or a hand-held homogenizer equipped with a Teflon pestle. If the sample is freeze-dried to obtain a dry weight, the initial homogenization is carried out with $CHCl_3$–CH_3OH (2:1) containing 5% H_2O. The insoluble residue is filtered with suction on a sintered glass filter of medium porosity, then re-extracted with 10 volumes of $CHCl_3$–CH_3OH (2:1). After filtration, a final extraction is carried out with 10 volumes of $CHCl_3$–CH_3OH (1:2) in order to achieve quantitative extraction of gangliosides.

Separation of Gangliosides and Other Lipids

The method chosen for the separation of gangliosides from other, less polar, lipids is often the classical, solvent-partition method of Folch.[1] However, for

LINDA M. HOFFMAN AND LARRY SCHNECK. Kingsbrook Jewish Medical Center and State University of New York, Downstate Medical Center, Brooklyn, New York.

certain determinations, column rather than partition methods of separation may be more desirable, particularly when the loss of less polar gangliosides upon partition is anticipated.

If the solvent-partition method is chosen, the combined crude lipid extracts are adjusted to 2:1 in $CHCl_3$–CH_3OH, or if it is more convenient, the extracts may be evaporated almost to dryness on a flash evaporator, then made up to a desired volume with $CHCl_3$–CH_3OH, 2:1. This total crude lipid extract is partitioned in order to separate gangliosides from other, less polar, lipids. A 0.2 volume of 0.1 M aqueous KCl is added, and the mixture shaken vigorously and then centrifuged to effect complete separation of the upper and lower phases. If a large volume of solution is used, the two phases are separated by letting the emulsion stand at 4°C overnight. The lower phase is washed, a first time with 0.4 volume of theoretical upper phase ($CHCl_3$–CH_3OH–0.1 M aqueous KCl, 3:48:47), then a second time with 0.4 volume of theoretical upper phase which does not contain salt ($CHCl_3$–CH_3OH–H_2O, 3:48:47). The combined upper phases containing ganglioside are dialyzed against several changes of tap water for 24 hours and then against distilled water for an additional 24 hours. The material remaining in the dialysis bag is lyophilized and dissolved in $CHCl_3$–CH_3OH–H_2O (60:30:5); it may be used for the analysis of gangliosides by thin-layer chromatography.

A number of methods have been described which employ column chromatography rather than solvent partition for the separation of gangliosides from other lipids. Ledeen and co-workers[2] have employed DEAE-Sephadex A-25 to separate gangliosides and other acidic lipids, e.g., sulfatides, from neutral lipids. The column is prepared from 2.2 g of DEAE-Sephadex A-25 (Pharmacia Fine Chemicals, Piscataway, N.J.) which has first been equilibrated with Solvent I ($CHCl_3$–CH_3OH–0.8 M aqueous NaOAc, 30:60:8) and then washed with Solvent II ($CHCl_3$–CH_3OH–H_2O, 30:60:8) before it is poured into the column. The total lipid extract (1 mg/ml of up to 200 mg of lipid) is slowly applied to the column. Elution is first carried out with 200 ml of Solvent II to provide a fraction containing neutral lipids. The gangliosides and other acidic lipids are eluted with Solvent I. Isolation of a pure ganglioside fraction requires the additional steps of alkaline methanolysis and the separation of gangliosides from other acidic lipids, e.g., sulfatides and fatty acids, on a Unisil column.

Alternatively, the column-chromatography method of Rouser and co-workers[3] using Sephadex G-25 may be used to separate gangliosides from other lipids. The gel is equilibrated in CH_3OH–H_2O (1:1), poured into a column, and then washed with the sequence of solvent mixtures to be used in the sequential elutions. These solvent mixtures are:

1. $CHCl_3$–CH_3OH (9:1) saturated with H_2O (about 5 ml/liter)

2. $CHCl_3-CH_3OH$ (9:1), 850 ml; glacial acetic acid, 170 ml; H_2O, about 42 ml (added to point of saturation)
3. CH_3OH-H_2O (2:1)

Columns 1 cm in diameter and 10–30 cm high may be used for resolving 250 mg of sample. For larger samples, columns 2.5 cm ID and 30 cm high are recommended. For a column of the latter size, 500, 1000, and 1000 ml of Solvents 1–3, respectively, are used for elution. Most lipids are eluted with Solvent 1, while the gangliosides are eluted in Solvent 2. Water-soluble nonlipids, such as salts, sugars, etc., are eluted with Solvent 3.

Further Purification of the Ganglioside Fractions by Alkaline Methanolysis

The ganglioside fractions obtained from the Folch partition or from DEAE-Sephadex A-25 column chromatography are usually contaminated with phospholipids. A mild alkaline hydrolysis may be carried out in order to reduce the phospholipid contamination. Up to 10 mg of material may be dissolved in 10 ml of 0.6 N sodium methoxide which is prepared by dissolving sodium metal in cold, dry CH_3OH. The reaction mixture is permitted to stand at room temperature for 30 minutes and is then neutralized with methanolic HCl. After neutralization, the sample is placed in a prewashed dialysis bag and then dialyzed against several changes of tap water for 24 hours, followed by distilled water for 24 hours. The contents of the dialysis bag are lyophilized to yield gangliosides of reduced phospholipid contamination.

It should be kept in mind, when carrying out quantitative determination of gangliosides, that the loss of ganglioside does occur when mixtures of gangliosides are present in the dialysis bag at low concentrations, i.e., at concentrations less than 150 μg/ml.[4] When such low concentrations are being analyzed, alternatives to dialysis include desalting on a Sephadex G-25 column or phosphotungstic acid precipitation of the gangliosides.[5]

Thin-Layer Chromatography of Gangliosides

The separation of the various gangliosides may be carried out on commercially available Silica Gel G plates. The plates should be washed overnight with, e.g., $CHCl_3-CH_3OH-H_2O$ (100:50:6), prior to use in order to remove organic contaminants which are found on the plate. The ganglioside sample is spotted on a plate which has been activated for 1 hour at 110°C, and is then run in a solvent system comprising $CHCl_3$–CH_3OH–2.5 N NH_4OH (60:35:8) for 18 hours. After drying the plate, the gangliosides may be visualized with a resorcinol spray which is specific for the sialic acid found in gangliosides.[6] The spray is made by preparing a solution comprising 80 ml of concentrated HCl, 10 ml of 2% aqueous resorcinol solution, 0.63 ml of 1% $CuSO_4$, and enough water to make a total of 100 ml of solution. The ganglioside thin-layer plate is sprayed lightly with this solution, covered tightly with a glass plate of the same size, and then placed in an oven at 110°C for 15 minutes. The gangliosides are visualized as purple bands which are suitable for quantitation by densitometry. Alternatively, ganglioside bands may be visualized with a nondestructive spray, e.g., Rhodamine 6G or bromthymol blue.

Silicic Acid Column Chromatography

An acid-washed silicic acid column, e.g., Unisil silicic acid (Clarkson Chemical Co., Williamsport, Pa.), is used to separate the neutral lipids, glycolipids, and phospholipids[7] obtained in the lower layer of the Folch partition. The silicic acid is activated at 80°C in an oven overnight, cooled, and then packed in a column as a slurry in ether. The adsorbent is then washed with several bed volumes of $CHCl_3$ until it turns translucent. Five grams of Unisil will form a column 15-cm × 1-cm ID, which is adequate for the fractionation of approximately 250 mg of lipid. The major lipid extract from the Folch lower phase is applied as a slurry in $CHCl_3$ to the top of the column. The column is eluted sequentially with 100 ml of $CHCl_3$, providing a neutral lipid fraction, 200 ml of acetone–CH_3OH (9:1) which elutes hexosylceramides and sulfatides, and finally with 100 ml of CH_3OH which removes phospholipids from the adsorbent. The ideal amount of solvent used in each elution step varies with the type of tissue being assayed. However, the amounts mentioned will serve as a general guide. The completeness of each elution step may be monitored by thin-layer chromatography.

Further Purification of the Glycolipid Fraction

The glycolipid fraction which is obtained from silicic acid columns is usually somewhat contaminated with phospholipids. The phospholipids may be removed by carrying out an alkali-catalyzed methanolysis under mild conditions. This treatment is accomplished by dissolving 1–10 mg of the dried glycolipid fraction in 1.0 ml of $CHCl_3$ and 1.0 ml of 0.6 N sodium methoxide prepared by dissolving sodium pellets in cold, dry methanol. The reaction mixture is allowed to stand at room temperature for 1 hour. It is then neutralized with 0.5 N methanolic HCl, and made up to 2:1 $CHCl_3$–CH_3OH by the addition of $CHCl_3$. A 0.2 volume of water is added, followed by thorough mixing. Centrifugation gives separation into two layers. The lower layer is washed three times with CH_3OH–H_2O (1:1). The resulting lower layer is suitable for use in the thin-layer chromatography of glycolipids.

Thin-Layer Chromatography of Hexosylceramides

The individual hexosylceramides are separated on commercially available Silica Gel G plates which have been washed overnight in the eluting solvent comprising $CHCl_3$–CH_3OH–H_2O (100:42:6). The plates are activated in an oven at 100°C for 2 hours before use. This thin-layer system separates mono-, di-, tri-, and tetrahexosylceramides, while gangliosides remain at or near the origin. The individual glycolipids may be visualized as blue bands by utilizing diphenylamine spray and then heating for 10 minutes at 100°C. The distribution of the various hexosylceramides may be quantitated by densitometry. Alternatively, the thin-layer plate may be sprayed with a nondestructive spray, such as Rhodamine 6G, if the individual bands are to be recovered.

Thin-Layer Chromatography of the Phospholipid Fraction Obtained from Silicic Acid Chromatography

The phospholipids may be spotted on a prewashed, activated, commercially made Silica Gel G plate and eluted with $CHCl_3$–CH_3OH–acetic acid–H_2O (50:30:8:4) or with $CHCl_3$–CH_3OH–2.5 N NH_4OH (65:35:8). The separated phospholipid bands are detected with an ammonium molybdate spray.[8] The individual bands may best be quantitated by scraping them off the plate and then assaying for phosphorus according to the method of Bartlett.[9] As little as 0.7 μg of an individual phospholipid may readily be determined if the phosphorus content of plate blanks are taken into account.

Further Characterization of Glycosphingolipids by Gas–Liquid Chromatography

Gas–liquid chromatography (GLC) is a powerful tool for analysis of the component parts of glycosphingolipids. The lipids may be cleaved by methanolysis in 0.5–1.0 N methanolic HCl, whereby the fatty acid methyl esters and methyl glycosides are obtained. Further products of the methanolysis are the sphingolipid bases and O-methyl derivatives of the bases. The fatty acid methyl esters and methyl glycosides may be separated and analyzed by GLC.[10] However, the sphingolipid long-chain bases are best determined after hydrolysis in an aqueous system,[11] whereby only the long-chain bases, rather than a mixture with their O-methyl derivatives, are obtained.

Methanolysis Conditions

The glycosphingolipid (100–1000 μg) is placed in a disposable· or solvent-washed screw-capped culture tube equipped with a Teflon-lined cap. Methanolic 0.5 N HCl is prepared by bubbling dry gaseous HCl into dry CH_3OH which has been distilled from magnesium and iodine. Then, 2 ml of the methanolic HCl is added to the lipid and heated at 80°C for 12–16 hours.

Separation of fatty acid methyl esters from the methyl glycosides is accomplished by extracting the fatty acid methyl esters into hexane three times, using 2 ml of hexane for each extraction. It is essential that the hexane be freshly redistilled to minimize the appearance of artifacts in the GLC analysis of fatty acid methyl esters. The CH_3OH layer is used in the analysis of the methyl glycosides.

GLC of Fatty Acid Methyl Esters

The hexane extracts are evaporated to dryness under nitrogen and then made up to 30 μl with redistilled hexane. An aliquot of 1–3 μl is chromatographed on a 6-ft. × 4-mm-ID glass column packed with 10% DEGS on 80/100 mesh Supelcoport or 10% DEGS on 80/100 mesh Chromosorb W AW. These columns are commercially available. Fatty acid methyl esters ranging from C_{14} to C_{24} may be separated isothermally at

180°C. Operating parameters on an F&M Hewlett–Packard 400 gas chromatograph equipped with a flame ionization detector include: injection port, 200°C; flame ionization detector, 250°C; nitrogen carrier gas, 40 ml/min; hydrogen, 45 ml/min; air, 220 ml/min.

Preparation of Methyl Glycosides for GLC

The CH_3OH layer containing the methyl glycosides is first mixed with a pinch of silver acetate to neutralize the HCl. During the methanolysis procedures, N-acetylamino sugars are deacetylated to some extent. In order to reacetylate them, 0.5 ml of acetic anhydride is added to the CH_3OH solution. Reacetylation of the amino sugars is carried out for at least 6 hours, or overnight. The AgCl precipitate is then centrifuged down and the supernatant is removed to another culture tube. The precipitate is washed at least three times with 2-ml portions of CH_3OH and the washings are added to the original supernatant. The CH_3OH solution of the methyl glycosides is then evaporated to dryness under nitrogen and treated with 50–100 μl of silylation mixture, comprising hexamethyldisilazane, trimethylchlorosilane, and pyridine (dry, redistilled from BaO) in the ratios of 3:1:9. Such mixtures are commercially available in 1-ml sealed ampules or the mixture may be made up in larger volumes and stored in a desiccator for up to two weeks.

GLC of the Trimethylsilyl Derivatives of Methyl Glycosides

The methyl glycosides of L-fucose, D-galactose, D-glucose, N-acetyl-D-galactosamine, and N-acetylneuraminic acid may be converted into their trimethylsilyl derivatives and separated on a 6-ft. × 4-mm-ID glass GLC column comprising 3% SE-30 or OV-1 on an 80/100 or 100/120 mesh support such as Gas-Chrom Q or Supelcoport. Typical conditions of GLC runs on a Hewlett–Packard 7620A gas chromatograph equipped with flame ionization detectors are: temperature program of 120–250°C at 4°C/min; injection port, 200°C; flame ionization detector, 275°C; nitrogen carrier gas, 40 ml/min; hydrogen, 30 ml/min; air, 220 ml/min.

A pattern of more than one peak is obtained for the methyl glycosides of each sugar. These peaks represent a mixture of the α- and β-methylpyranose and the furanose ring forms which exist at equilibrium. This pattern of peaks is helpful in the recognition of each sugar during a programed run.

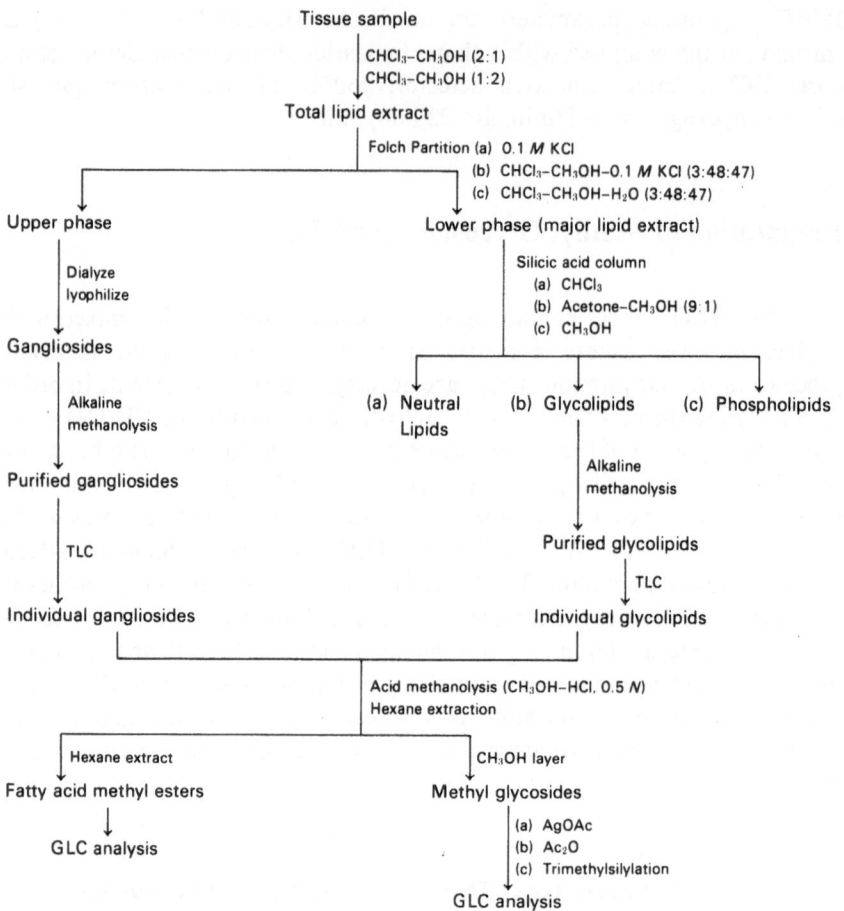

FIGURE 1. Flow diagram of the procedures for sphingolipid analysis.

The pattern obtained may be used to determine the ratio of sugars in a given glycosphingolipid. The total amount of each sugar which is present is proportional to the combined areas under the peaks which represent each sugar. Also, the number of nanomoles of a glycosphingolipid in an injected aliquot may be determined by relating the peak areas of individual sugars to a standard curve.[12] The standard curve is drawn by subjecting nanomole amounts of individual sugars or a pure ganglioside, such as G_{M1}, to the same steps, starting with methanolysis, as the sample, then plotting the GLC peak areas of the methyl glycosides of each sugar vs. nanomoles of the sugar.

The analytical procedures described above are outlined in the flow diagram shown in Figure 1.

References

1. Folch-Pi, J., Lees, M., and Sloane-Stanley, G. H., A simple method for the isolation and purification of total lipides from animal tissues, *J. Biol. Chem.* **226:**497 (1957).
2. Ledeen, R. W., Yu, R. K., and Eng, L. F., Gangliosides of human myelin: Sialosylgalactosylceramide (G₇) as a major component, *J. Neurochem.* **21:**829 (1973).
3. Rouser, G., Kritchevsky, G., and Yamamoto, A., Column chromatographic and associated procedures for separation and determination of phosphatides and glycolipids, in: *Lipid Chromatographic Analysis*, G. Marinetti, ed., Marcel Dekker, New York, pp. 99–162 (1967).
4. Kanfer, J. N. and Spielvogel, C., On the loss of gangliosides by dialysis, *J. Neurochem.* **20:**1483 (1973).
5. Dunn, A., Brain ganglioside preparation: Phosphotungstic acid precipitation as an alternative to dialysis, *J. Neurochem.* **23:**293 (1974).
6. Svennerholm, L., Quantitative estimation of sialic acid. II. Colorimetric resorcinol–hydrochloric acid method, *Biochim. Biophys. Acta* **24:**604 (1957).
7. Vance, D. and Sweeley, C. C., Quantitative determination of the neutral glycosyl ceramides in blood, *J. Lipid Res.* **8:**621 (1967).
8. Vaskovsky, Y. E. and Kostetsky, E. Y., Modified spray for the detection of phospholipids on thin-layer chromatograms, *J. Lipid Res.* **9:**396 (1968).
9. Bartlett, G. R., Phosphorus assay in column chromatography, *J. Biol. Chem.* **234:**466 (1959).
10. Clamp, J. R., Dawson, G., and Hough, L., The simultaneous estimation of 6-deoxy-L-galactose (L-fucose), D-mannose, D-galactose, 2-acetamido-2-deoxy-D-glucose (*N*-acetyl-D-glucosamine) and *N*-acetylneuraminic acid (sialic acid) in glycopeptides and glycoproteins, *Biochim. Biophys. Acta* **148:**342 (1967).
11. Carter, H. E. and Gaver, R. C., Improved reagent for trimethylsilylation of sphingolipid bases, *J. Lipid Res.* **8:**391 (1967).
12. Dijong, I., Mora, P. T., and Brady, R. O., Gas chromatographic determination of gangliosides in mouse cell lines and in virally transformed derivative lines, *Biochemistry* **10:**4039 (1971).

METHODOLOGY: ENZYME CHEMISTRY

GUTA PERLE AND ABRAHAM SAIFER

Methods for the Pre- and Postnatal Detection of TSD Heterozygotes (Carriers) and Homozygotes (Patients) by Means of Hexosaminidase Analysis of Their Biological Fluids and Tissues

Collection and Preparation of Biological Fluids for Hex A Analysis

Serum

1. Draw 8–10 ml of venous blood and allow it to clot in a refrigerator (5°C).
2. Centrifuge it at 3000 rpm for 15 min at 0°C in a refrigerated centrifuge.
3. Pour the serum into another clean tube and centrifuge again for 15 min at 3000 rpm.

GUTA PERLE AND ABRAHAM SAIFER. Isaac Albert Research Institute of the Kingbrook Jewish Medical Center, and Touro College, Brooklyn, New York.

4. Pour the clear serum into a properly labeled and dated tube.
5. Stopper the tube and freeze the serum until it is used, or refrigerate it at 5°C if it is to be run within a 10-day period.

The enzyme in serum is stable at room temperature for 1 day, at 5°C for about 2 weeks, and for at least 6 months when kept frozen at −20°C.

Leukocytes

1. Collect 8–10 ml of venous blood into two "Vacutainer" tubes containing sodium citrate solution (blue top, No. 3204 W, Becton-Dickinson, East Rutherford, N. J.). Invert the tubes several times and allow them to stand at room temperature for 1–1½ hours.
2. Centrifuge the tubes in a refrigerated centrifuge (0°C) at 1200 rpm for 5 min.
3. With a capillary pipet, transfer the plasma into one clean tube and the buffy layer (leukocytes) into another tube.
4. Respin the plasma tube at 1200 rpm for another 5 min at 0°C and add any sediment to the tube containing the buffy layer.
5. Wash the leukocytes by adding 8 ml of hypotonic saline (1 vol 0.9% $NaCl$ + 3 vol H_2O), gently inverting the tube several times, and centrifuging the sediment at 800 rpm for 5 min at 0°C.
6. Remove and discard the supernatant solution and repeat the washing step until all red blood cells are lysed and a water-clear wash solution is obtained.
7. Wash the leukocytes with 8 ml of saline–phosphate buffer (9 vol 0.9% $NaCl$ + 1 vol 0.1M phosphate buffer, pH 7.0) and spin down the sediment at 800 rpm for 5 min at 0°C.
8. Remove the supernatant fluid and drain off the excess by inclining tube onto a gauze pad.
9. Suspend the leukocytes in 0.5 ml of the saline–phosphate buffer and mix well.* Freeze and thaw the suspension five times.
10. Centrifuge the tube at 14,000 rpm for 10 min at 0°C.
11. Transfer the supernatant fluid to a clean test tube labeled with name, contents, and date, and keep it in a freezer (−20°C) until it is assayed.
12. If the total hexosaminidase activity of the leukocyte extract is higher than the 100% fluorescent working standard, the extract should be diluted with saline–phosphate buffer to an enzyme activity of 600–700 nmol/ml/h.

---

* For shipping to another laboratory for analysis, freeze the suspension and mail it in a styrofoam container with sufficient dry ice to last for 48 hours.

Amniotic Fluid

1. A minimum of 30–40 ml of amniotic fluid is collected aseptically in sterile tubes with leakproof closures.
2. A 10-ml aliquot of the amniotic fluid is centrifuged at 3000 rpm for 15 min in a refrigerated centrifuge at 0°C.
3. The clear fluid is transferred into three clean plastic tubes, tightly sealed, and frozen until assayed.
4. The remainder of the amniotic fluid (20–30 ml) is used for tissue culture.

Cultured Amniotic Fluid Cells

1. The flasks in which the cells are grown should contain at least 10^6 cells in total.
2. The culture flasks are washed 3 times with 5 ml of saline–phosphate buffer.*
3. The cells are then scraped into a 15-ml centrifuge tube and centrifuged at 800 rpm for 5 min at 0°C in a refrigerated centrifuge.
4. Decant the supernatant fluid and suspend the sediment in 0.5 ml of saline–phosphate buffer and mix well. Freeze and thaw the suspension five times.
5. Continue the procedure as described under "Leukocytes" beginning with step 10.

Tissue Homogenates

1. Weigh the tissue specimen on Parafilm with an analytical balance.
2. Transfer the tissue to a suitable homogenizing tube and add sufficient cold 0.9% NaCl (5°C) to make a 10% (wt/vol) homogenate.

* When less than 10^6 cells are available for analysis, an increased yield may be obtained by washing once with 1.0 ml of a trypsin–versene solution (0.1% EDTA in 0.1% trypsin solution). Decant the wash solution and add 0.5 ml of fresh trypsin–versene solution. Incubate the flask at 37°C for 1–2 min to release the cells. Add 10 ml of saline–phosphate buffer and transfer the cell suspension to a 15-ml centrifuge tube. Centrifuge at 800 rpm for 5 min at 0°C and decant the supernatant. Add 5.0 ml of saline–phosphate buffer and resuspend the sediment. Centrifuge again as above, decant the supernatant fluid, and suspend the cells in 0.5 ml of saline–phosphate buffer. The cells can either be disrupted by freezing and thawing five times or, if time is a factor, by sonification as follows: The cells, after the final centrifugation, are transferred to a clear, plastic, 12-ml centrifuge tube and suspended in 1.0 ml of saline–phosphate buffer and the tube packed in ice. The Sonifier Cell Disrupter (Model W-185-C, Heat Systems Co., Plainview, N. Y.) is set at about ⅓ full scale and the sonification performed in 5 or 6 short bursts (~1 sec) allowing time for the temperature to return to 0°C before the next burst. The degree of cellular disruption should be checked by a microscopic examination.

3. The tube containing the tissue is placed in an ice bath and, when at 0°C, it is homogenized under ice with a motor-driven pestle.
4. The tissue is homogenized for about 1 min using 10- to 15-sec challenges and is allowed to cool down to 0°C between each application. The appearance of the homogenate should be examined after each challenge since some tissues, e.g., brain, are easily homogenized; while others, e.g., liver, heart, and skin, may require additional periods of homogenization.
5. Centrifuge the homogenate in a centrifuge tube at 16,000 rpm for 10 min at 0°C.
6. Pour the supernatant fluid into a clean, labeled test tube and freeze it until it is assayed.
7. Assay the fluid for total hexosaminidase activity and dilute it to an activity of 600–700 nmol/ml/h with 0.9% NaCl prior to analysis.

Hex A Analysis of Biological Fluids with the Heat-Fractionation Method for the Detection of TSD Heterozygotes and Homozygotes*

Reagents

1. Citrate-phosphate buffer, 0.04 M citric acid, pH 4.45: 40 ml of 1 M citric acid and 319 ml of 0.2 M Na_2HPO_4 are transferred to a 1-liter volumetric flask and diluted to mark with distilled water. Check and adjust the solution to pH 4.45.
2. Propanol stopping buffer, 0.02 M, pH 10.3: Dilute 13.3 ml of 2-amino-2-methyl-1-propanol solution (221-Buffer, Sigma Chemical Co., St. Louis, Mo.) to 1 liter with distilled water.
3. Human serum albumin: 0.75 g% solution of albumin (Kabi, Stockholm, Sweden) in 0.04 M citrate–phosphate buffer.
4. Substrate: 1 mM solution of 4-methylumbelliferyl-2-acetamido-2-deoxy-β-D-glucopyranoside (Research Products International, Elk Grove Village, Ill.) in 0.04 M citrate–phosphate buffer. Dissolve 3.4 mg of the substrate in 10 ml of buffer.
5. Fluorescent standard: Prepare a stock standard solution of 1.3×10^{-4} M 4-methylumbelliferone (Research Prod. Intl.). Dilute 0.1 ml of the stock standard with 10.0 ml of 0.02 M propanol buffer. This diluted standard (1.3×10^{-6} M) is used to set the Beckman fluorometer to 100%.

* After O'Brien et al.[1]

Method

1. 100 μl of serum is diluted with 900 μl of 0.04 M citrate–phosphate buffer (leukocytes, amniotic fluids, and cultured cell and tissue extracts are diluted 1 : 10 with the albumin solution).
2. A 50-μl aliquot of the diluted serum is pipetted into each of seven test tubes (13 $\times$ 100 mm) with an accurate micropipet.
3. A 50-μl aliquot of the albumin solution is pipetted into a test tube to serve as a reagent blank.
4. Three of the seven serum tubes (t_0) and one blank tube (Bl) are tightly stoppered and placed in a freezer.
5. The four remaining tubes are tightly stoppered and placed in a water bath at 50°C.
6. After 3 h in the 50° bath, two tubes (labeled 3 h) are removed and placed in the freezer.
7. After 4 h in the 50° bath, two more tubes (labeled 4 h) are removed to an ice bath (together with the t_0, 3 h, and Bl tubes).
8. After 10 min in the ice bath, 100 μl of substrate is added to each tube and all the tubes are placed in a 37°C water bath for 1 h.
9. The tubes are then removed to an ice bath and 5.0 ml of propanol stopping buffer is added to each tube to stop the enzyme reaction and to develop fluorescence.
10. The Beckman Dual Beam Ratio fluorometer is set at 0% with the stopping buffer and at 100% with the diluted 4-methylumbelliferone (1.3 $\times$ 10^{-6} M) standard using 7-37 (primary) and 2A (secondary) filters.
11. The fluorescent reading of the reagent blank tube (Bl) is subtracted from the average readings of the three (t_0) tubes and the two 3 h plus two 4 h tubes.

Calculations

1. Total Hex (nmol umbelliferone released/ml/h), average (t_0) reading $\times$ 1340.
2. Hex B (nmol umbelliferone released/ml/h), average of 3 h and 4 h readings $\times$ 1340.
3. Hex A (nmol umbelliferone released/ml/h), total Hex − Hex B = Hex A, or

$$\% \text{ Hex A} = 100 - \left[\frac{\text{heat-stable Hex reading}}{\text{total Hex reading}} \times 100 \right]$$

Normal Ranges

1. Serum (as % Hex A) = 57–78.
2. Leukocytes (as % Hex A) = 62–80.
3. Amniotic fluid (as % Hex A) = 9–35.
4. Cultured amniotic cells (as % Hex A) = 45–72.

Pregnancy Range

1. Serum (as % Hex A) = 26–62.
2. Leukocytes (as % Hex A) = 57–84.

Heterozygote (Carrier) Range

1. Serum (as % Hex A) = 28–56.
2. Leukocytes (as % Hex A) = 42–61.

Homozygote (TSD Children) Range

1. Serum (as % Hex A) = 0–15.
2. Leukocytes (as % Hex A) = 2–25.
3. Amniotic fluid* (as % Hex A) = 2–19.

Serum Hex A Analysis with the pH-Inactivation Method for the Detection of TSD Heterozygotes and Homozygotes**

Reagents

1. Glycine–HCl buffer: 0.5 M glycine, pH 2.80. 75.0 g/liter glycine = 1 M solution. 86 ml conc. HCl diluted to 1 liter with distilled water = 1 M HCl. 50 ml 1 M glycine and 14 ml 1 M HCl are diluted to 100 ml with distilled water. Check and adjust to pH 2.80 $\pm$ 0.05.
2. Sodium citrate buffer: 0.1 M, pH 4.5. 54 ml of 1 M sodium citrate and 46 ml of 1 M citric acid are diluted to 1 liter with distilled water. Check and adjust to pH 4.5.
3. Substrate: 30 mg 4-methylumbelliferone-2-acetamido-2-deoxy-D-glucopyranoside (Research Prod. Intl.) is dissolved in 15 ml of sodium citrate buffer. This reagent should be freshly prepared before use.

* Fluids obtained from mothers with predicted Tay–Sachs fetuses.
** After Saifer and Rosenthal.[2]

4. Stopping buffer: 0.02 M, pH 10.3. Dilute 13.3 ml of 2-amino-2-methyl-1-propanol solution (Sigma 221-Buffer) to 1 liter with distilled water.
5. Fluorescent standard: same as for heat-fractionation method.

Method

1. Prepare, in duplicate, tubes labeled B and W. Add 0.25 ml glycine–HCl buffer into the B tubes and 0.25 ml of H_2O into the W tubes (set 1).
2. Add 0.20 ml of substrate into a second set of tubes labeled exactly as the first set (set 2).
3. Place both sets of tubes in 37°C bath for 5 min to reach temperature.
4. At 30-sec intervals, pipet 50 μl of serum into each tube of set 1 and mix well.
5. Incubate for exactly 5 min at 37°C, and at 30-sec intervals remove a 50-μl sample from each tube of set 1 and add it to the corresponding labeled substrate tube of set 2 and mix well.
6. After 20 min remove tubes of set 2 from the 37°C bath at 30-sec intervals and stop the reaction by adding 5 ml of propanol stopping buffer and mixing by inversion.
7. Read the fluorescence of each tube in a Beckman ratio fluorometer against a methylumbelliferone (1.34×10^{-6} M) standard set at 100%.

Calculations

$$\% \text{ Hex A} = 100 - \left[\frac{p\text{H-stable Hex}}{\text{total Hex}} \times 100\right]$$

where Total Hex = average reading of W tubes and pH-Stable = average reading of B tubes.

Normal Range

Serum (as % Hex A) = 61–79.

Heterozygote (Carrier) Range

Serum (as % Hex A) = 37–60.

Homozygote (TSD children) Range

Serum (as % Hex A) = 1–20.

Leukocyte, Amniotic Fluid, and Amniotic Cell Hexosaminidase A Analysis by Acrylamide Gel Electrophoresis for the Detection of TSD Heterozygotes and Homozygotes*

Reagents

1. Lower buffer for electrophoresis. (a) Stock buffer. Dissolve 60.5 g tris(hydroxymethyl)aminomethane (Tris, Sigma) in 250 ml of 1 N HCl and dilute to 500 ml with distilled water. Adjust to pH 8.1 $\pm$ 0.2 at 25°C. (b) Working buffer. Dilute stock buffer 1:10 with cold (5°C) distilled water, filter, and refrigerate.
2. Upper buffer for electrophoresis. (a) Stock buffer. Dissolve 20.0 g Tris and 36.1 g Tricine [N-tris(hydroxymethyl)methylglycine] (Sigma) in 500 ml of distilled water. Adjust to pH 8.1 $\pm$ 0.2 at 25°C. (b) Working buffer. Dilute stock buffer 1:10 with cold (5°C) distilled water, filter, and refrigerate.
3. Tris buffer: 0.18 M, pH 6.3. Dissolve 2.06 g Tris in 16.8 ml of 1 N HCl and dilute to 100 ml with distilled water, filter, and refrigerate.
4. Acrylamide solution: Dissolve 30 g purified acrylamide and 0.8 g methylene N,N'-bisacrylamide (Eastman Chemicals, Rochester, N. Y.) in 100 ml of distilled water, filter, and refrigerate.
5. Flavin mononucleotide: (a) Stock solution, 5 mM solution FMN (Sigma). Dissolve 239.2 mg of FMN in 100 ml of distilled water. Divide into 1.0-ml aliquots in small vials and freeze. (b) Dilute stock solution 1:100 with distilled water, filter into an amber bottle, and refrigerate.
6. N,N,N',N'-tetramethylenediamine (Eastman Chemicals). Dilute 0.1 ml to 1.0 ml with distilled water just before use. *Do not pipet by mouth; this substance causes skin irritation and is harmful if inhaled.*
7. Sucrose solution: 40 g dissolved in 100 ml water.
8. Bromophenol blue: 100 mg dissolved in 100 ml water.
9. Substrate: Dissolve 60.0 mg of 4-methylumbelliferyl-2-acetamido-2-deoxy-β-D-glucopyranoside (Research Prod. Intl.) in 100 ml of 0.1 M sodium citrate buffer, pH 4.5 (see p. 238).

Equipment

1. Acrylamide gel electrophoresis apparatus (Model 1200, Canalco, Rockville, Md.).
2. Fluorescent light, 15 W.
3. Fluorometer with TLC scanner (Model III, G. K. Turner Assoc., Palo

* After Friedland *et al.*[3]

Alto, Calif.) coupled to a recorder (Model EU-A-20-1, Heath Co., Benton Harbor, Mich.).

4. Constant current power supply, Duostat (Beckman, Fullerton, Calif.).

Method

1. One-step acrylamide gels are prepared by adding 6 ml each of working solutions 3, 4, and 5 above to 6 ml of distilled water in a 125-ml suction flask.
2. Add 0.15 ml of solution 6 to the flask and de-aerate with suction to prevent bubble formation during polymerization.
3. Add about 0.25 ml of 40% sucrose to each of the rubber-stopper wells mounted on a wooden block.
4. Insert the gel tubes (7.5 × 0.7 cm, OD) firmly into each rubber stopper.
5. Carefully layer the gel solution over the sucrose in each tube and fill to the top.
6. Add a drop of water to the top of each gel.
7. Illuminate the tubes with the fluorescent lamp for about 1 h, until the gels polymerize.
8. Leukocytes, amniotic fluid,* amniotic cells, or tissues are prepared as described on pages 234–236, and the total hexosaminidase activity of each preparation is determined as described on page 237. Each sample is then diluted to an activity of about 800 nmol 4-methylumbelliferone/ml/h with saline–phosphate buffer solution.
9. Wash the gel tubes free of sucrose with distilled water and insert the tubes, gel side down, into the holes of the upper reservoir of the electrophoretic apparatus.
10. Immerse the tubes completely in the cold (5°C) lower buffer.
11. Mix 0.3 ml of each sample, e.g., leukocytes, with 0.15 ml of the 40% sucrose solution and apply 0.15 ml of the mixture to the top of a gel.
12. Layer the cold (5°C) upper buffer over the samples and then fill the upper reservoir with buffer.
13. Add 2 drops of the bromophenol blue solution to the upper buffer as a tracking dye.
14. Electrophoresis is carried out at 5°C in a cold room for 5 min at 1 mA/tube and then for 1 hour and 25 minutes at 3.0 mA/tube, migrat-

---

* For amniotic fluid analysis, mix 2 vol amniotic fluid with 1 vol 40% sucrose and add 0.15 ml of the mixture to a gel. Prior to the application of the 0.15-ml sample (page 241, 11) to a gel, add 2 drops of a Sephadex suspension (G-100 superfine) to the top of each gel. The Sephadex suspension is prepared by adding a small amount of powder to a flask and adding 5 mM (in phosphate) Tris–phosphate buffer (pH 7.3) in small increments until a viscous, homogeneous solution is obtained. This solution tends to separate into 2 phases on standing and should be well mixed before use.

ing toward the anode, for leukocytes, amniotic cells, and tissue extracts, and for 1 hour and 35 minutes at 3.5 mA/tube for amniotic fluid.

15. Loosen the gels by injecting cold (5°C) 0.1 M, pH 7.0 phosphate buffer along the inside rim of the tube with a pressure gel remover (No. 1806, Canalco).
16. Submerge the gels in the substrate (see page 240) in a covered shallow glass dish and place in an incubator for 1 h at 37°C.
17. Remove the gels from incubator, pour off the substrate, keep the gels moist at 5°C in a covered dish, and scan each gel in the fluorometer without delay.
18. Place each gel in a small (80 × 5 mm, ID) cylindrical quartz cuvette (SDA 322A, Schoeffel Instruments, Westwood, N. J.) and fill cell with cold (5°C) 0.1 M, pH 4.5 citrate buffer so as to remove all air bubbles.
19. Mount the cell on the door of the Turner automatic scanning unit using 7-60(primary) and 3-73 (secondary) filters at 30 × sensitivity with a 6- to 7-mm slit width and scan the gel according to the manufacturer's instructions. The scan of the fluorescent bands are recorded as peaks on the Heath recorder.
20. Quantitate the area under each curve by triangulation or planimetry.

Calculations

$$\% \text{ Hex A} = \frac{\text{area under Hex A curve}}{\text{total area (Hex A + Hex B)}} \times 100$$

Normal Ranges

1. Leukocytes (as % Hex A) = 52–86.
2. Amniotic fluid (as % Hex A) = 6–35.
3. Cultured amniotic cells (as % Hex A) = 30–66.

Pregnancy Range

Leukocytes (as % Hex A) = 57–87.

Heterozygote (Carrier) Range

Leukocytes (as % Hex A) = 31–61.

Homozygotes (TSD Children) Range

1. Leukocytes (as % Hex A) = 0.
2. Amniotic fluid* (as % Hex A) = 0.
3. Cultured amniotic cells* (as % Hex A) = 0.

* Fluids obtained from mothers with predicted Tay–Sachs fetuses.

Automated Determination of Serum Hex A by *p*H Inactivation for the Detection of TSD Heterozygotes and Homozygotes*

Reagents for the *p*H-Inactivation Procedure

1. Sodium citrate buffer, 0.5 *M*, *p*H 4.5: Add 280 ml of 1 *M* sodium citrate and 220 ml of 1 *M* citric acid to a 1-liter volumetric flask, dilute to mark with distilled water, and mix. Adjust to *p*H 4.5 $\pm$ 0.05 and store at 5°C when not in use.
2. Glycine hydrochloride buffer, 0.5 *M*, *p*H 2.80: Add 500 ml of 1 *M* glycine solution and 140 ml of 1 *M* HCl to a 1-liter volumetric flask, dilute to mark with distilled water, and mix. Adjust to *p*H 2.80 $\pm$ 0.02 and store at 5°C when not in use.
3. Fluorogenic substrate: Dissolve 100 mg of 4-methylumbelliferone-ace-tamido-2-deoxy-D-glucopyranoside (Research Products International Corp., Elk Grove Village, Ill.) in 100 ml of the sodium citrate buffer. This solution should be prepared just before using.
4. Glycine carbonate buffer, 0.5 *M*, *p*H 10.0: Dissolve 37.6 g of glycine and 53.0 g of anhydrous sodium carbonate in a 1-liter volumetric flask containing 900 ml of distilled water, dilute to mark with distilled water, and mix. Adjust to *p*H 10.0 and store at 5°C when not in use.

Reagents for the Total Hexosaminidase Procedure

Sodium citrate–glycine hydrochloride buffer mixture (2:1 by vol): This reagent is a mixture of the sodium citrate and glycine hydrochloride buffers above. Mix two volumes of the sodium citrate buffer with one volume of the glycine hydrochloride buffer in sufficient volume for each run.

All other reagents are the same as those described above for the *p*H-inactivation method. Add 0.5 ml of Brij-35 (Technicon Instrument Corp., Tarrytown, N. Y.) per liter of solution to all reagents used for the automated procedures.

Fluorescent Standards

1. Stock standard, 4-methylumbelliferone, 1 mmol/liter: Dissolve 17.6 mg of 4-methylumbelliferone (Research Prod. Intl.) in 100 ml of the glycine–carbonate buffer in a volumetric flask.
2. Working standards: From the stock standard, prepare solutions containing 200, 150, 100, 75, 50, and 25 nmol/ml by diluting with the glycine–carbonate buffer.

* After Saifer and Perle.[4]

Equipment

The equipment used for the Hex A assay is the Autoanalyzer II system (Technicon) designed for hexosaminidase analysis. It consists of a Sampler IV with a 60 sample/h (1:1) cam, a Proportioning Pump III, a Fluoronephelometer with flowcell (No. 126-BO14-02), primary filter (355 nm, No. 7-60) and secondary filter (460 nm, No. 48 plus 426 nm, No. 3-73), and a single-pen AutoAnalyzer Recorder modified for fluorometric measurements. The flow diagram of the manifold for the automated system used for the pH-inactivation (Hex B) assay is illustrated in Figure 1. The same manifold is used for the total hexosaminidase assay except that the mixed-buffer reagent is substituted for the pH 4.5 and 2.8 buffer.

Method

1. Bring the sodium citrate and glycine hydrochloride buffers to room temperature and check and adjust pH of glycine hydrochloride buffer to pH 2.80 + 0.05.

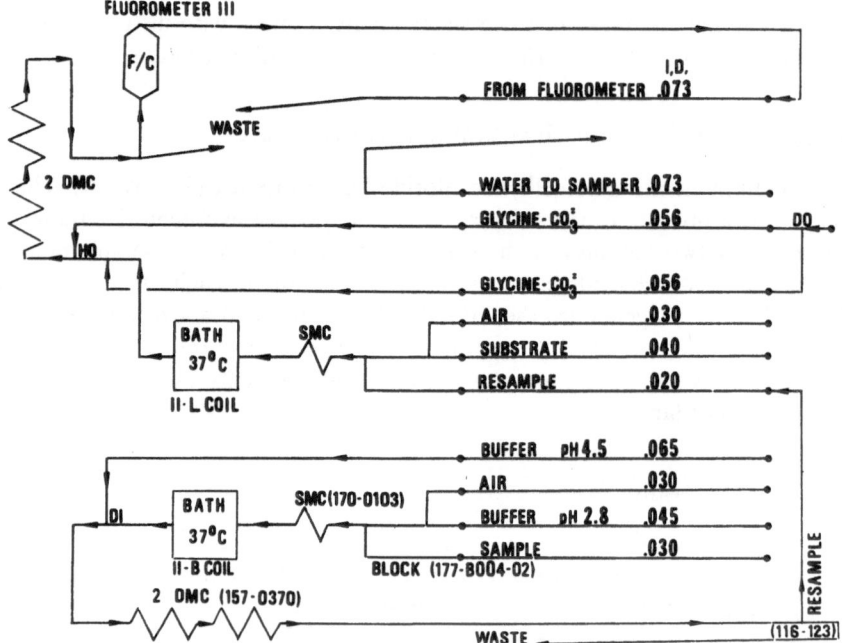

FIGURE 1. Flow diagram for measurement of N-acetyl-β-D-hexosaminidase B (Hex B) activity by pH inactivation. The same manifold is used for the total hexosaminidase method except that the mixed-buffer reagent is substituted for the pH 4.5 and 2.8 buffers.

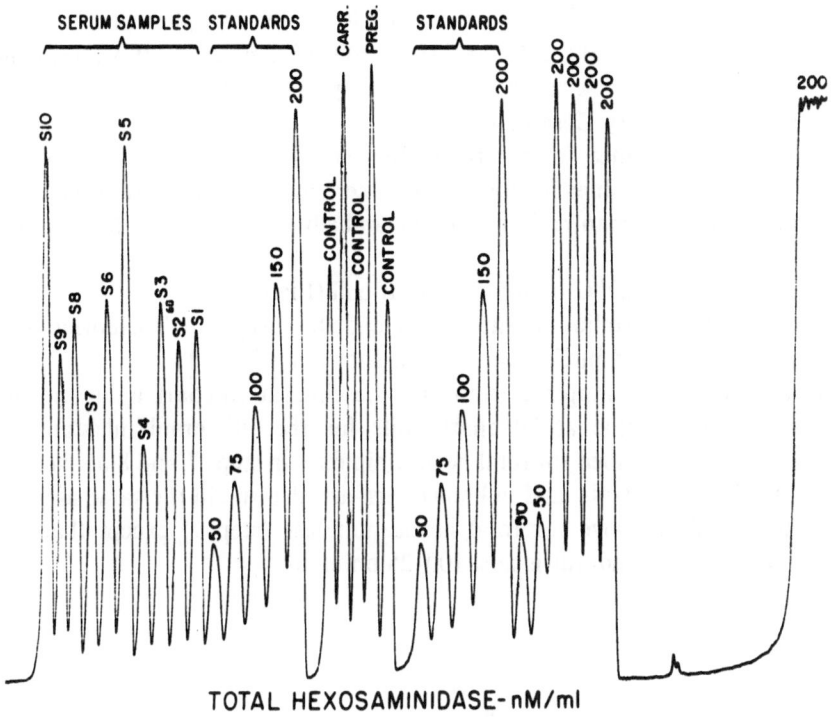

TOTAL HEXOSAMINIDASE-nM/ml

FIGURE 2. Recorder tracings obtained in experimental run with the automated total hexosaminidase procedure. Sera are designated S, other numbers are standards in nmol/ml.

2. Disconnect the 37°C bath for the II-B coil, turn on fluorometer, and pump water through entire system for at least 20 min.

3. Set the reference aperture at 2 and sample aperture at 1. The flow cell should be peaked according to the manufacturer's operating instructions, but once set, it need not be reset for subsequent runs.

4. Prepare the fluorogenic substrate as described on page 243.

5. Prepare mixed (sodium citrate–glycine hydrochloride) buffer as described on page 243.

6. Remove the pump lines from water and place them in the appropriate reagents for the total hexosaminidase procedure (see page 243).

   Make certain that the mixed-buffer reagent is pumped through the pH 4.5 and pH 2.8 lines shown in Figure 1.

7. After 20 min with all reagents pumping, set the fluorometer standard calibration control to 4.00 and adjust the reading on the recorder chart to 10 chart units with the baseline control knob.

8. Aspirate the 200 nmol/ml standard for 10 min and adjust the steady-state value to 90 chart units with the standard calibration control.

9. Place a series of fluorescent standards on the sampler wheel in the following order: 200, 200, 200, H₂O, 200, 150, 100, 75, 50, water, control serum, and a series of unknown samples interspersed with a control serum after every 12 samples.

10. Readings obtained for the fluorescent standards are plotted on graph paper and the values for the unknown sera are calculated from the standard curve in nmol/ml of 4-methylumbelliferone released (see Figure 2).

11. Reconnect the 37°C bath for the II-B-coil (Figure 1).

12. Substitute the sodium citrate buffer and the glycine hydrochloride buffer for the mixed-buffer reagent as is shown in Figure 1.

13. With reagents pumping, establish a baseline at 10 chart units and the steady-state value at 90 chart units for the 100 nmol/ml standard exactly as described for total hexosaminidase in steps 7 and 8 above.

14. Standards, controls, and unknown sera are also run in the same manner as described above for total hexosaminidase (step 9) except that the range of the standards is now 100–25 nmol/ml.

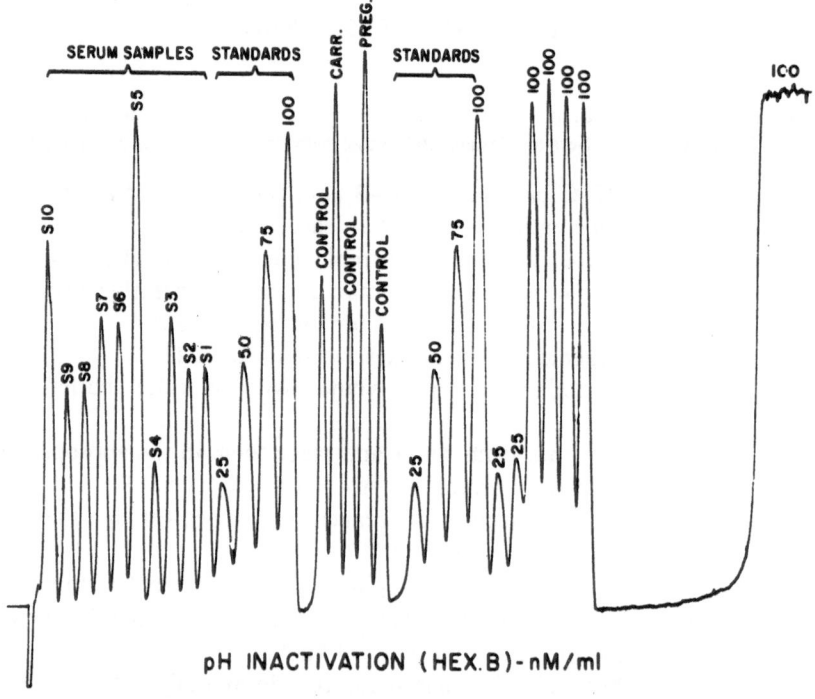

FIGURE 3. Recorder tracings obtained in an experimental run with the automated pH-inactivation (Hex B) procedure. Sera are designated S, other numbers are standards in nmol/ml.

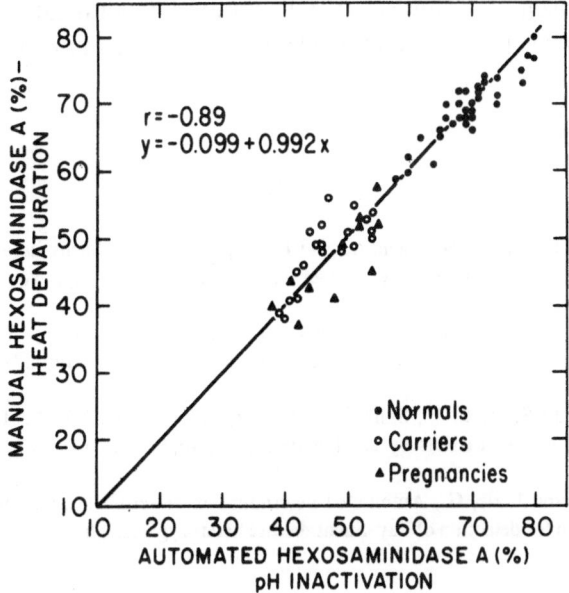

FIGURE 4. Comparison of Hex A data obtained by automated pH-inactivation and manual heat-denaturation methods from normal persons, carriers, and pregnant women.

15. Plot the values of the standards in terms of nmol/ml of 4-methylumbelliferone released and calculate the values of the unknown sera from the standard curve (Figure 3).
16. After completion of the pH run, wash the entire system with 1 M NaOH for 5 min and then with 0.1 M methylaminopropanol buffer, pH 10.4 (Sigma) for 10 min and with distilled H_2O for 20 min before performing subsequent runs.

Calculations

$$\text{Hex A (\%)} = 100 - \left[\frac{\text{Hex B}}{\text{total Hex}} \times 100 \right]$$

Normal Range

Serum (as % Hex A) = 58–79.

Heterozygote (Carrier) Range

Serum (as % Hex A) = 39–59.

Homozygote (TSD Children) Range

Serum (as % Hex A) = 0–27.

Comparison of serum Hex A data obtained by automated pH-inactivation and manual heat-denaturation methods are shown in Figure 4.

References

1. O'Brien, J. S., Okada, S., Chen, A., and Fillerup, D. L., Tay–Sachs disease: Detection of heterozygotes and homozygotes by serum hexosaminidase assay, *New Engl. J. Med.* **283**:15 (1970).
2. Saifer, A. and Rosenthal, A. L., Rapid test for the detection of Tay–Sachs disease heterozygotes and homozygotes by serum hexosaminidase assay, *Clin. Chim. Acta* **43**:417 (1973).
3. Friedland, J., Schneck, L., Saifer, A., Pourfar, M., and Volk, B. W., Identification of Tay–Sachs disease carriers by acrylamide gel electrophoresis, *Clin. Chim. Acta* **28**:397 (1970).
4. Saifer, A. and Perle, G., Automated determination of serum hexosaminidase A by pH inactivation for detection of Tay–Sachs disease heterozygotes, *Clin. Chem.* **20**:538 (1974).

METHODOLOGY: HISTOCHEMISTRY

MASAZUMI ADACHI AND BRUNO W. VOLK

Lipids

Sphingolipids

Modified Periodic Acid Schiff Method[1,2]

1. Fix the tissue in 1% calcium acetate–10% formalin solution.
2. Mount frozen sections on slides previously coated with chrome–gelatin and dry them in air. (Prepare the chrome–gelatin slides by dipping slides in a mixture of 1% gelatin–0.05% chrome potassium alum.)
3. Optional stage to remove phosphoinositides: Hydrolyze the sections with 2 N NaOH for 1 h at 37°C, wash them in water, and rinse them in 1% acetic acid.
4. Deaminate the sections with a 10% aqueous solution of chloramine-T at 37°C for 1 h.
5. Wash the sections rapidly in a large volume of water. It is necessary to rinse them rapidly to prevent the tissue from swelling in water, with the resulting loss of the section from the slide.

MASAZUMI ADACHI AND BRUNO W. VOLK. Isaac Albert Research Institute of the Kingbrook Jewish Medical Center and State University of New York, Downstate Medical Center, Brooklyn, New York.

6. Oxidize the sections with performic acid for 10 min. [Prepare performic acid by adding 4.5 ml H_2O_2 (30% = 100 vol) and 0.5 ml of conc. H_2SO_4 to 45 ml formic acid (98%). Let this solution "mature" for about 1 h and then stir it well with a glass rod before use. The solution remains active for about 24 h.]
7. Wash the sections in water.
8. Treat them with saturated 2,4-dinitrophenylhydrazine in 1 N HCl at 4°C for 2 h.
9. Wash them thoroughly for 10 min.
10. Stain the sections with the standard (McManus) PAS method (see Carbohydrates, McManus Periodic Acid Schiff Method, page 249).
11. Rinse the sections in 3 N HCl and then wash them well in tap water.
12. Mount the sections in glycerine jelly.
13. Duplicate sections are extracted with chloroform–methanol (2:1 vol/vol) at 20–25°C at 2–18 h before step 3.
Result: Cerebrosides and protein-bound gangliosides stain pink to red. The color is extracted by chloroform–methanol.

Nile Blue Sulfate Method[3]

1. Fix the tissues in formol–calcium solution (see Modified Periodic Acid Schiff Method, page 249) for 6–12 h.
2. Prepare frozen sections without embedding in gelatin or carbowax.
3. Stain the sections for 90 min at 60°C in 500 ml saturated aqueous Nile blue sulfate with 50 ml 0.5% H_2SO_4 (boil for 2 h before use).
4. Rinse the sections in distilled water.
5. Place them in acetone heated to 50°C.
6. Remove the acetone from the source of heat and allow the sections to remain in it for 30 min.
7. Differentiate the sections in 5% acetic acid for 30 min.
8. Rinse them in distilled water.
9. Differentiate them again in 0.5% HCl for 3 min.
10. Wash them in distilled water and mount in glycerine jelly.
Result: Phosphoglycerides and sulfatides stain blue.

Various Luxol Dyes[4,5]

1. Fix small blocks of tissue in 10% neutral formalin solution.
2. Prepare frozen or paraffin sections cut at 6-μm thicknesses.
3. Use Luxol dyes (MBS, MBSN, G, AR, ARN, and L) as 0.1% in 95% ethanol solution; stain for 16 h.
4. Rinse the tissue in 70% ethanol.

5. Differentiate it in lithium carbonate.
6. Rinse it in water.
7. Mount the tissue in Paragon water-miscible, frozen-sections mounting medium.

Result: Nonspecific reaction; perhaps, protein-bound lipids stain blue.

Smith–Dietrich Method (after Kaufman and Lehmann[6])

1. Add 1% calcium chloride to 10% formalin and neutralize it with suspended calcium carbonate. Fix the tissue in this fixative for 3 days.
2. Embed the tissue in 25% gelatin, or, if thinner sections are desired, evaporate if for 30 h in a desiccator over anhydrous calcium chloride at 37°C, stopping the evaporation while the gelatin solution is still liquid.
3. Then cool the sections in a refrigerator, cut out the tissue block, and harden one day in formalin solution (1 g calcium chloride and 1 g cadmium chloride in 100 ml 10% formalin solution).
4. Prepare frozen sections at 15 μm from the 25%-gelatin-embedded tissue.
5. Attach the sections by floating them onto slides previously coated with 2.5% gelatin; drain and dry.
6. Expose the slides to the fumes of concentrated formalin for 10 min to harden the gelatin.
7. Wash the slides for 3 min in water.
8. Place them in cold 5% potassium bichromate solution in a Coplin jar and place the jar in an oven at 60°C for 48 h.
9. Lift the slides out of the solution several times during the first few hours to eliminate air bubbles.
10. Take the jar out and allow it to cool.
11. Wash the slides in several changes of distilled water.
12. Stain for 5 h in a modified Kulschitzky's hematoxylin solution (1 g hematoxylin, 98 ml distilled water, 0.2 g sodium iodate, and 2 ml glacial acetic acid) at 37°C.
13. Differentiate the tissue in solution (2 ml 5% borax and 0.1 g of potassium ferricyanide in 38 ml of distilled water for 15 h).
14. Wash the slides for 5 min in running water and mount them in glycerine jelly.

Result: Phospholipids stain black.

Modified Acid Haematein Method (after Adams[7])

1. Fix the tissue in 1% calcium acetate–10% formalin solutions.
2. Mount frozen sections on glass slides.

3. After thoroughly drying the sections on the slides, immerse them in 5% potassium dichromate-1% aqueous calcium chloride for 18 h at room temperature and then for an additional 24 h at 60°C.
4. After thoroughly washing the slides, stain them in acid haematein for 5 h at 37°C. [Prepare acid haematein by adding 1 ml of 1% sodium periodate (NaIO$_4$) to 50 ml of 0.1% haematoxylin. Heat just to boiling and, after cooling, add 1 ml of glacial acetic acid. The solution should be freshly made each day.]
5. Wash the slides thoroughly and differentiate in solution (0.1 g of potassium ferricyanide and 2 ml of 5% aqueous tetraborate in 38 ml of distilled water) for 18 h at 37°C.
6. After washing them in water, mount the sections in glycerine jelly.
Result: Lecithins and sphingomyelins stain blue to black.

Phosphomolybdic Acid–Stannous Chloride Method (Landing et al.[8])

1. Place frozen sections on gelatinized slides; drain, blot, and expose them to formalin vapor for 10–15 min.
2. Allow the sections to dry thoroughly and dip them into 50/50 acetone–ether.
3. Transfer the slides to 1% phosphomolybdic acid in 50/50 ethanol–chloroform for 15 min.
4. Rinse them in ethanol–chloroform, then in chloroform, and then dry them.
5. Dip the slides into 1% aqueous stannous chloride in freshly made 3 N HCl.
6. Wash them in water.
7. Counterstain with 1% aqueous eosin.
8. Dehydrate, clear, and mount the slides in Canada balsam.
Result: Lecithins and sphingomyelins stain in molybdenum blue shades.

Okamoto's Mercury Diphenylcarbazone Method (after Ueda[9])

1. Fix the tissue in 10% neutral formalin solution.
2. Place frozen sections (6–10 μm) in acetone containing 0.65% magnesium chloride for 48 h at 22°C.
3. Place them in ether for 48 h at room temperature.
4. Rinse the sections thoroughly in acetone.
5. Wash them thoroughly in water.
6. Treat them with 5% KI for 4–5 min.
7. Wash them in water for 10 min.
8. Treat them with 2% sodium acetate for 10 min.

9. Place them in saturated diphenylcarbazone in 90% alcohol for 10 min.
10. Wash them thoroughly in water and mount in glycerine jelly.
Result: Sphingomyelins and lecithins stain blue-violet.

Performic Acid Schiff Method[10]

1. Fix the tissue in formol–calcium solution (see Modified Performic Acid Schiff Method page 249).
2. Mount frozen sections on chrome–gelatin slides and dry them in air. (Prepare chrome–gelatin slides by dipping them into a mixture of 1% gelatin–0.05% chrome potassium alum.)
3. Treat the slides with performic acid for 10–20 min. Prepare performic acid by adding 4.5 ml H_2O_2 (30% = 100 vol.) and 0.5 ml of concentrated H_2SO_4 to 45 ml formic acid (98%). Let this solution "mature" for about 1 h and then stir it well with a glass rod before use. It remains active for about 24 h.
4. Wash the slides in tap water for 5 min.
5. Stain them in Schiff's solution for 20 min.
6. Wash them in running tap water for 20 min.
7. Mount them in glycerine jelly.
Result: Phospholipids and cerebrosides with unsaturated bonds stain pink to purple.

Osmium Tetroxide Method[11]

1. Fix the tissue in formol–calcium (see Modified Performic Acid Schiff Method page 249).
2. Mount frozen sections on slides or stain them free floating.
3. Immerse them in 1% OsO_4 for 2–18 h. The container should be air-tight to reduce vaporization of OsO_4.
4. Wash the sections in running tap water for 20 min.
5. Mount them in glycerine jelly.
Result: Unsaturated lipids stain black.

Toluidine Blue Method (after Pearse[12])

1. Deparaffinize and hydrate the sections.
2. Stain the sections in 0.5% aqueous toluidine blue for 4–6 hr.
3. Rinse them in distilled water.
4. For histochemical purposes, examine the sections immediately in water.
5. Mount them in glycerine jelly.
Result: Mainly sulfatides and some mucopolysaccharides stain red to violet.

Cresyl Violet–Acetic Acid Method[13]

1. Fix the tissue in formol–calcium (see Modified Performic Acid Schiff Method page 249).
2. Frozen sections are stained in 0.02 g cresyl violet in 100 ml of 1% acetic acid for 10–30 min.
3. Wash the sections well in tap water and mount them in glycerine jelly.

Result: Sulfatides stain brown.

Sterols

Perchloric Acid–Napthoquinone Method[14]

1. Fix the tissue in 10% neutral formalin or formol–calcium (see Modified Performic Acid Schiff Method page 249).
2. Frozen sections are left free floating in the formalin solution for at least a week, preferably longer, to allow preliminary atmospheric oxidation of cholesterol to occur.
3. Mount the sections on slides and dry them in air.
4. Heat the sections, lightly painted with reagent, at the bottom of an oven or on a hotplate at 60–70°C for 5–10 min, until the red color which first appears turns dark blue. Care must be taken not to overheat, and thus carbonize, the tissue. The reagent is 0.1% 1,2-naphthoquinone-4-sulfonic acid in a mixture of ethanol–perchloric acid (60%)–formaldehyde (40%)–water (2:1:0.1:0.9 vol/vol).
5. Place a drop of 60% perchloric acid on the section and lower a coverslip into position.

Result: Cholesterol and cholesterol esters stain dark blue (the color is stable for a few hours and then gradually turns gray-black. The color is not stable in either water or glycerine).

Schultz Method (after Weber et al.[15])

1. Fix the tissue in 1% calcium acetate–10% formalin solution.
2. Wash frozen sections (20–30 μm) for 24 h in distilled water (several changes).
3. Treat them with 2.5% ferric ammonium sulfate in 0.2 M acetate buffer at 37°C for 7 days. (It is recommended that the buffer be adjusted to pH 3 by mixing 2 ml of 0.2 M sodium acetate with 98 ml of 0.2 M acetic acid. The final pH is about 2.)
4. Wash the sections for 1 h each in 3 changes of acetate buffer.

5. Rinse them in distilled water and transfer them to 5% formalin for 10 min.
6. Mount the sections on slides and remove excess water by blotting the edges. Do not dry the sections.
7. Place a drop of a mixture of equal parts of sulfuric and acetic acid on a coverslip. Invert the slide and apply even pressure to the coverslip so as to flatten the section. Grasp the coverslip at the corners and oscillate it several times.

Result: Cholesterol and cholesterol esters appear pale violet or red, turning rapidly to green within a few seconds. The color remains stable for 30–50 min.

Feigin Method[16]

1. Immerse formalin-fixed frozen sections in a 0.5% solution of digitonin in 40% ethanol for 3 h at room temperature.
2. Drain and immerse the sections in a mixture of equal parts of absolute ethanol and ether for 3 h at room temperature.
3. Drain and immerse the sections, together with an untreated control section, in 2.5% aqueous iron alum at 37°C for 2–4 days.
4. Drain, dry, and carry out step 7 of the Schultz method.

Result: Cholesterol esters are extracted by the alcohol–ether mixture and stain only in the control section. The free cholesterol–digitonin complex is not extracted and, therefore, stains in both test and control sections.

Triglycerides, Fatty Acids, and Other Lipids

Sudan Black B Method[17]

1. Fix the tissue for 1–5 weeks in a solution of 1 g cobalt nitrate in 80 ml distilled water with 10 ml 10% $CaCl_2$ and 10 ml commercial (40%) formalin.
2. Dehydrate the tissue blocks in 3 changes of acetone, each of $\frac{1}{2}$-hour duration, and place them directly in molten paraffin wax. (This procedure seems to have no advantage over the routine methods of embedding, especially if postchroming has been carried out.)
3. Bring the sections to 70% alcohol.
4. Stain them for 30 min at room temperature in saturated Sudan black B in 70% alcohol. (Longer times are advisable in case the tissue is fixed in other than formol–calcium solutions and for tissue which has not been postchromed.)

5. Remove the excess dye by rinsing the sections quickly in 70% alcohol.
6. Wash them in running water.
7. Counterstain them in 1% aqueous neutral red for 1 min.
8. Wash them in water and mount in glycerine jelly.

Result: Unsaturated triglyceride esters, unsaturated free fatty acids, unsaturated cholesterol esters, glycolipids, and phospholipids stain black to blue.

Oil Red O Method[18]

1. Fix the tissue in 10% neutral formalin solution.
2. Stain frozen sections, after rinsing them in water and then in 60% isopropanol, in freshly filtered oil red solution for 10 min. (Prepare the stock solution by adding 0.5 g oil red 0 to 100 ml 98% isopropanol. For use, dilute 6 ml of that solution with 4 ml of water, let it stand for 24 h, and then filter. Use this filtrate as a stock staining solution. Filter through Eaton-Dikman No. 610 paper for immediate use.)
3. Differentiate the sections briefly in 60% isopropanol (keep tightly stoppered or make up fresh).
4. Wash them in water.
5. Stain them for 5 min in Mayer's hematoxylin.
6. Wash in running water for at least 10 min.
7. Mount in glycerine jelly or gum syrup.

Result: Unsaturated triglyceride esters, unsaturated cholesterol esters, unsaturated free fatty, acid and cerebrosides stain red. Phospholipids do not stain.

Carbohydrates

Orcin–Sulfuric Acid Test[19]

1. Mounted frozen or paraffin sections are moistened with 2–3 drops of a solution consisting of 1 ml 2% aqueous orcin solution and 10 ml 2 N H_2SO_4.
2. Place the sections in an incubator.
3. The reaction appears within 2–5 min at 90–100°C.

Result: Pentoses and hexoses stain red to blue-red.

McManus Periodic Acid Schiff Method[17]

1. Deparaffinize and hydrate the sections.
2. Oxidize them for 10 min in 1% aqueous periodic acid.

3. Wash them in running water for 5 min.
4. Immerse them in Schiff's reagent 10 min.
5. Wash them in running water for 5 min.
6. Counterstain them with Mayer's hematoxylin for 5 min.
7. Differentiate them if necessary in 1% acid alcohol followed by thorough washing in running water.
8. Dehydrate them in alcohol, clear in xylene, and mount in a suitable synthetic medium.

Result: Polysaccharides, mucopolysaccharides, steroids, fatty acids, phospholipids, and glycolipids stain red to purplish-red.

Alcian Blue Method[20]

1. Deparaffinize and hydrate the sections.
2. Stain them in a freshly filtered 1% solution of Alcian blue 8GS in 3% acetic acid for 10–30 min.
3. Rinse them in distilled water.
4. Counterstain them in 1% neutral red for 30 sec.
5. Rinse them in tap water.
6. Dehydrate them through alcohol, clear in xylene, and mount in Canada balsam.

Result: Acid mucopolysaccharides stain clear blue-green.

Proteins

Coupled Tetrazonium Reaction (after Pearse[12])

1. Fix the tissue in 10% neutral formalin and embed it in paraffin.
2. Deparaffinize and hydrate it.
3. Immerse it in freshly tetrazotized benzidine at 4°C for 15 min. (The solution consists of 3 ml of a 2% suspension of benzine in 2 N HCl at 4°C; add 8 drops of cold, fresh, 5% sodium nitrite; agitate rapidly for 10 minutes; add 1 ml 5% cold ammonium sulfamate and 10 ml of cold, saturated, aqueous sodium carbonate. As effervescence ceases and the solution becomes alkaline, it changes to a clear dark yellow. Add water to 50 ml. This solution deteriorates rapidly even at 4°C and should be used within an hour after preparation.)
4. Wash the tissue in water.
5. Rinse it in veronal acetate buffer at pH 9.2 three times (2 min in each change).
6. Immerse it in a saturated (1 g in 50 ml) solution of HCl in veronal acetate buffer at pH 9.2 for 15 min.

7. Wash it in water for 3 min.
8. Dehydrate it in alcohol and clear in xylene.
9. Mount it in balsam.

Result: Aromatic and heterocyclic amino acids (tyrosine, tryptophan, histidine) stain reddish brown.

Millon Reaction (after Pearse[12])

1. Fix the tissue in 10% neutral formalin and embed it in paraffin.
2. Deparaffinize and hydrate it.
3. Place the sections in a small beaker containing the Millon reagent and boil gently. (The reagent contains 10 g H_2SO_4 in 100 ml 10% H_2SO_4. Heat the mixture until it is dissolved, make volume up to 200 ml, and add 0.5 ml 0.25% $NaNO_2$ to 5 ml of above solution.)
4. Stop heating and allow the solution to come to room temperature.
5. Remove the sections and wash them 3 times in distilled water (2 min each wash).
6. Mount the sections in glycerine jelly.

Result: Tyrosine-containing proteins stain red, pink, or yellow-red.

Benzoylation Method (after Pearse[12])

1. Fix the tissue in Carnoy's fixative (60 ml absolute alcohol, 30 ml chloroform, and 5 ml glacial acetic acid) for 3 h.
2. Immerse the paraffin sections in light petroleum (petroleum ether) for 3 min.
3. Remove them and allow them to dry in air.
4. Place the dry sections in 10% benzoyl chloride in dry pyridine for 10–16 h at room temperature. (This solution lasts for about 1 month, but rapidly loses strength if water is allowed to contaminate it. Pyridine should be dried by disstillation over barium sulfide.)
5. Rinse the sections in absolute acetone.
6. Immerse them in absolute alcohol.
7. Take the sections to water.
8. Continue with the Coupled Tetrazonium Reaction, step 3. (page 257).

Result: Histidine-containing proteins stain purple to reddish brown.

Ninhydrin Schiff Method (after Yasuma and Itchikawa, quoted by Pearse[12])

1. Fix the tissue in Zenker, with and without acetic acid, or absolute alcohol.
2. Deparaffinize it and hydrate it.
3. Treat the sections with 0.5% ninhydrin in absolute ethanol for 16–20 h at 37°C.

4. Wash them gently in running water for 2–5 min.
5. Immerse the sections in Schiff's reagent for 15–25 min. (full-strength Schiff reagent should be used).
6. Wash them in running water for 10 min.
7. Counterstain the nuclei, if required, in Mayer's hematoxylin; wash and differentiate in 1% acid alcohol.
8. Dehydrate, clear, and mount the tissue in a synthetic resin.

Result: Proteins stain pinkish red to magenta if they contain a sufficient number of reactive NH_2 groups.

Modified Bial Method (after Diezel[19])

1. Place air-dried frozen sections, or paraffin sections from which the paraffin has been removed in acetone for 1 h at 60°C and in ether for 1 h (this step is essential in the case of brain-tissue sections to remove interfering phosphatides and cerebrosides).
2. Spray the dried sections with Bial's reagent (40.7 ml concentrated HCl, 0.1 orcin, 1 ml 1% $FeCl_3$ solution) until the section has become moistened. Drain off the surplus reagent from the section.
3. Pour about 20 ml conc. HCl into a glass container approximately 30 cm in height and 12 cm in width which can be hermetically sealed. Then place the sections into the glass container so that they are suspended over the HCl in a glass frame, the upper surface of the sections facing downward, whenever possible. The HCl fumes should pass closely over the tissue sections.
4. Place the sealed glass container in the incubator at 60°C for 30 min to 1 hr. Meanwhile, the resulting reaction may be observed through the glass. It is advisable initially to add a test section known to contain a large quantity of neuraminic acid (e.g., cerebral cortex obtained in a case of Tay–Sachs disease or paraprotein secretions in amyloid degeneration).
5. Remove the sections and air dry them.
6. Clear them in xylene and mount them in balsam.

Result: Neuraminic acid stains red. Red-violet shades of color are conclusive evidence of a particularly high concentration of neuraminic acid in tissues. After 12 h, the color slowly fades.

References

1. Adams, C. W. and Bayliss, O. B., Histochemical observations on the localization and origin of sphingomyelin, cerebroside and cholesterol in the normal and atherosclerotic human artery, *J. Pathol. Bacteriol.* **85**:113 (1963).

2. Adams, C. W., Bayliss, O. B., and Ibrahim, M. Z. M., Modifications of histochemical methods for phosphoglyceride and cerebroside, *J. Histochem. Cytochem.* 11:560 (1963).

3. Menschik, Z., Nile blue histochemical method for phospholipids, *Stain Technol.* 28:13 (1953).

4. von Drews, G., Über Ergebnisse mit dem Phosphatidnachweis nach Menschik, *Acta Histochem.* 3:72 (1956).

5. Landing, B. H., O'Brien, J. S., and Wilcox, L. G., Luxol-dye staining in lipid storage diseases, in: *Inborn Disorders of Sphingolipid Metabolism,* S. M. Aronson and B. W. Volk, eds., Pergamon Press, Oxford, pp. 121–128 (1967).

6. Kaufman, C. and Lehmann, E., Sind die in der histologischen Technik gebräuchlichen Fettdifferenzierungsmethoden spezifisch? *Virchows Arch. A.* 261:623 (1926).

7. Adams, C. W. M., Acid hematein method (modified after Baker) in: *Neurohistochemistry,* C. W. M. Adams, ed., Elsevier, Amsterdam, p. 51 (1965).

8. Landing, B. H., Uzman, L. L., and Whipple, A., Phosphomolybdic acid as staining reagent for lipids, *Lab. Invest.* 1:456 (1952).

9. Ueda, M., Histochemical studies of lipids: Histochemical examination of Gaucher's disease, *Hyogo J. Med. Sci.* 1:117 (1952).

10. Lillie, R. D., Ethylenic reaction of ceroid with performic acid and Schiff reagent, *Stain Technol.* 27:37 (1952).

11. Adams, C. W. M., A histochemical method for the simultaneous demonstration of normal and degenerating myelin, *J. Pathol. Bacteriol.* 77:648 (1959).

12. Pearse, A. G. E., *Histochemistry,* Little, Brown & Co., Boston Vol. 1 (1968).

13. Hirsch, T. V. and Peiffer, J., A histochemical study of the prelipid and metachromatic degenerative products in leucodystrophy, in: *Cerebral Lipidoses: A Symposium,* L. van Bogaert, J. N. Cumings, and A. Lowenthal, eds., Blackwell, Oxford, pp. 68–76 (1965).

14. Adams, C. W. M., A perchloric acid–naphtoquinone method for the histochemical localization of cholesterol, *Nature (London)* 192:331 (1961).

15. Weber, A. F., Phillips, M. G., and Bell, J. T., An improved method for the Schultz cholesterol test, *J. Histochem.* 4:308 (1956).

16. Feigin, I., A method for the histochemical differentiation of cholesterol and its esters, *J. Biophys. Biochem. Cytol.* 2:213 (1956).

17. McManus, J. F. A., Lipoid morphology of the tubercle, *Nature (London)* 157:772 (1946).

18. Lillie, R. D., Various oil soluble dyes as fat strains in supersaturated isopropanol technic, *Stain Technol.* 19:55 (1944).

19. Diezel, P. B., Histochemical study of primary lipidoses, in: *Cerebral Lipidoses: A Symposium,* L. van Bogaert, J. N. Cumings, and A. Lowenthal, eds., Blackwell, Oxford, pp. 11–31 (1957).

20. Steedman, H. F., Alcian blue 8GS: A new stain for mucins, *Q. J. Microsc. Sci.* 91:477 (1950).

METHODOLOGY: ELECTRON MICROSCOPY

MASAZUMI ADACHI AND BRUNO W. VOLK

Tissues

Preparation of Solutions

3% Glutaraldehyde Solution with Cacodylate Buffer[1]

Chemicals: 2.14 g cacodylic acid (dimethylarsinic acid), 2.7 ml 0.2 M hydrochloric acid, 6.25 ml 50% glutaraldehyde solution.

1. Mix 2.14 cacodylic acid, 50 ml distilled water, and 2.7 ml 0.2 M hydrochloric acid.
2. Remove and discard 2.7 ml of this solution.
3. Add an additional 50 ml distilled water.
4. Adjust to pH 7.4
5. Take 93.75 ml of this buffer solution and mix it with 6.25 ml 50% glutaraldehyde solution.

MASAZUMI ADACHI AND BRUNO W. VOLK. Isaac Albert Research Institute of the Kingbrook Jewish Medical Center and State University of New York, Downstate Medical Center, Brooklyn, New York.

1% Osmium Solution[2,3]

Note: All work must be done under an evacuation hood, since osmium vapor is toxic. Chemicals: 1.9 g crystalline sodium acetate, 2.88 g barbital sodium (sodium diethylbarbituate), 0.5 g osmium capsule, 2.25 g sucrose, 8 ml 0.1 N hydrochloric acid.

1. Prepare veronal acetate: Dissolve 1.9 g crystalline sodium acetate and 2.88 g barbital sodium in 100 ml distilled water.
2. Prepare the osmium solution: Dissolve a 0.5-g capsule of osmium crystals in 25 ml distilled water. Break the capsule in water using a glass rod. Do not attempt to remove crystals from the glass capsule until water has dissolved them. Aid the dissolving process by shaking the water-containing glass capsule. Once the crystals are dissolved, add them to above prepared osmium buffer solution. Adjust to pH 7.4–7.5. Keep the solution under refrigeration and seal the bottle to prevent escape of the vapor.

Alcohol Solution

Prepare solutions of 30%, 50%, 70%, 80%, 95%, and 100% ethyl alcohol.

Epon [4]

Chemicals: 100 ml dodecenylsuccinic anhydride, 89 ml nadic methylanhydride, 162 ml Epon 812.

1. Mixture A is prepared by mixing 100 ml dodecenyl succinic anhydride and 62 ml Epon 812.
2. Mixture B is prepared by mixing 89 ml nadic methylanhydride and 100 ml Epon 812.
3. The final mixture is a 6:4 ratio of mixtures A and B.
4. Place the final mixture in an electric mixer and mix at medium speed for approximately 30 min.
5. At that time, add 0.6 ml DMP (1.5 ml/100 ml Epon).
6. Make sure that the DMP is thoroughly mixed into A and B.

Tissue Preparation, Embedding, and Stains

1. Immediately after the specimen is obtained, dice the tissue in cold (4°C) 3% buffered glutaraldehyde solution, then fix it for three h in the solution.

2. Mince postfixed tissue in cold (4°C) 1% buffered osmium solution for 1 h.
3. Rinse it in distilled water. From here on, all processes are performed at room temperature.
4. Dehydrate the tissue in graded series of ethanol: 30% alcohol solution for 10 min, 50% alcohol solution for 15 min, 70% alcohol solution for 15 min, 80% alcohol solution for 10 min, 95% alcohol solution for 15 min, 100% alcohol solution for 10 min (three times), and propylene oxide for 10 min (twice).
5. Place the tissue in mixture of propylene oxide and Epon (5:5) for 40 min.
6. Place the tissue in mixture of propylene oxide and Epon (2:8) for 40 min.
7. Place the tissue in plain Epon for 25 min, twice.
8. For embedding the tissue, arrange gelatin capsules in a holder. Identification numbers, written on small slips of paper using a brush or a pointed instrument, may be inserted into the capsule. Place one piece of tissue at the bottom of the capsule. Fill up capsule with fresh Epon.
9. Leave all capsules in a 60°C oven for 3 days, until they become hard.
10. Sections are obtained on ultratomes using glass or diamond knives.
11. Sections are stained with either lead hydroxide[5,6] or uranyl acetate.[7]

Uncultured Cells from Amniotic Fluid

Preparation of Solutions

Prepare 6% buffered glutaraldehyde and 1% buffered osmium solutions by methods similar to those given on pages 261–262.

Cell Preparation and Embedding

1. Obtain 40 ml of amniotic fluid.
2. Fix in 40 ml of 6% buffered glutaraldehyde solution for 1 h at room temperature.
3. Centrifuge the solution at 800 rpm for 5 min.
4. Remove the supernatant fluid.
5. Rinse it in 0.25 M sucrose with the buffered solution (three times) with a pipette.
6. Postfix in 1% buffered osmium solution for 1 h at room temperature. (During steps 2 to 6 use the centrifuge tube. Do not shake.)

7. Dehydrate the cells (using methods similar to those used for tissues, page 263).
8. Embed the cells (use a 5:5 ratio of mixture A and B Epon and cut with a diamond knife).

Cultured Cells from Amniotic Fluid

Preparation of Solutions

Prepare 3% buffered glutaraldehyde and 1% buffered osmium solutions by methods similar to those given on pages 261, 262.

Cell Preparation and Embedding

1. Remove the culture medium from the culture dish.
2. Add new culture medium (2 ml) in the dish.
3. Scrape the cultured cells from the dish with a hard rubber stick.
4. Centrifuge at 800 rpm for 5 min.
5. Remove the supernatant fluid.
6. Add 3% buffered glutaraldehyde solution (3 ml) and fix for 1 h at room temperature.
7. Continue with steps 3–8 given above for "Cell Preparation and Embedding of Uncultured Cells from Amniotic Fluid."

References

1. Sabatini, D. D., Bensch, K., and Barrnett, R. J., Cytochemistry and electron microscopy: The preservation of cellular ultrastructure and enzymatic activity by aldehyde fixation, *J. Cell Biol.* **17**:19 (1963).
2. Palade, G. E., A study of fixation for electron microscopy, *J. Exp. Med.* **95**:285 (1952).
3. Caulfield, J. B., Effects of varying the vehicle for OsO_4 in tissue fixation, *J. Biophys. Biochem. Cytol.* **3**:827 (1957).
4. Luft, J. H., Improvements in epoxy resin embedding methods, *J. Biophys. Biochem. Cytol.* **9**:409 (1961).
5. Millonig, G. A., A modified procedure for lead staining of thin sections, *J. Biophys. Biochem. Cytol.* **11**:736 (1961).
6. Watson, M. L., Staining of tissue sections for electron microscopy with heavy metals. Applications of solutions containing lead and barium, *J. Biophys. Biochem. Cytol.* **4**:727 (1958).
7. Watson, M. J., Staining of tissue sections for electron microscopy with heavy metals, *J. Biophys. Biochem. Cytol.* **4**:725 (1958).

METHODOLOGY: CELL CULTURE

DANIEL AMSTERDAM AND STEVEN E. BROOKS

Culture of Amniotic Fluid

Collection and Shipment of Amniotic Fluid

1. A minimum of 25–40 ml of sterile amniotic fluid collected aseptically in a sterile tube with a leak-proof closure is required.
2. A 10-ml aliquot of the fluid should be separated, and centrifuged, and the supernatant should be frozen. (This is for direct enzymatic analyses.)
3. The remaining fluid is refrigerated but *not frozen.*
4. If sample is to be mailed, the collection vessel should be well secured, taped closed, and packed in ice in an insulated mailing container so that a minimum amount of jostling results. Mark outside of package *HUMAN FLUID SAMPLE (KEEP REFRIGERATED)–DO NOT DELAY.*
5. The rapidity with which culture results are obtained are proportional to the number of and viability of the cells at the time they reach the culture initiation point. Hence, any contamination of the fluid with blood, or lesser volumes than those requested, will interfere with optimum results.

DANIEL AMSTERDAM AND STEVEN E. BROOKS. Isaac Albert Research Institute of the Kingsbrook Jewish Medical Center, Brooklyn, New York.

Initiation of Culture

1. Aseptically transfer 10–20 ml of amniotic fluid (AF) into a sterile conical centrifuge tube. Centrifuge AF at 800 rpm (75–100 g) for 5 min. For fluids contaminated with blood, see special procedures below.
2. Decant AF from the cell pellet.
3. For each 8–10 ml of initial AF centrifuged, add to the cell pellet 2.0 ml of McCoy's basal medium plus 30% fetal calf serum (FCS) containing 100 units/ml penicillin and 100 μg/ml streptomycin.
4. Disperse the cells in the medium by gently pipetting up and down; aliquot 2.0 ml/T-30 flask.
5. Adjust the pH by bubbling sterile 5% CO_2:95% air into the flask or by exhaling into the flask through a cotton-tipped pipet. Incubate, with a loosened cap, at 37°C in a 5% CO_2:95% air humidified environment.
6. After 5–7 days incubation, decant the medium containing unattached cells, and replant it in another T-30 flask. Refeed the original flask with 3.0 ml McCoy's medium.
7. Refeed all flasks at 3-day intervals (twice a week) with 3.0 ml McCoy's medium.
8. After 2–3 weeks, or when clones have reached a significant size (4–6 mm in diameter), they are dispersed and passed (see the section on "Passage" below).
9. If cells are passed at a 1:2 split ratio, then the contents of one flask serves as the inoculum for two new flasks.

Bloody Fluids (after Lee *et al.*[1])

1. Centrifuge AF at 800 rpm for 5 min.
2. Discard the supernatant AF and any red blood cells (RBC) which remain suspended.
3. Add 1.0 ml Hanks balanced salt solution (HBSS) plus 10–15 ml of sterile 0.83% solution of ammonium chloride. Incubate at 4°C for 3 min.
4. Add 3.0 ml McCoy's medium and centrifuge for 5 min at 4°C. Addition of the serum-containing medium inhibits the lytic reaction.
5. If large number of RBCs remain, repeat the procedure.
6. Wash the pellet once with complete McCoy's medium containing 30% FCS and proceed as in step 3 of "Initiation of Culture," above.

Disaggregation of Cells for Subculture (Passage)

1. Decant the nutrient medium.
2. Wash the monolayer twice with 2.0 ml of a mixture of 0.1% trypsin–0.1% EDTA (Versene) in GIBCO solution A (Grand Island Biological Company, Grand Island, New York).
3. Incubate the drained, moist flask at 37°C for 1–3 min.
4. Tap the flask firmly several times against a hard surface to facilitate removal of cells.
5. Add sufficient fresh nutrient medium and dispense cells at the desired split ratio into new flasks.
6. Incubate each flask for one week, or until a confluent monolayer is obtained. Continue feedings at 3-day (twice a week) intervals.

Harvesting Confluent Flasks for Enzymatic Analysis

1. Wash the flask three times with phosphate-buffered saline (PBS) pH 7.1.
2. Rinse the flask twice with trypsin–EDTA solution.
3. Incubate the drained flask at 37°C for 2 min.
4. Add 10.0 ml PBS to the cells and centrifuge at 800 rpm, at 4°C for 5 min.
5. Decant the PBS and add 10.0 ml fresh PBS; centrifuge and collect the pellet.

Primary Explant Technique

For Skin Biopsy, Surgical Specimens, Autopsy, and Fetal Tissue

All specimens must be handled with aseptic techniques and sterile instruments. Skin surfaces should be scrubbed well with 70% ethanol. Several rinses in balanced salt solution may be necessary to remove RBCs.

1. Collect tissue in a sterile container containing HBSS pH 7.1.
2. Mince the tissue in HBSS into fragments approximately 1- to 2-mm square.
3. Add 2.0 ml MEM (Earle's salts) containing 10% FCS; nonessential

amino acids; and antibiotics, 100 units/ml penicillin, 100 μg/ml streptomycin, and 1.25 μg/ml fungizone to a 25-cm² Falcon T-30 plastic
flask.

4. Place about 5 tissue fragments in each flask and incubate at 37°C in 5%
CO_2:95% air.
5. Do not disturb explants for several (4–7) days so that they can adhere.
6. After this period, flasks can be examined with the use of the inverted
microscope. Medium may be added if care is taken not to dislodge the
explant.
7. In approximately 2–3 weeks cellular outgrowth should be sufficient for
passage at a 1:2 split ratio.
8. Pass culture by disaggregation, as discussed previously.

Preservation of Cells for Long-Term Storage in Liquid Nitrogen

Cryoprotectant Medium

This medium contains MEM (Hank's BSS) without antibiotics; FCS,
10%; and DMSO (dimethylsulfoxide), 15%.

Preparation and Freezing Procedures

1. Disperse the cells from monolayer in the usual manner.
2. Suspend the cells in an equivalent volume of cryoprotectant medium.
3. Centrifuge at 600–800 rpm at 4°C for 5 min.
4. Decant the medium and resuspend cells in cryoprotectant medium to a
concentration of 1.0–2.0 × 10⁶ cells/ml.
5. Add 2.0 ml of cell suspension to sterile, labeled, freezing ampules.
6. Freeze the ampules slowly; a controlled drop of 1°C/min to −40°C is
recommended. Use the BF-5 Biological Freezer (Union Carbide) cover
fitting the Linde (Union Carbide) LR-50 liquid nitrogen refrigerator.
7. When ampules are frozen, transfer them to labeled canes in the liquid
nitrogen refrigerator.

Defrosting Procedure

1. Remove the selected ampule from the cane while wearing safety gog-
gles.

2. Inspect ampule to make sure that no liquid nitrogen has seeped into container. If liquid nitrogen is present, allow to evaporate slowly.
3. Plunge the ampule into a 37°C water bath and agitate it rapidly until it is defrosted.
4. Remove 1.0 ml from the ampule with a Pasteur pipet; transfer to a culture flask (T-30) containing 4.0 ml of nutrient medium, pH 7.0.
5. Refeed with fresh nutrient medium when cells adhere (2–4 hrs).

Enumeration of Viable Cells

1. Suspend the cells in a known volume and remove 0.5 ml.
2. Add 0.1 ml GIBCO 0.4% trypan blue and allow the mixture to stand for at least 5, but not more than 15, minutes.
3. Place a drop of the mixture on an alcohol-washed counting chamber (Neubauer Brightline hemocytometer).
4. If 8–10 cells/box are present, count only five diagonal boxes; otherwise count all 25 boxes. Only unstained cells are viable; record dead (stained) cells separately.
5. Count at least 4 loadings of the chamber and take an average.
6. Calculate the total number of viable cells/ml (Nv):

$$Av = \text{average number of viable cells counted}$$
$$\text{for 25 boxes, } Nv = Av \times \tfrac{6}{5} \times 10^4$$
$$\text{for 5 boxes, } Nv = Av \times 5 \times \tfrac{6}{5} \times 10^4$$

7. The total number of cells (T) can be calculated by the above formulae if the total count (viable and dead cells) is substituted for Av.
8. The percentage of viable cells (% V):

$$\%V = \frac{\text{viable count}}{\text{total count}} \times 100$$

Roller Culture for Mass Growth of Diploid Cells

Cells in monolayer can be grown on the inside surface of large bottles when rolled at low speeds. The glassware and equipment are available from Bellco, Vineland, N. J. The procedure is economical in terms of culture vessels and media required to achieve large yields.

1. A-2000 ml roller vessel, 840-cm² growth area is seeded with 3–4 confluent T-75 flasks (6.0–8.0×10^6 cells).

2. Add 50 ml Eagle's MEM medium as described under "Primary Explant Techniques For Skin Biopsy, Surgical Specimens, Autopsy, and Fetal Tissue," step 3.
3. Gas the vessel with 5% CO_2:95% air and seal it.
4. Rotate the culture vessel at 0.5 rpm at 37°C for 24 h, until cells attach to glass surface. After 24 h, increase rotary speed to 1 rpm. If culture becomes alkaline, check the seal and regas the culture.
5. Medium changes are indicated when medium becomes acid, usually twice a week.
6. When the culture vessel is confluent, harvest the cells by washing once with 0.1% trypsin–versene (5 ml) followed by incubation with 5.0 ml trypsin–versene at maximum rotary speed until cells become dislodged.
7. Cells may be harvested or subcultured at the appropriate split ratio.

Reference

1. Lee, C. L. Y., Gregson, N. M., and Walker, S., Eliminating red blood cells from amniotic fluid samples, *Lancet* 2:316 (1970).

CONCLUSIONS

The lay public and even the medical profession may justifiably wonder why a group of rare, untreatable, and uniformly fatal disorders has so captured the public's imagination and generated so much interest in the scientific community. The question has been partially answered by Bernsohn and Grossman in their preface to the book *Lipid Storage Diseases*. They point out that "these groups of diseases present an almost idealized progression of research process in medicine." Structural and biochemical pathologic delineating rapidly lead to the identification of the enzymatic deficiency. The basic research information was immediately applied to amelioration of the medical problems. At present, treatment is at best preventive and involves mass screening of ethnic groups to detect high-risk pregnancies and the antenatal detection of the affected fetus. The ability of influencing human heredity and reproductive biology has understandably created new ethical and social problems which have already affected future research trends. The availability of animal models should further facilitate research in both the fetal and adult stages of the diseases.

Ultrastructural studies, employing freeze-etching and scanning electron microscopy, could provide new insights into the role of these lipids in various membrane systems. Direct enzyme replacement in certain disorders such as Fabry's disease appears promising. Enzyme replacement by means of enzyme-containing liposomes or enzyme induction by virons is under active investigation. The application of microfluorometric enzyme assay to single mammalian cells will provide immediate identification of enzymatically abnormal amniotic-fluid cells. Cell culture systems are now being used to study the physiology, biochemistry, and genetics of cells. With regard to the nervous system, further work is needed to culture and identify groups and individual cell types and to study their interrelationships. An apparently healthy Tay–Sachs disease carrier has been identified with a complete absence of Hex A in the white cells and blood. Tallman *et al.* have suggested that Hex A and B represent different conformational states of the same enzyme. Immunochemical and physicochemical analytic techniques combined with somatic-cell hybridization may answer some of the problems involved in enzyme–substrate interaction and the genetic and structural relationships between various isoenzymes. One can, with confidence, predict the discovery of new phenotypic and genotypic subtypes of the monosialogangliosidoses. The polysialogangliosidoses may prove lethal to the developing embryo or fetus. The Editors hope that this book has provided the reader with an overall view of the field and acquainted the research specialist with related investigative trends.

B. W. V.

L. S.

INDEX

273